SOUL
MACHINE

ALSO BY GEORGE MAKARI

Revolution in Mind:
The Creation of Psychoanalysis

SOUL MACHINE

The Invention of the Modern Mind

George Makari

W. W. NORTON & COMPANY

Independent Publishers Since 1923

New York · London

For information about permission to reproduce selections from this book,
write to Permissions, W. W. Norton & Company, Inc.,
500 Fifth Avenue, New York, NY 10110

For information about special discounts for bulk purchases, please contact
W. W. Norton Special Sales at specialsales@wwnorton.com or 800-233-4830

Manufacturing by Quad Graphics Fairfield
Book design by Ellen Cipriano Design
Production manager: Julia Druskin

ISBN 978-0-393-05965-6 (hardcover)

W. W. Norton & Company, Inc.
500 Fifth Avenue, New York, N.Y. 10110
www.wwnorton.com

W. W. Norton & Company Ltd.
Castle House, 75/76 Wells Street, London W1T 3QT

1 2 3 4 5 6 7 8 9 0

For my parents, Jack and Odette Makari,
and especially, for Arabella

Contents

PART IV. THE SERPENT THAT ATE ITS TAIL

Prologue

IMAGINE A TIME in the future when your mind might travel. Perhaps it would enter a different torso or a foreign face. Would you still possess the same self, the same being? Our minds, most of us would agree, define us; they carry our personhood, and where they go, we go too. In Western culture, much depends upon this belief; it underpins a great deal of our literature, art, politics, and jurisprudence. It is the foundation of the commonsense psychology so crucial to social life. The concept of the mind is everywhere, and yet at the same time, it is strangely nowhere. The most powerful arbiter of truth in contemporary life, natural science, refuses to ratify this belief. While our own psyches seem abundantly clear to us, attempts to objectively establish their existence have been mired in seemingly insoluble problems. And so, while the mind remains central to 21st-century Western thought, a number of prominent neuroscientists and philosophers inform us that it surely does not exist.

Soul Machine is an attempt to untangle these contradictions by returning to their origins, the beginning of the modern age, when religious beliefs, philosophy, medicine, science, and political power were all in flux. The emergence of the mind as a formative, if always embattled, belief, cannot be understood outside this historical context; it was never the result of a timeless debate in which Plato, Kant, and Wittgenstein argued over dinner. Instead, this book recovers a lost lineage, parts of which have been long discarded as embarrassing, wrongheaded, or irrelevant. This collective forgetting has led to impoverished, skewed discussions among different specialists, and no broad, historical account of how the modern mind emerged.

The invention of the mind was not the result of sedate academic debate. The mind was a radically destabilizing, heretical idea that grew out of intense, often violent, conflict. Far from being a story of scholarship alone, this history begins and ends in bloodshed. Characters in this account include thinkers writing at their desks, but also wild-eyed prophets, doctors whose spare rooms were littered with carcasses, political spies, bitter refugees, witches, quacks, and pornographers. This story takes place in universities, courts, hospitals, London coffeehouses and Paris salons, but also on battlefields, in lunatic asylums, poorhouses, and prisons. For better or worse, advocates and enemies of the mind were not sequestered in their studies. Often they could be found at the barricades.

Any history of the modern mind must begin with its ancient origins. By the time Socrates lifted the chalice of poison to his lips, over two centuries of thought about the immortal soul had preceded him. Later when ancient Greek thought merged with the Christianity of the Church Fathers, a soul-based view of human nature became one of the ruling conceptions of Western belief. In Christendom, the soul was the "knot of the universe," the unifying link between nature, man, and God, and the single most prized human attribute. It provided believers with universal dignity, repose before a bewildering, brutal world, and consolation in the face of death.

By the middle of the 17th century, however, these same beliefs were seen as a rich source of corruption, unceasing strife, terrorism, and cruelty of vast dimensions. For decades, Christian sects waged war with each other over competing claims regarding the soul and its salvation. Emerging challenges from natural science combined with long-standing political instability to create a crisis. While the soul and the psyche were once understood to be synonymous, some thinkers now advanced a radical idea. What if the mind was not so much spirit as it was bodily? What if thinking matter existed *within* human flesh? An object, this mind would still somehow house human subjectivity. Endowed by God, it still would be material, and therefore sicken and die. A naturalized mind first emerged wrapped in these enigmas.

Once modernity gave birth to the theory of an embodied mind, the implications were grave. If it wasn't the soul but rather a fallible mind that made men and women think, choose, and act as they did, then long-standing beliefs were erroneous. Convictions regarding truth and illusion, innocence and guilt, health and illness, the rulers and the ruled, and the roles of the individual in society would need to change. Not surprisingly, therefore, from its inception this concept was considered scandalous. Early advocates surrounded themselves in clouds of ambiguity; they published anonymously and when discovered, quickly fled from red-faced censors and mobs. Monarchs and theologians decried these heretics and roused their forces against them. Most natural scientists also opposed this bizarre notion. For if human agency and intention emerged from within matter, than their own mechanistic beliefs about the natural world were surely wrong.

Considered both heretical and unscientific, this idea still did not die. After 1700, the mind took hold among thinkers in England, Scotland, Holland, France, Switzerland, the American colonies, and the Austrian and German territories. Over the next century, as the feudal order crumbled, theories of mental life bloomed along with liberalism, egalitarianism, hedonistic ethics, individualism, political toleration, and the rational logic of the Enlightenment.

During the second half of the 18th century, a further shift took place in this emerging, often clandestine discourse. If our mental activities were truly part of bodily processes, then they needed to be studied not just by ethicists and philosophers, but also physiologists, anatomists, and doctors. Hybrid discourses began to appear as medically sophisticated *philosophes* and philosophical physicians offered bio- and psychopolitical theories for their rapidly changing world. New experts generated novel, if highly unstable, fields of inquiry, such as animal magnetism, phrenology, anthropology, human science, psychology, mental medicine, and psychiatry.

As the general prestige of science rose, these would-be Newtons of mental life sought to link data from experience and introspection with revelations about anatomy—nerves, twitching muscles, and brain structures. New taxonomies for mental differences and diseases were created. Once the province of theology, ethical and behavioral norms began to be codified in medical terms, a process that continues to this day. As these beliefs spread through the broader population, alongside Christians who feared for their souls, there now stood those jittery moderns who faced the terror of losing something that not long ago they did not know they possessed, their minds.

During the 18th century, the idea of an embodied mind supported belief in the rule of reason, liberty of conscience, the contingency of human knowledge, self-governance, and the personal pursuit of happiness, as well as man's vulnerability to bias, error, mania, and delusion. With the French Revolution, these notions burst out into the open and were freely pursued more than ever before.

Only a few decades later, this era ended. After the defeat of Napoleon, the first wave of mentalism receded and a period of reaction began. Nonetheless, between 1640 and 1815, a tradition had been created that would not be fully lost. Humans, it had been said, possessed something that was part soul and part machine, but fully neither. It was a strangely active kind of thinking and willing interior entity called a mind. For decades during the middle of the 19th century, that conception of humankind fell quiet, a bomb with a long fuse. When it blew again, the second great wave of debates over the mind commenced, and since then, they have never ceased.

THE MODERN MIND was constructed during the Enlightenment, a defining if now controversial period of Western history. Some have questioned whether such an epoch ever existed and have argued instead for numerous, different national enlightenments. This book moves from the English and Scottish enlightenments to the French and German ones, but as we shall see, these varied intellectual communities were deeply intertwined. While powerfully influenced by local differences, their theories of the mind also represent chapters in one interconnected European story.

In addition, the meaning of this historical period has been challenged. Once hailed as a great epoch of human progress, the Enlightenment has lost much of its luster. For critics, like the widely cited Michel Foucault, this period became one of insidious social control, brute prejudice masked as science, bureaucratically normalized terror, and internalized censorship. While these scholars cannot be wholly discounted, this book does not follow their lead. Writing in the wake of the Holocaust, many of these thinkers overreached in their attempts to find the origins of, not the Enlightenment, but rather the horrors of 20th-century totalitarianism. At the same time, it would be impossible to return to the cheery narratives promulgated by earlier historians, who created a timeline of steady advancement and dismissed the pernicious aspects of this era.

In an effort to integrate these opposed narratives, this history departs from the influential, now much criticized trajectory mapped out by Foucault, while at the same time adopting some of his assumptions. There can be no question that the rise of faith in the mind, in rational citizenry, and in individuals as moral and political agents, necessarily became linked to deep concerns about the potential for irrationality and mental instability. The Age of Reason, as Foucault aptly noted, was also the Age of Unreason. I have sought to grasp these and other complexities, historical conflicts in which toleration necessarily begat new prohibitions, where radical materialism inadvertently sustained spiritual belief, and where reason and madness, like shadow and light, defined each other.

However, to follow Foucault and argue that the phenomena associated with the modern mind were always, only constructed as a means of social and political control, would be—as historian Roy Porter and others have shown—wrong. It would also close off the very debates that animate this work. What do we mean by the mind? Is it a necessary theory, a physical thing, a language game, or a deep-seated prejudice? I have used the term "invention" in my title to frame these questions, for along with its contemporary meaning, that word once denoted a process of uncovering. In this dual sense, then, the invention of the mind allows us to freely consider what was made and what was found.

Such openness is required because *Soul Machine* is a history of critical contests that helped define modern Western culture, not because they came to any decisive conclusion but because they did not. Modernity has answered many questions, but it has never found a way to fully reconcile the complex triumvirate of body, soul, and mind. Instead, it has left us haunted, divided, with competing histories, values, and rationales that have been at odds ever since.

PART I

THE LOST SOULS OF MODERNITY

For what shall it profit a man,
if he shall gain the whole world
and lose his own soul?

—ST. MARK

Dare to know.

—HORACE

1

A Soirée with Mr. Spirit and Mr. Flesh

O N MAY 29, 1660, King Charles II rode into London, the capital he had fled as a boy after the decapitation of his father. The streets were thick with welcoming crowds, tired of Puritan rule. Two or three days later, by the gate of Little Salisbury House, Charles tipped his hat to an aged well-wisher in the throngs; it was his old math tutor from Paris, one of the oddest fellows he had ever met, a Mr. Thomas Hobbes.

The melancholic, timorous Hobbes had been urged by his hard-drinking buddy, John Aubrey, to hasten in from Derbyshire, greet his former student, and perhaps win his favor. Protection of this sort was something old Hobbes could badly use. At seventy-two years of age, his longevity was already astonishing given the fearlessness of his pen: by all odds, his ideas should have left him dangling under a gallows tree years earlier. Hobbes had survived thanks to some fancy footwork, a quick dash to Paris when he infuriated English parliamentarians, then a sprint back to London when his writings enraged French Catholics.

Hobbes's trip into London proved fortuitous: he was awarded a pension and free access to the king. With Charles II enthroned, this infamous philosopher, whose name was routinely spat out as a curse, would run no more. His disturbing beliefs would need to be rebutted by words, not the tip of a sword. He would be scorned, lampooned, and refuted, but through it all he would remain free, and serve as a symbol of the fledgling kind of tolerance for moderate, "rational" dissent that marked Restoration England and led to the staging of some of the great debates that would begin to forge the modern world.

By the time of the Restoration, over two decades had passed since Hobbes had taken up a crisis that lingered over Western Christendom. Centuries of certitude—about nature, ethics, medicine, law, politics, and God—had become shaky. Thomas Hobbes was one of a loose confederation of 17th-century wanderers who moved about in search of a safe haven where they could freely consider long-forbidden, but increasingly critical new problems. Outcasts, freethinkers, libertines, and itinerant natural philosophers, they were members of an invisible tribe, the Republic of Letters, as they were dubbed by Pierre Bayle. These men made their way without support from clerically dominated universities; those that were not independently wealthy got by as tutors, doctors, clerics, and minor officials. Clandestinely, they passed about their unsigned tracts that questioned long-standing beliefs about Nature and God; political, social, and ethical life; art; math; the heavens; and the body. And at the heart of many of these controversies lurked this question: what was the human soul?

A TRANSLATION OF the Greek *psyche,* the Latin *anima,* and the Hebrew *nepesh,* the soul was an Old English word that carried a complex history. Its origins in the Western world dated back to the Homeric epics of 8th century B.C., in which a dead man's psyche was said to take up residence in Hades as a ghostly double, a shade. In this way, the soul became entwined with notions of the spirit (Greek *pneuma,* Latin *spiritus),* which referred to the wind or breath of life. Two hundred years later, pre-Socratic philosophers began to add attributes to the psyche, including an infinite capacity for understanding. By the 5th century B.C., the Greeks had amassed other, often contradictory, beliefs about the soul. Orpheus and his cult believed it was one's essence, imprisoned in the body and in need of liberation. Followers of Pythagoras considered the psyche to be a daemon cast out of heaven, sentenced to subsist in a chain of material bodies.

For Plato, the soul was our immortal, spiritual essence. The rational component was like a charioteer that drove a cart pulled by two winged horses—one noble, the courageous soul, and the other wild, the passionate soul. All thought, feeling, and passion were in *psyche*'s realm, beyond the natural world. However, as the heated debates around Socrates' death demonstrated, controversy existed over this belief. Various philosophers claimed that the soul was made of fire or air, water or blood. In that case, what Socrates and Plato both deemed eternal would perish.

Aristotle took stock of these wide-ranging positions and presented a powerful synthesis in *De anima*. By then, Greek thought

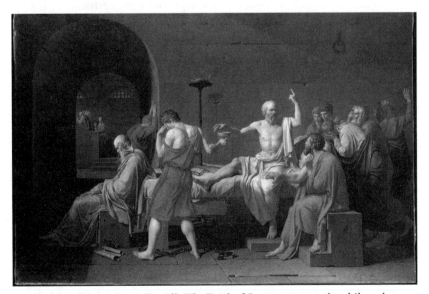

Figure 1. Jacques Louis David's *The Death of Socrates* portrays the philosopher preparing to die after beating back arguments against the soul's immortality.

included beliefs that the soul was the vital spark, the eternal being of the afterlife, the source of human reason, and the cause of bodily motion. To integrate all these meanings, Aristotle divided the soul into two forms that were material and one that was immortal. The vegetative soul was required for all life and passed away with it. The sensitive soul was the force that caused animal movement and action; it too was of matter. Only the rational soul, equated with the intellect, was eternal and divine.

Some of Aristotle's complex assemblage of meanings overlapped with the revealed truths of the Judaeo-Christian tradition. In Genesis, the soul was that which gave life to man. However, biblical notions of life after death included eternal judgment and therefore placed the battle over one's soul firmly at the center of Christian ethics and metaphysics. It was not until the 13th century that a full integration of ancient Greek and Christian notions was created by the Dominican friar Thomas Aquinas. The masterful Aquinas unified Christian theology with Aristotle, as well as that of Ptolemy and Galen. For four centuries, his integration mostly held.

At the center of the Thomist vision was a conception of the soul that proved malleable enough for classical Greek and Christian worldviews. There were three souls (or perhaps one split in three parts—the distinction kept metaphysicians up at night). Living things like trees were distinguished from dead matter by the possession of a nutritive soul. The appetitive or sensitive soul allowed for movement and was the source of the driven hungers found in animals alone. Lastly, the rational soul was exclusively human; while authors argued about its faculties, they were most often considered to be memory and reason. Throughout much of the Renaissance, this highly theorized soul united scholars and theologians. For university students, the final step in their training was the study of Aristotle's *De anima* as recontextualized by Christianity.

In Aquinas's hands, Aristotle's rational soul happily meshed with the Christian one; it distinguished humans from those they might enslave and kill, like pigs and cows. It linked men and women to the afterlife and wedded the material with the immaterial.

Thanks to these three different souls, everything from stones to beasts to angels had a place in the order of things. The medieval hierarchy known as the Great Chain of Being ranked each of God's creations. Nature began with the soulless and dead—things like rocks. Next came the most primitive living beings, plants from lowly green fungi to many-armed oaks. Animals with their striving appetites rose in complexity from oysters to lions and elephants, the reputed kings of the animal world. Lastly, above all these things, living and dead, towered one. Humans alone possessed a soul that granted them reason and thus a taste of godly power.

Reason. The capacity to think and freely act. That lifted men above passion-ridden beasts. It made humans half planted in the earth and half hovering with the seraphim. Made of flesh, torn by desire, humans alone held some of that heavenly power to think and not be ruled by their passions.

And so for the orthodox, all that was needed to be known was known. Everything had its place in the deep order willed by the Creator. Nature was as it should be, the angels and devils and stars were in place, and so too was man, from his inner being down to his social, ethical, and political world. For among humans, there was a God-given hierarchy of souls. The divinely chosen king was closest to God, followed by nobles, then lastly, the peasantry. Society and the divine were in concert, pieces of one grand system hinged on different inner essences.

Then starting almost imperceptibly in the middle of the 16th century, the scholastics' mansion of universal knowledge began to crack and fall down. And hammering away at the fissures were a growing band of rebels who called themselves modern, men such as the king's old tutor, Mr. Thomas Hobbes.

HOBBES WAS WIDELY detested. However, the task he took upon himself was acknowledged to be a great one. He was among a tiny group
of intellectuals who believed the past could no longer be relied on,
that tradition, orthodoxy, and the word of their venerated fathers
had failed them. Some, like Bernard de Fontenelle, dared to dismiss
all scholastic learning as no more than a mass delusion. A new way
of conceptualizing nature, man, and society was needed, one that
allowed for God, but was not solely based on the dictums of the
Ancient World. For the truths that had long given meaning to men
and women as they stared up at the stars and watched the seasons
change, those secure beliefs that succored them as they faced illness and sought direction in their everyday lives, this revered net of
meaning seemed to possess a growing defect: it was wrong.

Or rather, traditional claims of Aristotle, Aquinas, and their
stalwart students increasingly faced contradictory factual assertions.
And since the schoolmen's system was so deeply interconnected, one
false note, it was feared, would spread far and wide. Doubt on a
miniscule matter might raise questions regarding Aristotelian logic,
Galenic medicine, Ptolemaic cosmology, human exceptionalism,
transsubstantiation, baptism, miracles, angels, witches, Heaven,
Hell, and lastly, God Himself. Scholastics became known for dogmatically defending even the most trivial metaphysical matters. For
those intent on preserving this interdependent structure, no argument was too small.

At the same time, throughout the 16th century, scholastic thinkers
repeatedly failed to accommodate these challenges. Famously, Nico-
laus Copernicus and Galileo Galilei refuted Ptolemy's claims about
the movement of the heavens, thus upsetting God's resting place.
While this may have disturbed the repose of some elites, many others glimpsed the failure of the old beliefs when they grew ill. When

Galenic doctors arrived with their lancets, many poor beings quaked with fear and prepared to witness firsthand the failures of tradition.

Around 1600, Western medicine was still a by-the-book affair, and its authority was in serious decline. The grand humoral tradition established in the 2nd century A.D. by Galen had resisted any significant reform for an astonishing period, over 1,300 years. However, as the 17th century commenced, throughout Europe everyday impotence before the galloping rampages of disease led to an increasingly popular belief that doctors were know-nothings and money-hungry frauds, and that their traditional remedies only hastened one's doom. In addition, since the Renaissance, anatomists like Vesalius and then William Harvey had found serious errors in Galen's anatomy. With the Greek physician's loss of prestige, competition emerged from untrained empirics, barber-surgeons, apothecaries, clergymen, midwives, and alternative healers who employed astrology, folk herbal methods, magic, alchemy, and secret potions.

Alongside this uncertainty in traditional Galenic medicine, the physicians of the soul had also fallen into discord and confusion. After the Reformation, the realm of the soul had been a bloody one. Religious warfare throughout Christendom was almost unending. Challenges to papal authority led one holy truth to cross swords with another revealed truth, grossly demonstrating that earthly power alone would decide which truth prevailed. In 1648, the Peace of Westphalia put an end to the Thirty Years War. The conclusion reached was simply that there could be no real conclusion in the violent struggle for supremacy among Christian sects. Which elect, which vision of redemption, and which caste of holy men were the true ones?

When Charles II returned to England to oust the Puritans and reestablish Anglican rule, he faced a Babel of contrary beliefs. Any one creed stood in opposition to a swarm of others, ranging from radical Protestants to Jansenists, Jesuits, and Ultramontanes. Without certainty regarding the one true and Holy Word of God, political authority itself was shaken, since monarchs across Europe took their authority from divine right. As monarchs from opposite camps claimed *their* divine right, Europe itself seemed like a madhouse where a host of inmates all claimed to be Christ. While some, like Charles II, would vainly attempt to hold together this crumbling order, others like his ambitious tutor would recognize that the Old World had already shattered. Hobbes would sift through the fragments, so as to build a different system, which unified matter, man, and society. Turning away from the scholastics and the Ancients, this was a new worldview that would be called modern.

Grandiose ambition of this sort should not have been expected from Thomas Hobbes. True, he studied at Oxford and befriended the illustrious founder of empiricism, Sir Francis Bacon, for whom he took dictation. However, during his early years, Hobbes failed to originate much. After publishing a translation of Thucydides, he fell silent for decades. However, during this period of quiescence, new ideas were building inside him. By the late 1620s, Hobbes had discovered geometry and became obsessed with the idea that mathematics might be the key to . . . well, everything. Traveling along with his aristocratic patron William Cavendish to Paris in 1634, Hobbes fell in with a circle of French thinkers who were also committed to using mathematics and other methods to create a new, comprehensive, and unified view of the world.

At the center of this community was the unlikely impresario of early modern thought, the erudite, inquisitive monk Marin Mersenne. Far from taking a vow of silence, Father Mersenne kept up a tireless chatter as he promoted modern views through gatherings and incessant correspondence. He became the unofficial secretary of the Republic of Letters and formed the link between otherwise scattered thinkers like Galileo, Descartes, Hobbes, and Pascal. However, Mersenne was not just a facilitator, a conduit for others. Having studied with the Jesuits at La Flèche, he was a fierce defender of the faith who concluded that Aristotle and Aquinas no longer served that purpose. They were crumbling idols. To the circle of freethinkers who gathered around him at the Minim Friars' convent off the Place Royale, Father Mersenne communicated his conviction that the dogmas of old, so violently defended in universities and churches, were done. They had failed and could not withstand the assaults of skeptics or, worse, the heretical doctrines of Renaissance naturalists.

The receding authority of scholasticism, Mersenne believed, exposed Christianity to the risk that the void left behind would be filled by notions of Nature that were laced with occult mystery and magic, a bevy of Platonic, Cabalistic, alchemical, and esoteric ideas, all heresies that replaced the central authority of God with a world soul or a God-like force in Nature. Renaissance "animists"—those who believed the spiritual world existed within the material one—were the heretics he most despised. For over a century, Italy had produced a number of such thinkers: Pietro Pomponace, a doctor condemned by the Inquisition, claimed miracles were simply hard-to-fathom natural occurrences. Girolamo Cardano, a physician and mathematician, believed the stars could dictate human actions. The most famous of these pagan challengers, the Dominican Giordano Bruno, was burned at the stake in 1600 for his pantheism. In England, fears of such conjurers had been stoked by the English playwright Christopher Marlowe's *The Tragical History of Dr. Faustus*, in which he retold the story of a scholar, astrologer, and magician, whose intense desire to know the powerful magic within nature led him to trade his soul to the Devil. Over the next three decades, legends accrued about this play, and it was said that during its performance, members of the audience saw demons, while others simply became mad.

Marin Mersenne loathed these heresies. And he feared them. By 1624, the friar began to search for a new way to replace scholasticism and simultaneously discredit those animistic naturalists, those Cabalists who placed the soul in the stars and in potions, and in the whole of the Earth. An alternative was needed that preserved the categorical

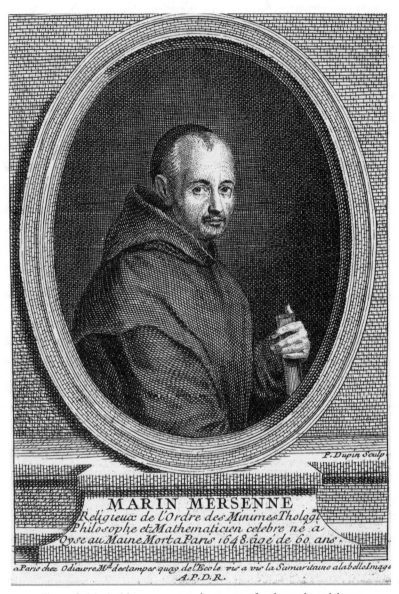

Figure 2. Marin Mersenne sat at the center of early modern debates
on the soul and Nature.

distinction between man's soul and Nature, a line heretics like Bruno
blurred or denied. Mersenne found his answer in the emerging new
philosophy based on an improbable prototype: machines.

Nature could be conceived of as a grand machine, a mechanism that yielded its secrets if one simply analyzed it as bodies in motion. This mechanical philosophy did not originate with the Minim friar. A number of early 17th-century thinkers had also fastened on mathematics, geometry, and physics to develop a mechanistic understanding of Nature. The most famed, Galileo Galilei, conducted decisive studies of mass in motion on the Earth, the seas and in the skies. Mersenne became a great supporter of the embattled Italian even after the Inquisition condemned him to house arrest. In Paris, the friar dared to promote Galileo's work and became his French translator. Mersenne added his own commentary and published *The Mechanics of Galilei* in 1634, then four years later *The New Thought of Galilei*.

Thereafter, Mersenne took up an almost evangelical belief in mechanics as the science of appearances, the outer dance of Nature. And his campaign would be so effective that a few decades later one of his former acolytes, Christiaan Huygens, now the leader of French science, proclaimed that the only true philosophy of nature was mechanical.

Father Mersenne was excited by both the strengths *and* the failings of this new philosophy. Mechanics disrupted the tired dogmas and allowed for an exciting, skeptical investigation of Nature. At the same time, this view undermined animistic and magical beliefs. While Renaissance naturalism had undercut biblical ideas of divinity and Christian ethics by making all of the soul, even the rational soul, a part of living, breathing Mother Nature, mechanics did precisely the opposite. It yanked the soul out of the Earth, the stars, and our bodies. Magical spirits and life forces were nonsense. Matter in motion explained Nature's workings. Mechanics dictated a cool analysis of actions and reactions in matter. By this reasoning, astrology eventually would become astronomy, and alchemy would transform into chemistry.

At the same time, Mersenne's Christian soul could rest easy. For machines, even glorious, ingenious machines, could only do so much. If Nature was a clock, as the common analogy declared, then something would always be missing. No clock built itself: it required a watchmaker. Moving matter could not decide or will or think. The springs and gears of a machine might record time. However, gears could never, ever contemplate time. Thus, the limits of mechanics happily made way for God. Mechanics required higher properties of human experience, which would rest on biblical revelation. If Nature was only matter in motion, then the soul would remain in another realm, forever divine.

Once he envisioned this forked path forward, Marin Mersenne promoted it tirelessly. As his Minim convent became renowned as the center of debate on the new natural philosophy, Mersenne entertained a wide array of anti-Aristotelian skeptics. He displayed no tolerance for animistic naturalists, whom he believed were blasphemers. When Tommaso Campanella, an astrologer who defended Galileo, fled Italy for France, he presented himself at the Minim convent. Father Mersenne turned him away. Astrologers were sinners and false prophets. Nature was not the realm of the miraculous, but rather the merely mechanical.

As he was waging this battle to redefine the boundaries of science and religion, Mersenne met the brilliant Pierre Gassendi. A Catholic priest who counted one of France's great libertines as a friend, Gassendi's thought was never easy to pigeonhole, a problem that may have contributed to his relative disappearance from history. Nonetheless, in the 17th century, Pierre Gassendi was a giant, a thinker whose efforts to redefine Nature and the soul would be greatly influential, if often unacknowledged.

A young prodigy born in Provence, Gassendi received his doctorate, became ordained, and seemed destined to devote his life to the Church. However, in 1617 he applied for and received a professorship in philosophy at Aix-en-Provence, where he was entrusted with passing on the Aristotelian dogmas he had already grown disenchanted with, thanks to his reading of classical sources like Cicero,

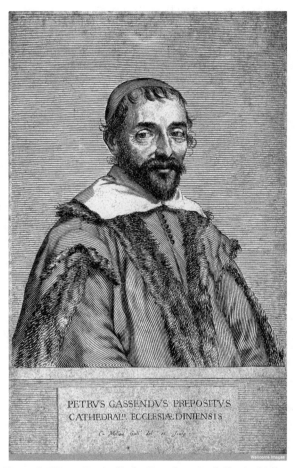

PETRVS GASSENDVS PREPOSITVS
CATHEDRAL. ECCLESIÆ DINIENSIS

Figure 3. Pierre Gassendi, the French anti-scholastic thinker.

Horace, and Lucretius, as well as modern authors like Michel de Montaigne. While Gassendi dutifully trained his students in scholastic thought, he also developed numerous stinging critiques of his forebearers. Not surprisingly, this questioning scholar was sacked after Jesuits took over the university in 1622.

Two years later, the former professor let out a howl of protest. *Exercitationes paradoxicae adversus Aristoteleos* was a no-holds-barred assault on the status quo. This scathing attack included the promise of seven more books to come, each intended to be another nail in old Aristotle's coffin. This first book would take up the philosopher's dogmatism, the second his dialectic, the third his physics, and so on. The fifth volume, he announced, would tear up false beliefs regarding the nature of life, as well as erroneous notions of reason and the soul. Following volumes would rewrite metaphysics and moral philosophy. In short, the blustery Gassendi announced a revolution. And he gave his enemies advanced warning of his battle plans.

In 1625, the provincial author traveled to Paris and discovered the old order was ready to greet him. Two months before Gassendi's arrival, the powerful theology faculty at the Sorbonne instigated legal changes in the Parlement that criminalized the promulgation of anti-Aristotelian ideas. Three renegade thinkers had been fingered and one arrested. As the scholastics clamped down, the young priest introduced himself to Father Mersenne, who took the young man in and urged him to let the diseased Aristotle die of his own accord. Attacking the flailing schoolmen was foolhardy and unnecessary. However, the times badly required the creation of a new foundation for the study of nature, one that would also be a bulwark for Christianity.

Gassendi took Mersenne's advice to heart; the next volume of his proposed polemic against the scholastics would only appear after its author's death. The other volumes would never be written. In 1630, when asked why he discontinued his criticism of Aristotle, Gassendi confessed it had become a matter of safety; the publication of the first volume almost led to what he vaguely referred to as a "tragedy," no doubt his own.

Nonetheless, while he would be careful about what he published, Pierre Gassendi did not fully retreat. Instead, he adopted a credo from Horace that would come to be a calling card for the self-proclaimed enlightened over the next 150 years: "*Sapere aude*"—Dare to know. He left Paris and for the coming years scraped by as an itinerant scholar who relied on wealthy patrons. And though he called off his duel with the Sorbonne theologians, Pierre Gassendi did boldly propose a new worldview. If Thomas Aquinas wove together Aristotle with the Scriptures, this priest believed the ancient philosopher Epicurus could provide a more stable foundation for our understanding of the natural world, ethics, and Christianity.

The choice was inexplicable, horrifying, and outrageous. A reviled heretic despised by Church Fathers, Epicurus never had been reconciled with Christianity. Widely believed to be an atheist and a lowdown hedonist, he won a special spot deep down in Dante's *Inferno*:

> *In this dark part are entombed*
> *Epicurus and all his followers,*
> *who made the soul die with the body.*

Epicurus's conception of Nature meant terrible things for a Christian. Nature, *in toto*, was made of atoms, the material *minima* of the world, thus there was no Providence. And since these infinite bits of matter made everything, that included man's soul, which meant that the soul would suffer the same rotten fate.

To make matters worse, Epicurus ascribed to hedonistic principles that were scandalous: ethics, he had argued, were based on the human search for pleasure and the avoidance of pain. Some have called the tradition of philosophy a history of creative or polemical misunderstandings; this was clearly Epicurus's fate. For upon inspection, a reader easily discovers that for him, the serenity of the soul was the highest pleasure of all. Thus, the Greek philosopher was skeptical about immediate kinds of hedonistic and sexual abandon, for he thought those spasms of joy might roil the soul for years to come. Epicurus and his followers actually were said to live rather ascetic lives. Nonetheless, their ethic was caricatured by rivals from the Stoics to the early Christians, as nothing more than a pig philosophy devoted to wild, orgiastic gratification. The Church Fathers denounced Epicureans, such as the brilliant Lucretius, as lechers, heathens, and anarchists. This was the Epicurus that Pierre Gassendi had nominated to be the bedrock of a new Christian worldview. Dare to know, indeed.

And yet, Gassendi saw that this ancient Athenian philosopher and his followers offered something important. The view that Nature was made up of small atoms in motion cohered nicely with the study of matter and motion, the mechanical philosophy the priest had adopted thanks to his reading of Galileo and the urging of Mersenne. Gassendi himself took up serious observation of the stars and planets, and sought to contribute to this field. And like Mersenne, he sought to discredit Renaissance naturalists with their animistic spirits, and even wrote a diatribe against the English astrologer Robert Fludd. In this struggle, Epicurus was a powerful ally, for he envisioned Nature as solid matter, which made no space for heretical notions like world souls, mystical natural forces, Platonic *anima mundi*, or other such heresies.

Still, any Christian follower of Epicurus faced deep trouble, for his philosophy suggested that the soul's rewards or punishments in Heaven and Hell were based on a lie. Souls made of atoms must perish. Undeterred, the Catholic priest hoped to rehabilitate a modified Epicurus and penned a glowing biography, a project that then grew into a full exposition of the man's thought. Rather than accept a universe of random atoms in motion, Gassendi argued that God had given atoms their first push. Since the Heavenly Father originated all motion, His presence and care hovered over all.

AS PIERRE GASSENDI began to work on a modern version of Epicurean thought, Thomas Hobbes arrived in Paris. Mersenne likely introduced the Englishman to Gassendi's belief in atomism and materialism. Soon, Hobbes returned to his homeland intent on pressing these ideas into his own fearless *summa*, a complete, universal mechanistic and materialist philosophy of nature and man. Like Epicurus, whose philosophy covered physics, logics, and ethics, Hobbes divided his unified theory into three: physics and the universe, psychology and the workings of inner man, and finally the political order. All these would be woven into a grand tapestry. If the scholastic vision had cracked, Hobbes planned to reunify all knowledge through his use of the same, simple building blocks—matter and motion. And so, he ruthlessly followed mechanics to quite shocking conclusions. There were no supernatural forces, no shift in kind from inert object to human beings to the divine. Matter structured the natural world, and it made man, his soul, and his God. Ghosts, angels, immaterial thoughts, and ethereal spirits were delusions, a kind of communal nightmare.

Hobbes hoped that his first volume of mechanics would demonstrate that the physical world was based entirely on lawful motion. The second would take up the soul and its passions "from their original causes," by which he meant their material basis. Memory, dreams, ideas, and hallucinations would not be accounted for by the soul, but would be understood as mechanical disturbances in the brain. The connection between soul and body would also be explained; ideas from the brain generated action in the heart, which made for pleasure or pain. Sad imaginations could affect the spleen, and strong spleens in turn could cause fearful dreams. In the third and final volume of this work, Hobbes would detail the way his materialist framework unveiled the true nature of ethics. He would create a science of politics, based on underlying mechanics of the natural world and the inner being of man.

In 1640, a draft of this unified worldview was completed; Hobbes was fifty-two years old. But as he continued work on his magnum opus, England began to teeter on the edge of civil war. His country began to "burn with questions of Sovereignty and the due obedience of citizens." As a defender of the Stuart monarchy, long in the employ of the wealthy polymath William Cavendish, the Earl of

Newcastle-upon-Tyne, Hobbes took time out from his loftier ambitions to write an anonymous pamphlet filled with Royalist convictions. When unmasked, Hobbes became a marked man. He fled to Paris and there seemed to abandon his dream of a unified synthesis of physics, psychology, and ethics.

Hobbes rejoined Father Mersenne's illustrious group at the Minim friars' convent, a vibrant community of doctors, aristocrats, and clergymen who shared a passion for geometry, mechanics, and a rational rewriting of Nature. By 1641, Hobbes had befriended Gassendi. The two developed a close bond, which was only heightened by a common enemy. Both thinkers had become embroiled in bitter quarrels with another luminary in Mersenne's circle, another man who aspired to be the modern answer to Aristotle, the vain, brilliant, and reclusive René Descartes.

Born in 1596, the son of a minor French noble, René studied at La Flèche, the same rigorous Jesuit academy that produced Mersenne. Afterward, he embraced military life and volunteered for battle. In the course of his adventures, the young man met Isaac Beeckman, a devotee of natural philosophy, who introduced the swashbuckler to the beauties of geometry and thereby ignited his dream of using mathematics to create an "opus infinitum." One cold November night, Descartes had a series of three dreams that fostered an epiphany of how spatial problems could become algebraic, which crystallized a vision of a natural world underwritten by mathematical laws. It was the sort of insight that had the power to change a man's life, and it did. Over the next decade, Descartes devoted himself to this grand, unifying project.

In 1628, during a public lecture in Paris in which an alchemist critiqued Aristotle, Descartes publicly revealed some of the fruits of this labor. He rose from the audience to dispute the veracity of this theory. His belief was that better methods and principles must be used to establish sound knowledge. Skepticism could be coupled with a process of breaking down problems into their smallest parts and building up conclusions from there. In the audience, Cardinal de Bérulle immediately grasped the power of Descartes's proposals. He became the patron of the thirty-two-year-old in the hope that his ideas would lead to practical advances and reform old fields, such as one close to Descartes's heart, medicine.

After he secured the cardinal's support, René took off for Holland, where he lived in seclusion for all but the last two years of his life. His destination was no accident. By the 17th century, the Dutch had won a reputation for harboring freethinkers and minorities from the Marrano Jews of Spain and the French Huguenots to whoever happened to be out of power in England. Descartes needed that freedom, but he also wanted to disappear. A loner who never married, he moved periodically from village to village so as to ensure his solitude; Mersenne was one of very few to reliably know the thinker's whereabouts. Deeply devoted to his studies, Descartes's quarters included a garden to observe plant life and a room suitable for dissections. And through these studies, he sought to establish a new view of the cosmos and man, all to be put forth in a book he planned to call simply, stunningly, *The World*.

An ardent believer, Descartes sought to remake the study of Nature while upholding the Christian faith. And following Mersenne, he had a ready solution. One could rid oneself of dogmatic scholasticism with all its unproven, hairsplitting doctrines by viewing Nature as a massive mechanical object. Thus, everything under and above the sun would be open for skeptical inquiry. At the same time, there would be an impassable boundary. Mechanical explanations would be helpless before questions regarding any higher-level actions, anything directed, willful, and purposeful. Hence, this framework liberated science to discover all it could about the Nature-machine, while preserving God's necessary place in human life. Nature was passive matter buzzing about in motion, but the Deity and his representative in humans, the soul, remained the Prime Mover, the only active force of life. By 1628, Descartes shared his views with Mersenne, whose powerful advocacy would soon be his.

The World would cover nature, the human body, and the soul. In the first section, Descartes, like Hobbes, accounted for nature as simple matter in motion. He proposed a theory of corpuscles in which different-sized objects moved in vortices and complex geometric patterns that made up the celestial world. Nature from the stars to the smallest pebble could be explained through predictable, lawful, interrelated causal actions.

By late 1632, Descartes moved on to the second section, which would be published as *Treatise of Man*. Here he dismissed the scholastic division of three souls animating plants, animals, and man and declared all of creation, every wiggling and purposeful thing, to be soulless except for mankind. Dogs and tigers were machines like the automata Descartes witnessed in the water fountains of the royal gardens of Saint-Germain-en-Laye. There an ingenious Italian craftsman had created hydraulically powered statues that whirled, slayed dragons, and to the audience's great astonishment, blared on trumpets. Impressed by this display, Descartes began to consider animals as machines of a similar sort.

Could the same be true of the human body? Descartes had been seriously studying anatomy and physiology for years; in Amsterdam in 1635, he was delighted to rent a home near the local butchers, where he often watched the slaughter and rescued discarded cow organs to dissect in peace at home. He devoured William Harvey's revolutionary book on blood circulation, another blow to Galen. And he began to imagine a mechanical physiology that did away with the humors.

The philosopher's entry into medicine was not unusual. In the 17th century, universities had only three realms of advanced study—theology, law, and medicine. Thus, the study of human nature fell to gentlemen trained in medicine as well as educated amateurs. Descartes was of the latter group, though one dead serious about his

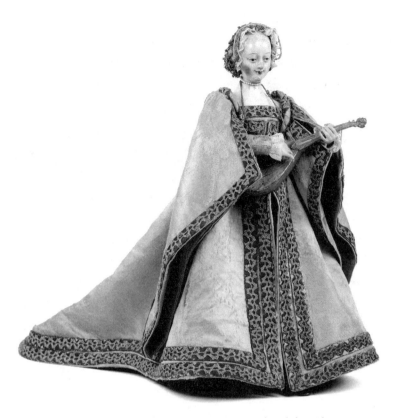

Figure 4. This 16th-century automaton played the zither,
and turned its head as it moved.

research. At the conclusion of his revolutionary 1637 *Discourse on the Method of Properly Conducting One's Reason and of Seeking Truth in the Sciences*, the Frenchman confided that his ardent desire was to secure pragmatic knowledge of a specific sort. The rest of his days, he announced, would be devoted to acquiring "some knowledge of Nature, which may be such as to enable us to deduce from it rules in medicine." This overriding interest would guide him to the exclusion of "all other sorts of projects."

Descartes considered himself a doctor of sorts. The grandson of two physicians, he knew the most potent form of proof for his own physiological theories was whether they cured or prevented illness. Not burdened by modesty, he declared that despite his own weak constitution—as a child, doctors had predicted his early demise—he would live more than a century, as long he perfected his medical theories. A few years later, Descartes revealed his investigation into the erroneous ways that people lived; from these studies, he promised to construct a medical compendium that would serve as his own "stay of execution." He let it slip that he considered the life span of the biblical patriarchs, recorded in the Book of Genesis as over nine centuries, within his grasp. Among the cognoscenti of Europe, word spread that Descartes had solved the riddle of mortality. Letters began to arrive that asked him for medical advice, and Descartes did not hesitate to prescribe treatments. In the end, he was confident that a radically new Cartesian medicine would prove its merits.

Next, Descartes prepared to write the last section of *The World* on the soul. In November of 1633, however, he was stunned to discover that Galileo had been condemned by the Inquisition for his heliocentric views. Frightened, he contemplated burning all his papers. He put aside *The World* forever.

⌒

SEVEN YEARS LATER, on November 11, 1640, Descartes informed Mersenne that a Dutch emissary, Constantijn Huygens, would be arriving in Paris with an untitled manuscript. Descartes hoped the friar would distribute this short series of meditations to both the conservative Theology Faculty at the Sorbonne as well as those free-thinkers within his circle. When the pages arrived, Mersenne opened them and discovered *Meditations on the First Philosophy in Which the Existence of God and the Real Distinction Between the Soul and the Body of Man Are Demonstrated*. The work adopted the literary conceit of following a philosopher during six straight days of contemplation. The association with Genesis was perhaps inadvertent, but readers throughout Europe would conclude that during those six days, Descartes had done something astonishing.

First published in Latin in 1641, the *Meditations* were translated and published in French in 1647, alongside a number of objections orchestrated by the Minim maestro, written by him as well as Pierre Gassendi, Thomas Hobbes, and others. Despite the many contradictions and doubts these interlocutors hurled in its way, Descartes's tour de force quickly won devotees. For while dismissing the Old Order in favor of skepticism, freedom of inquiry, and a mathematical, rule-based approach to natural philosophy, the *Meditations* absolutely affirmed Christianity. The thinker had lifted the skeptics' sword and at the last moment turned it against them, thereby cutting a path for devout, natural philosophers.

In solitude, Descartes had struggled with the terrible problem that faced the moderns and what was called their *philosophie nouvelle*. In his *Discourse on Method*, he told his own coming-of-age story, one that rang true for many early savants. He had devoted himself to garnering knowledge at the Collège de La Flèche, one of the great educational institutions in Europe, and at the end of his rigorous studies, concluded that he knew nothing. He expected little more from books, for now he could see that the best minds created nothing more than opinions. Thus, the graduate set out to study the book of the world; he traveled, went to war, and discovered to his dismay that under the guise of common sense and custom, much that passed for truth was absurd. Surrounded by a rotting orthodoxy, many of his educated readers would have agreed.

Descartes sought to subject everything to doubt, and as he did so, he wondered where it would end. If received wisdom was little more than misguided custom, if reason was stuffed full of false ideas, one should be skeptical of one's own thought. While Aristotle compared perception to the faithful imprint an object made on wax, for Descartes, like Hobbes and Gassendi, that was quite naïve.

Perception was often demonstrably false, and therefore clearly not based on a direct imprint. Seeing and hearing and feeling only led to mediated and questionable information. And once such doubt resided within perception, absolute truth vanished.

However, in the *Discourse on Method*, the narrator had proposed a solution that he had developed in the *Meditations*. Of all that he might doubt, one reality seemed indubitable if ironic: he was now doubting. Famously in 1637 he wrote: "Cogito, ergo sum"—I think, therefore I am. In the *Meditations*, Descartes returned to the bottom floor, the solid place from which other undeniable truths might be

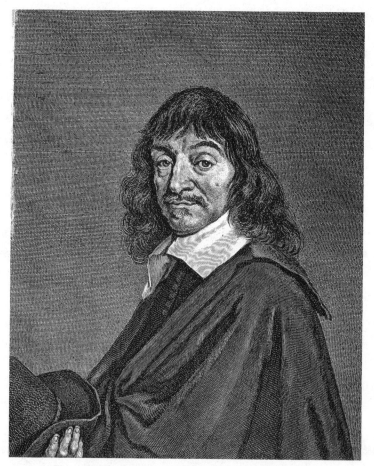

Figure 5. The brilliant, reclusive René Descartes, 1649.

built. Only one reality could not be questioned. "I am, I exist." I am therefore a "thing that thinks."

With this, Descartes expressed something that could not but resonate powerfully with his readers: inner experience was immediate, unquestionable, and utterly unique. Knowledge of our own thoughts was not like knowing whether the sun rose in the east or if all frogs were green. Thought presented itself with certainty; its immediacy and wholeness seemed to be a foothold in an otherwise shadowy world of perceptions and inferences, the dark world of Plato's cave.

In the *Meditations*, Descartes reached this philosophical terra firma by pushing his skepticism as far as it could go. Say the world was a dream, or God's cruel deception, or a massive delusion created by an evil demon. Even so, our own thought could not be unreal. To some of his contemporaries, Descartes's logic was odd, even a bit perverse. Pierre Gassendi urged his colleague to drop the rhetorical games. However, this Jesuit-trained thinker was quite serious: he believed he had embraced skepticism and then—almost magically—turned that traditional weapon against faith into a bulwark for believers. By relying on nothing more than questioning and analysis, he seemed to have proven that thought was the absolute foundation of being and knowledge.

And not just abstract thought, but a "thing that thinks," which must be the soul. Descartes dispensed with the other souls from Aquinas that he could not justify philosophically. He restricted that term to that immaterial aspect of human beings that can think. He dismissed sensitive and vegetative souls, dismissed a soul that gave life, and left only one. The soul thinks.

Thus, long histories attached to powerful words collapsed and became confused. The Latin *anima* and its French cognate, *âme*, were words that naturally referred to the "animating," life-giving soul. The Latin *mentis* from the Greek *menos*, was "mind" in English, a widely used synonym for not the entirety of the soul, but just the rational soul. It had no equivalent in French. One could refer to *mentalité* as an adjective, but the closest noun in French was *esprit*—spirit, which was loaded with religious connotations. For this term primarily denoted the immaterial spirit, the third part of the Trinity, and the spirit of angels and demons. Only secondarily did it refer to the soul's faculties of thought; a 1611 French-English dictionary gave those as the sixth and seventh possible meanings.

In early sections of the French translation of the *Meditations* that Descartes carefully revised and authorized, these same traditional, if shaky, distinctions remain. *Mentis* is rendered *esprit*, or mind, and *anima* becomes *âme*, or soul. However, later, especially in the Sixth Meditation, Descartes collapsed these distinctions. He approved the translation of the Latin word for "mind" with the French word for "soul," then zigzagged back and forth interchangeably using words for mind and soul. This was no error. Descartes exploited the ambiguity in French to unify the indisputable thinking being with that eternal life force and distinguish both from the material body. *Esprit* and *âme*, *mentis* and *anima*, mind and soul: all were one. The complex Thomist soul was sheared of its material and animal realms, and left to stand as pure, immaterial consciousness, God's gift to humankind, the very opposite of the body. After speaking at length of his mind, he concluded: "It is certain that this me, that is my soul, by which I am what I am, is entirely and truly distinct from my body." Before the razor of radical skepticism, only that remained. Like a modern Aquinas, Descartes believed he had found a way to merge the demands of skeptical naturalism with those of Christian belief. Through logic and doubt, he secured the immortal soul. Conscious thought, doubt, and reason stood at the center of what made us human.

Despite grave problems with this synthesis, the Cartesian split between the soul and Nature would spread. In part, it was old wine in a new bottle. Descartes preserved the most critical aspect of Thomist inner life, the rational soul, while he jettisoned the rest of scholastic biology along with its accounts of what distinguished the living from the dead, what made for action and will, what separated animals from man. He preserved the rational soul for believers who now reconciled themselves to life in an otherwise mechanical world. It was not folly for Descartes to hope that the Theology Faculty in Paris, to whom he dedicated this work, would be delighted.

However, to save the soul, Descartes had performed a radical amputation. And as with all such surgeries, there were grave side effects. The unified schema of Aquinas, honed over centuries, answered many questions that were now left in doubt. Though Descartes preserved the rational soul, he ripped up the Chain of Being and segregated humans from the rest of creation. In his view, there were two utterly divided domains: Nature was composed of passive matter and ruled by mechanical actions. Though its substance never fully disappeared, its elaborate constructions broke down and died. The soul, however, never decayed. It was linked to the realm of Heaven, and its sole function was the intellect, understanding, thought. Mankind was half matter and half spirit, part machine and part divine reason.

Mersenne had faith that mechanics required a place for God and this was his reward. Everything but the soul was mechanized, even life. With a few strokes of his pen, Descartes had desacralized the pulsing, hungry, and buzzing world. Only humans possessed a force capable of will and directed action. No *anima* made sense of flowers, bees, and bears. In Descartes's new model, the sky, the earth and all that lay in it comprised a grand, whirring machine. While his body remained part of that Nature-machine, man's Cogito stood outside of it; it was the children of God's sign of distinction, proof of their holy origins.

IN 1648, DURING a rare visit to Paris in which he hoped—in vain, it turned out—to win a pension from the Court, Descartes attended a gathering at the home of Thomas Hobbes's patron William Cavendish, the exiled Earl of Newcastle-upon-Tyne. There he came face-to-face with his two great rivals, Thomas Hobbes and Pierre Gassendi. The meeting could not have been comfortable. While Gassendi and Hobbes shared a loathing for Descartes, he felt contempt for his rivals. The Englishman and his sniping—which included a fifty-six page riposte attacking the *Discourse*—greatly annoyed him. Other than the publication *De cive*, this haughty English fellow had little to support such arrogance, though he could be congratulated on recently becoming the math tutor of his country's banished prince, the young Charles. In his letters, Descartes deemed Hobbes to be pernicious, childish, and ridiculous. His notions of a corporeal soul and a corporeal God were absurd.

Hobbes had been relatively gentle in his published criticisms of Descartes's *Meditations*, but even that did not mask their mutual dislike. Hobbes insisted that there could be no innate idea of the soul; furthermore, Descartes had not proven that the soul was incorporeal. In the end, Hobbes asserted that Descartes's soul, his basis for our very being, divorced as it was from the senses, rested solely on the conviction that the Heavenly Father would not delude his children. Hobbes mischievously added that a beneficent Lord might delude us for our own good. Descartes's attempt to know God and the soul through reason was risible, absurd. He would later tear into Cartesian phrases like "immaterial substance" and conclude they were ludicrous oxymorons.

With Pierre Gassendi, the quarreling was worse. His snide objections to Descartes's *Meditations* quickly descended into name-calling, finger-pointing, and bitter recriminations. Both thinkers were pushed to justify their differences: Gassendi would publish a rebuttal, which at over 300 pages was far longer than the book he would rebut. Descartes, in a later edition of *Meditations*, floated the accusation that the priest was behind a clandestine conspiracy against him.

Bubbling beneath Hobbes and Gassendi's anger was the belief that Descartes had sold out. He had pandered to ecclesiastic author-

ity. His attempts to justify the Catholic belief that the bread and wine
of communion were literally transformed into the body and blood
of Jesus, Hobbes privately concluded, was simply an act of bad faith,
a rationalization that revealed how badly this thinker strove to be
the Jesuits' intellectual savior. Hobbes complained that both he and
Gassendi had been forced to beat back Descartes's ghosts and had in
the process paid a heavy price.

For Gassendi, the cost of the fight was greatest. Around 1637, as he
went about integrating Catholicism with Epicurus, busily preparing a
chapter on fate and causality, he fell into a personal crisis. Materialism
had led him down a path and now he saw what lay ahead: atheism,
heresy. When Gassendi read Hobbes's *De cive*, his ally's materialism
seemed to dictate that we lived in a world in which God did not
intercede. Hobbes had created a system in which corpuscular physics
made human fate nothing more than motion and matter.

While Pierre Gassendi fought to be free from dogma, he was
also deeply committed to the freedom of individuals to pursue serenity and pleasure. A free God had made the world and passed this
capacity for liberty on to his children. His patron Nicolas-Claude
Fabri de Peiresc had introduced Gassendi to some of the great *libertins
érudits* of France, skeptics who pursued moral freedom like Gabriel
Naudé, Elie Diodati, and the tutor of Louis XIV, François de La
Mothe le Vayer. While scholars have suggested Pierre himself was
secretly a libertine, Gassendi's pursuit of liberty never overrode his
faith. Instead, the clash of these two imperatives created intense tension and paralysis, as he struggled to find a way to accommodate
contradictory beliefs.

In 1645, thanks to the brother of Minister Richelieu, Gassendi
garnered a professorial post in mathematics at the Collège Royal.
However, endless revisions and hesitancy continually held him back
from publishing. In 1647, he finally released his grip on a ten-year-
old manuscript, his admiring portrait of Epicurus. Then two years
later, after endless rewrites and a great deal of pressure from frus-

trated admirers, the reluctant philosopher released *Animadversione*, a three-volume work of more than 1,700 pages. Purported to be a translation of Diogenes, these books held reams of commentary. And smuggled into this wild tangle were hints of the philosopher's long-awaited synthesis. However, it was only in 1655, after his death, that the fruit of Pierre Gassendi's terrible inner struggles emerged.

Syntagma philosophicum was written during the last six years of Gassendi's life. In it, he reconciled doubt and faith, materialism and immortality, in a way that rejected the dogmas of the past as well as the modern dogmas of René Descartes. At the heart of his proposals was the conviction, expressed years earlier in his critique of the scholastics, that human knowledge was a highly limited enterprise. Knowledge was based solely on sensations and experience and therefore its truths were fallible and unsure. The professors at the Sorbonne eliminated uncertainty with doctrine. So too did Descartes with his creed that clear and evident ideas led to certain knowledge. Gassendi brushed aside Descartes's assertion that God would not delude us and acidly asked how Monsieur Descartes knew *that*?

Instead of such false certainty, Gassendi embraced epistemic modesty, the limits of human knowledge, and probability. If knowledge came from the processing of sensations, humans could know only so much. Claims that went beyond these boundaries were mere vanity. Where Descartes wrote "I am then absolutely a thing that thinks, that is to say a spirit, a soul, an intelligence, a reason," Gassendi found nothing but pomposity and a string of increasingly empty words.

Humans lived in an atomistic world, where sensations registered in the soul led to only highly partial, contingent understanding. Despite living in a mechanical world, human beings, as moral agents, were liberated to think and choose not between right and wrong, but rather between possibilities. If knowledge was partial, it could never be absolute or support tyranny. Skepticism led to liberty in thought and action. In this, Gassendi went far, though not as far as some skeptics like La Mothe le Vayer, who believed nothing could be truly known and therefore everything was permitted.

Readers had a right to be confused by some of these conclusions. If Gassendi claimed that the immortal soul registered half-truths and faulty impressions, how could it be God's gift to man? To solve this dilemma, Gassendi split the soul in half. Passive sensation was registered in a material soul, one common to brutes and humans. That soul performed tasks like simple apprehension, inference, and judgment, all of which were frail and imperfect. Another soul, however, was divine. This logic was transparently a matter of convenience; it covered the philosopher's flank. However, its results upset centuries of doctrine. For against Descartes and his immaterial Cogito, Pierre Gassendi had asserted that in some ways, *matter could think.*

With that, Gassendi pushed open a door that had been locked. He cleared the way for natural philosophers to consider a material, thinking soul. Still, he did not believe man was nothing but flesh. His second soul was also a seat of rationality, one that allowed for volition, abstract thought untied to sensation, and universal kinds of understanding. *That* soul could not be known through Descartes's cunning sophistry, but only through faith. And as for this soul's nature, its relation to the body, its substance and faculties, all those things were impossible to fathom.

While these positions were not fully in print until the priest had left this world, many of them had burst forth in his angry quarrel with Descartes. Gassendi mocked Descartes's claim to know the soul by tricks and derided his pretension of doubting everything and pretending reality was a dream. Did Descartes walk off cliffs without apprehension, since the cliff was a dream? He did not. To speak like this was ridiculous. Fed up, Gassendi addressed his foe as "Spirit, (or whatever name you want to go by!)" The comment enraged Descartes, who retorted that such a comment could only come from a being made only of matter, "Flesh (or whatever name you want to go by!)?"

As the exchange grew even more heated, the two men consolidated their positions and mocked each other with these new nicknames. Mr. Spirit and Mr. Flesh relentlessly struggled over great questions regarding how exactly the Moderns, advocates of the new natural philosophy, would define the soul, inner being, thought, and the body. Mr. Flesh sarcastically congratulated Mr. Spirit on his great discovery, *the mind thinks!* However, he adamantly rejected as utterly unproven the assertion that animals were unable to think, and that the body contributed nothing to thought. Committed to a broader notion of the soul, Gassendi pressed Descartes: "Stop right there, Spirit!" he demanded. Are you just a thinking thing? And if you are a mind, aren't you part matter? Descartes dismissed many of Gassendi's questions, but to this he replied that the meaning of the soul had grown so dirty that it needed a good bath. He himself had cleansed the word of many false meanings: it meant only one thing—thought. *Anima* was *mentis*, *esprit* was *âme*, the soul was the mind, and the mind was the immortal, rational soul.

The battle between Mr. Spirit and Mr. Flesh was nasty, and a prelude to centuries of argument to come. In this exchange, Pierre Gassendi pointed out Descartes's Achilles heel. Gassendi demanded to know how an immaterial soul could possibly affect a material body and vice versa. With this, Descartes fell silent. In a letter to a colleague, he quipped: "Ignorant people can in fifteen minutes ask more questions of *this* kind than a wise man could answer in a lifetime, and that's why I am not answering either of them."

<hr />

COMPETING MODERN VISIONS of the soul swirled about at the soirée hosted by the Marquess of Newcastle in 1647. For centuries, it seemed, humans had been deceived by Aristotle, Galen, and Ptolemy. The moderns believed they needed to be a new foundation for knowledge, one that took into account this lesson regarding false beliefs, and the imperfections of perception. Thus, new worldviews would end up resting rather perilously on fine points regarding how one knew and thought. By placing such weight on the workings of what was the rational soul, these moderns were forced to closely reconsider not just its immortality, but also functions like understanding, imagination, and thought as well as their shadows, illusion, hallucination, and delusion.

This dinner party would be the first and last time these three titans of early modernity would meet. Only a year later, the conductor of these great debates, Marin Mersenne, died with Father Gassendi by his side. Thus ended one of the most extraordinary intellectual communities of the time. A number of informal scientific groups rose up to fill the void. For example, two supporters of Hobbes and Gassendi, Samuel Sorbière and Abraham du Prat, created a salon for physicians, philosophers, and experimentalists in the home of Henri-Louis Habert de Montmor, which formed the nucleus that founded the Académie des Sciences in Paris in 1666.

By then, however, the two other titans who tried to pull together a modern synthesis for Nature, man, and God, also had ended their days. In 1650, René Descartes developed a fever, rejected the bleedings of a court physician, one of his personal enemies, and relied on his own medication, wine flavored with tobacco. When that failed, the patient who had hoped his research would grant him the life span of Abraham and Methuselah, consented to be bled and soon thereafter became nothing but Cogito. In 1655, Father Pierre Gassendi also left this earth; he too was hurried into God's arms by the bloodletting of his doctor.

Unlike the others, however, Thomas Hobbes was granted the gift of a long life. He used his extra time well. A year after that evening with Descartes and Gassendi, at the ripe age of sixty, Hobbes finally sat down to write a work that would justify the admiration he had won from a wide circle of savants. In 1651, *Leviathan; or, The Matter, Forme, and Power of a Common-wealth, Ecclesiasticall and Civill*

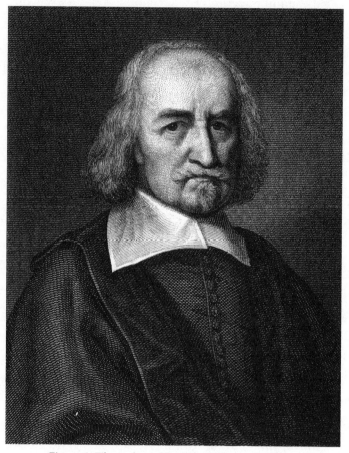

Figure 6. The author of *Leviathan*, Thomas Hobbes.

appeared: it offered a view of Nature and man that was materialist and mechanistic in the extreme. Matter made up humans, the
brain, and consciousness alike; individuals coalesced like particles
to form the body politic. There was no such thing as immaterial
substance.

Setting aside his earlier ambitions, *Leviathan* left physics and biology to the side and elaborated the author's views on human nature
and social life. Distressed by continual religious warfare, Hobbes's
aim was to create a science of politics, one in which natural law
established legitimate political authority. Often intended to under-

mine divine right, natural law was developed by, among others, the Dutch jurist Hugo de Groot, who was horrified by the "orgy of bloodshed" shed by warring sects in Western Christendom.

After completing *Leviathan*, Hobbes presented a copy to his young charge, the exiled Charles II. The future King of England, as well as his cousin, Louis XIV of France, should have been delighted, for Hobbes had turned materialism to their use. He constructed an exhaustive case for absolute monarchy as the natural political order, one where the king was the guiding consciousness of the people. However, even this fidelity did not prevent Hobbes from nearly being imprisoned. The author of *Leviathan* had placed the state above the church and railed violently against the superstitions that elevated ecclesiastic authority. Hobbes scampered across the Channel, a step ahead of Catholic authorities.

And so, in the end, the dream of unified knowledge died. A number of 17th-century thinkers set out to replace Thomas Aquinas and erect a comprehensive worldview, but no one could seamlessly bridge atoms, body, mind, the universe, the sociopolitical world, and the spiritual one. Instead, different savants devised ways of dividing these domains, not because they were unconnected, but because no one could determine how to connect them. Thomas Aquinas's idea of the soul, which once united classical Greece and the Vatican, Aristotle and Christ, gave way. Among a small band of modern thinkers, attracted to materialism and mechanics but also firm believers in God, the old ties no longer held. The soul's vast imperium came undone and in the resultant fragmentation, its pieces would be fought over, renamed, and, in newer guises, reemerge somewhere between science and ethics, matter and society.

Once the "knot of the universe," the soul transformed from an all-purpose answer into a series of nearly impenetrable problems. Books, pamphlets, and lectures on the soul, from the vantage point of metaphysics, history, and theology proliferated in the last decades of the 17th century. Most of these works were apologetics intended to defend the disintegrating order, but the very need, felt by so many, to pen these defenses spoke volumes about a growing anxiety and confusion.

Among these many commentators, there stood three giants whose fates all differed. For the next century, Thomas Hobbes and his radical materialism became a dark symbol of atheism, a charge he steadfastly denied. Among the Anglican elite, the horror inspired by his philosophy outweighed his staunch monarchism. His dangerous beliefs would be spoken of in whispers, rarely cited, and considered blasphemous, even Satanic. Still, he remained *de rigueur* reading for forward-thinking men and women of the Republic of Letters.

Hobbes faced another source of resistance. His proposed solution for consciousness and free will in a deterministic world depended on a dogmatic faith in the superiority of the sovereign, a common if increasingly challenged belief. Ordinary men, made of matter, had no free will and were compelled to jostle and push each other so as to seek out their own urgent wants, making life a horror show of conflict. Plebeians could not manage ethics at all, but the sovereign, usually a monarch, could and therefore should act for all. God-anointed leaders were the rational soul in the body politic. Only they could think, will, and create. Hobbes's reliance on kings and princes to solve the problem of higher-order mental functions in a mechanical world would soon seem concrete, reactionary, and vacant. Even in the court of Charles II, the elderly philosopher was treated like a bear to be baited and tormented but not taken seriously. And if the philosopher expected the universities to alter his reputation after the Restoration, he would be disappointed. In 1683, four years after his death, Oxford paid homage to Thomas Hobbes by burning his books.

The reception of Pierre Gassendi in his home country was no less troubled. His rehabilitation of Epicurean hedonism encountered repulsion and disbelief. Furthermore, the great payoff for adopting Gassendi's philosophy—probability and uncertainty—was not exactly a full meal for those raised on scholastic certitude. With his hybrid notion of the soul, Gassendi seemed the lesser Christian in his debates with the more orthodox Descartes. And he didn't help himself. As a propagandist for his own cause, this ponderous scholar stuck to Latin and was no match against the sharp rhetoric of his adversary, whose powerful arguments found their way into the vernacular and transfixed French readers.

While in Montpellier and Paris Gassendi's philosophy of probability attracted a smattering of followers, they never coalesced into a devoted community. After the priest's death, Gassendi's reputation sagged, especially after 1656, when his personal physician and most ardent promoter, the Montpellier doctor François Bernier, took a job in the court of the Great Mogul of India and effectively dropped off the map.

Bernier shipped off as committed Cartesians in France and the Netherlands were massing. As early as 1637, a number of learned men began to take Descartes as their master. A professor of medicine in Utrecht, Dr. Henrick de Roy or "Regius" can be counted as one of the first diehard Cartesians. His promotional efforts helped get his hero's work banned in his hometown, but Regius would not be deterred and eventually recruited more followers. In France, Cartesianism became fashionable as the view of opposition aristocrats, those who rebelled against Louis XIV. In salons, religious orders, and schools, Descartes's writings began to be read. A papal edict against his works in 1663 and a royal decree a few years later could not hold back a rising tide that made this compromise popular.

René Descartes's dualism would move to the foreground in Catholic France. For while his thought ceded Nature to mechanical science, he preserved enough of the old soul to be theologically safe. With this doctrine, believers did not need to change their core views, for their immortal soul was left intact. As for Descartes's transformation of lions and elephants into machines, that mattered little, for his Cogito contained the supernatural beliefs of his creed. Counter-

Reformation Catholics could embrace this version of modernity without losing faith. His soul was packaged for the Catholic conscience, for it was the product of one. Increasingly, many adopted the Cartesian compromise with its red line between Nature and thought, mechanized bodies and immortal souls.

In scientific salons around France, Gassendi gave Descartes more of a fight. Epicurean notions were admired at Montmor's illustrious academy, and when Henry Oldenburg, the secretary of the Royal Society in England visited Paris, he reported that the academies seemed tilted toward the priest from Provence. For a short while, the Sun King's own Academy of Sciences in Paris took an anti-Cartesian stance; however, by 1700, the Academy followed the schools in France and became Cartesian.

For some skeptics, the early 18th century ascent of Descartes signified the victory of one dogma over another. The rise of this new Cartesian philosophy with its logical certainties continued despite stinging critiques that Cartesians never could answer. As Pierre Gassendi pointed out, no one could adequately explain how an immaterial Cogito could control a material body. In Cambridge, Henry More's enthusiasm for Descartes waned as he encountered this problem, and grew concerned that this philosophy made a mess of the soul's agency. Others mocked his notion that animals were machines. The French poet Jean de La Fontaine took up his pen and wrote fables with sophisticated animal characters that satirized Descartes's belief that beasts were windup toys. Nonetheless, the master's divisions continued to win ground. His segregations of Nature and the soul became a new faith, a new common sense. There could be no natural home for inner life and no Baconian study of the inner world. Mr. Spirit, it seemed, had won.

However, across the Channel in Oxford and London, Pierre Gassendi found a few converts in a small community of Protestant scientists, "natural philosophers" as they were then called, whose influence would become increasingly profound. While victorious

French Cartesians drove a stake in Mr. Flesh, they would find his ideas rising up to challenge them thanks to a new generation armed with scalpels and glass tubes filled with chemicals, men wrist-deep in brains and nervous juices who were not guided by the logic of "Cogito, ergo sum," but who rather eagerly pursued the anatomy of the soul compelled by the haunting proposition that matter alone could think.

Science and the Thing That Thinks

T HE RETURN OF Charles II and the end of Puritan rule led
to changes throughout England, including those bastions
of Royalist sentiment, Oxford and Cambridge universities. With
the Restoration of 1660, the Anglican dons collectively breathed
a sigh of relief and busily went about purging Cromwell's sympa-
thizers and redistributing prestigious lectureships to the faithful. In
Oxford, the inhabitant of the Sedleian Chair of Natural Philosophy,
Dr. Joshua Crosse, was accused of embezzlement and summarily
replaced by Thomas Willis, a doctor who had fearlessly conducted
secret, Anglican services in his Christ Church rooms during the
interregnum period.

Dr. Willis was expected to employ his lectureship as tradition
dictated. Just as the Regius Professor of Medicine at Oxford was
mandated to read twice weekly from Hippocrates and Galen, the
Sedleian Chair of Natural Philosophy was to read on Wednesday and
Saturday at 8 A.M. from anything at all, so long as it came from one
source. He could choose from Aristotle on physics, Aristotle on the
soul, or Aristotle on the laws of generation and disease in life forms.
However, despite being a staunch conservative in his politics and
religious beliefs, the new Sedleian lecturer did not want to return
to the ways of the scholastics. He had come to be part of an exciting

gathering of natural philosophers called the Oxford Experimental Philosophical Clubbe, men like those who surrounded Mersenne, who sought to break from the past and find a "modern" way.

This small group had gotten its start years earlier, bolstered by Oliver Cromwell's government, which tried to undermine monarchist sentiment at the university by hiring rebellious, antischolastic advocates of natural philosophy. These new professors based their principles on the skepticism and the empirical rules for knowledge laid out by Sir Francis Bacon.

In his *Novum organum*, Bacon opened with a salvo against those who believed all that could be known was known: "They who confidently or magisterially pronounce of nature, as of a thing already discovered, have highly injured philosophy and science, and had the success, not only to enforce a belief, but to stop further enquiry." In fact, since Adam and Eve were forced from Eden, mankind needed a cure for its mind's many delusions. Bacon went on to analyze how reason went wrong thanks to what he called the Idols of the Tribe, the Idols of the Den, the Idols of Commerce, and the Idols of the Theater. Vanity, habit, conformity, ill-regulated passions, and intemperate beliefs led to prejudice, obsession, false coherence when there was difference, and distorted perception. The Idols were passions and distempers of the mind that must be combatted by a widespread shift, a cultural cure. Bacon proposed a rigorous method to combat the Idols of the Mind and help men find truth: they should devote themselves to rigorous, careful fact-gathering that began with sensory experiences and then challenge those impressions through careful, experimental inquiry. Gradually, through this method, inferences might yield general principles.

This approach to Nature echoed Puritan convictions. Since Calvin, Protestants rejected guidance from the certainties of canonic law and scholastic theology: they sought to feel and experience God's presence firsthand. So too should it be with Nature, Bacon believed. Against Aristotle's syllogisms and deductions, Bacon proposed an unbiased method to establish facts. If widespread superstition, false beliefs, and obsessively held dogmas were the illness, then the treatment was this method, which would take the name of empirical science.

Inspired by Bacon, the Oxford *virtuosi*, as they were known, met in the High Street rooms of men like Dr. William Petty. They included doctors and divines such as Thomas Willis, John Wilkins, John Wallis, Christopher Wren, Robert Hooke, and Robert Boyle. While committed to Bacon's empirical approach, they also were sold on the mechanical views of Mersenne's group, with the group roughly split between adherents of Descartes and Gassendi. So when the Stuart reign resumed and the old guard at Oxford sought to return to scholasticism, the *virtuosi*, many of whom were also politically unassailable Royalists themselves, resisted.

The Experimental Philosophical Clubbe continued at Oxford, and some members left for London, where they were warmly welcomed at Gresham College. There a group had been quietly meeting since 1645. One recalled, "our business was (precluding matters of theology and state affairs) . . . to discourse and consider of philosophical Enquiries," by which he meant subjects like medicine, chemistry, physics, magnets, astronomy, and geometry. All questions would be fair game, except those that touched on Church and State.

The Restoration of the monarchy necessarily fostered some uncertainty among this growing network of moderns, but they could count among their supporters some with great power, wealth, and aristocratic lineage. One such follower, Robert Moray, prevailed directly upon Charles II, who blessed the natural philosophers' efforts. And so in the autumn of 1660, the Royal Society of London for the Promotion of Natural Knowledge was founded. At the center of the Society and its original thirty-nine members was another scion of privilege, one of the Oxford experimenters, Robert Boyle.

The fourteenth son of the Earl of Cork, Boyle was rich, passionate about natural philosophy, rigid, and sternly pious. His family had managed to be more flexible, at least when it came to their wealth: they played both sides of the civil war—serving Charles I, then Cromwell, then Charles II—and in the process preserved their fortune. Educated by a Calvinist tutor in Geneva, the sickly Robert became interested in medicine. Before he left Oxford for London and the Royal Society, he was even awarded an honorary medical degree, since much of his effort at the time went toward devising medicinal remedies, such as his cure for childhood convulsions—an ounce of earthworms washed in white wine and dried to a powder. Some of Boyle's therapeutic efforts were, it seems, also an effort to cure himself of an array of complaints and ailments. In 1653, Boyle had been diagnosed by one doctor as a hypochondriac.

This preoccupation with his own health and the failures of orthodox medicine likely encouraged Boyle to explore a dissident branch of Hippocrates' art—alchemy. Alchemists were renegades who rejected the four elements that were believed to be the critical building blocks for all of Galenic medicine. Instead, they believed sulphur, salt, and mercury were the three essential elements of the natural world. Their infamous apostle, Paracelsus, looked not to God but to mysterious forces within Nature to understand the alterations of these substances as they created life and disease. Reputed to be the model for mythical Dr. Faustus, Paracelsus spoke of occult forces, poisonous mysteries yet to be known, that had the power to restore health or kill. In 1599, Paracelsus's writings were promptly added to the Vatican's Index of heretical works; however, with the eroding credibility of Galenic medicine, his tantalizing claims for life-restoring elixirs held great allure.

In 1654, when Boyle first moved to Oxford, many of his fellow virtuosi disparaged alchemy. As mechanists and mathematicians, they disdained that field's association with murky forms of magic. Like Marin Mersenne, Oxford's natural philosophers were also disturbed by the threat animism posed for Christian belief, especially since during the interregnum period in England, beliefs of this sort seemed to be on the rise. Some radical Protestant sects embraced pantheistic notions in which the source of life was not believed to be God, but the mysteries of Mother Earth. Charles II would brutally suppress these sects, but he could not silence the whispers of miraculous alchemical potions and remedies.

At the same time, controversies over Gassendi's hero, Epicurus, swept through Oxford and Cambridge. Some rose up to denounce him as an atheist, but these charges were met by Walter Charleton, a physician to Charles I. In 1654, he penned a defense of the Greek thinker that was at the same time the first elaboration of Gassendi in English. By the late 1650s, Robert Boyle, intrigued enough to study atomism with trepidation, explored Democritus, Epicurus, and the "learned" Gassendi. In the margins of his notes on these authors, he scribbled: "These Papers are without fayle to be burnt." Nonetheless, by 1661, Boyle had become committed to atomistic notions, which he would feature in *The Sceptical Chymist*, the book that made his reputation. In it, the father of chemistry aggressively beat back scholastics and Renaissance alchemists in a way that would have made Mersenne smile. Chemistry, he insisted, must be based on elements, atomistic corpuscles. As for the life force and human consciousness, those were not due to alchemy, but rather to God.

A fierce defender of the Anglican faith, Boyle was eager to prove natural philosophy posed no threat to belief. This was a man so committed to his church that he learned Hebrew and Greek to better read the Bible and also funded a translation of the Good Book into Arabic in order to convert Muslims. He detested those who would have naturalism challenge the mysteries of Christianity.

The essence of any human being resided in their divinely endowed soul, Boyle proclaimed, "an immaterial spirit" and a "substance of so heteroclite a kind" that it would always remain mysterious. Natural philosophy could study God's first five days of work during creation. However it must lay down its arms during the sixth day when He made man. God granted us souls through supernatural intervention. These incorporeal spirits could move matter through divine intervention. Therefore, angels, nocturnal visions, and devils were real, deadly, and powerful.

In an essay written in 1665, "The Excellency of Theology Compar'd with Natural Philosophy," Boyle extolled natural philosophy's capacity to enrich our lives, but reminded his readers that those rewards were nothing compared to knowledge of God, the Resurrection, and transubstantiation, things to live by. All that was learned from the Scriptures and relied on faith. Boyle knew that even the great Descartes, the philosopher who had masterfully employed logic to preserve the soul, had, in private letters, conceded defeat with regard to proving the soul's immortality. So Boyle made no such pretenses: learned inquiry might illuminate the rational soul's "Existence/ Properties and Duration," but the nature of the soul, that "noble and more valuable Being, than the whole Corporeal World" came from faith alone.

In all this, Boyle had an archenemy, a thinker who gave succor to atheists, unreconstructed Epicureans, and Stoics—the now elderly Thomas Hobbes. Against this nemesis, Boyle asserted that once God made bodies, He attached a fully formed and indivisible soul, as written in the Bible. Boyle never tired of repeating that inner life was exactly where science ended and religion began. Apologetic works poured forth from his pen; he wrote: "Functions of the Rational Soul; such as, To Understand, and that so, as to form Conceptions of Abstracted things, of Universals, of/Immaterial Spirits, and even of that infinitely Perfect One, God himself . . . to express intellectual Notions . . . to exercise Free-will," all prove "the Rational Soul is a Being of an higher Order, than Corporeal." Virtuosi knew this better than even scholastics, who in their unified system endowed plants and animals with different souls, and confused what was immortal with what was not. Even Aristotle, Boyle declared, led to apostasy, for in that pagan's view, an ape can see, hear, imagine, and love. To that he answered, a hundred nos.

Boyle became a tireless advocate for two distinct cultures, divided between what Francis Bacon had called the Book of the Scriptures and the Book of Nature. Boyle employed the analogy of the two books as he attacked vulgar moderns like Thomas Hobbes, whose materialist conceptions supported the death of the soul and rank heresy.

As Robert Boyle's scientific stature grew, his vision of science and its limits became imprinted on the fledgling Royal Society. He became the champion of inductive logic, the accrual of solid facts, and experimentation. When challenged by old Hobbes, who argued that science was the study of causes, Boyle was scathing. It was man's destiny to discover laws through the interaction of speculative philosophy and experimentation. Experiments rectified the failures of human senses, determined doubts, confirmed truths, and corrected errors. Natural philosophy ascertained individual facts through "ocular demonstrations," repeated before others, so they too could see for themselves. If an experiment was successful, a new truth would be recorded by the members of the Royal Society. All the gentlemen of the Society abdicated the right to remain skeptical in the face of such visible demonstrations. Knowledge would no longer consist of opinions endlessly in dispute, but rather would be empirical facts, listed in the Society's *Proceedings*, which became, literally, the Book of Nature.

The Royal Society abided by its credo: *Nullius in verba*–Take no man's word for it. The phrase from Horace declared freedom from received authority. And so, the Society unleashed a bevy of exciting and imaginative experiments on metals, magnets, eclipses, glasses, worms, poisons, diving engines, springs, Saturn, the speed of sound, and first-person accounts of dying. And the cry that went forth when an astonishing claim came forward from one of the members was for a demonstration before the Society. *Nullius in verba*.

The well-bred, reasonable gentlemen of the Royal Society would freely examine all phenomena, except for that faculty which allowed them to think. Such questions would cross over into religion and politics. Nature was a mindless machine, inert matter in movement. The mind for the Christian virtuoso was no mystery; it was the miracle of the divinely endowed soul. And so, the Cambridge divine, Henry More, sang the praises of the Royal Society, for they were doing God's work.

THOMAS HOBBES WANTED to link the mechanics of Nature to ethical and political life. Unloved at home, Hobbes found admirers in Paris who championed his cause. For example, Samuel Sorbière and Abraham du Prat argued for his notion of science as a search for mechanical causes. However, by 1663 they had lost their battle, as their group was overrun by "zealots" who preached experimentation only.

One of these devotees was Christiaan Huygens. Nicknamed "the young Archimedes" thanks to his youthful prowess in mathematics, the Dutchman grew up surrounded by some of the greatest thinkers of his time. His erudite father, a Protestant secretary to the House of Orange, was a close ally of Descartes: it was he who personally delivered the *Meditations* to Father Mersenne in 1641. While the family business was politics, Christiaan showed such promise in math and science that in 1655 he came to Paris to devote himself to these studies. Deeply influenced by his father's friend, Huygens started out as a Cartesian but gravitated over time to the epistemological restraint and notions of probability championed by Gassendi. By the time he entered Montmor's home on the Rue Vieille du Temple, a mansion filled with fabulous mechanical inventions and Albrecht Dürer paintings, the young man was sophisticated beyond his years. Despite the dazzling surroundings, he was not cowed or much impressed with what he found. A lot of empty philosophizing, he concluded.

This might have been dismissed as extraordinary arrogance if

Huygens did not go on to discover Saturn's largest moon and its rings. Now a scientific hero in France, the young man traveled to London to investigate Gresham College and the Royal Society, then returned to Paris, a committed follower of Bacon and Boyle. In 1663, when Sorbière petitioned Louis XIV for a Royal Academy for natural philosophy and other scholarly endeavors, Huygens put forward a competing plan that explicitly would not study "the mysteries of religion or the affairs of the state." The king of France chose Huygens's proposal and lured the star-watcher into his services with an astronomical salary. Thus, the Academy of Sciences in Paris was founded in 1666 with two branches: one would be solely mathematical and the other experimental. French science would revolve around these realms. Academicians would dissect animals, stare at the night sky, examine perpetual motion machines, grind lens, employ burning mirrors, and forge new tools, but they would not cross over to the realms of the soul, politics, or ethics.

While he smuggled the shocking writings of the archmaterialist Baruch Spinoza into France, as a Dutch Protestant in Louis XIV's court, Huygens needed to be careful. He outwardly kept quiet about such interests. Then in 1672, his position in the Sun King's court became quite treacherous, since Louis along with England's Charles II had launched a war intended to destroy the Dutch republic, where Huygens's father and brother were prominent political figures. French opponents peered hard at this prodigy descended from a family of Dutch diplomats and political brokers and accused him of being a spy. By keeping his nose buried in firmly apolitical studies, Huygens saved himself. Throughout the conflict, he remained in Paris, a man who publicly at least, was solely devoted to science.

In London, members of the Royal Society found their notions of natural philosophy had spread to Paris, and then other outposts across western Europe and in the New World. Some of these groups were less tied to the government than the Royal Society, while others in Berlin, Stockholm, and St. Petersburg were state-run operations, committed to the service of their royalty. Some modeled themselves on the humanistic, Renaissance academies of Italy and incorporated arts and letters, alongside mechanics, anatomy, and astronomy, but most did not. These became outposts of the so-called Invisible College and remained linked through active correspondences and itinerant thinkers, as well as the spread of the first scientific journals, the *Journal des sçavans* in France and the *Philosophical Transactions of the Royal Society* in England.

Over the next century, these early scientific societies spawned ninety others. While the new societies posed a direct challenge to the scholasticism in the universities, they followed the rules laid down in London and Paris and did not challenge religious or political dogma. Consequently, in quite varied political climates, these small communities were welcomed by the status quo. Christians of many sorts—Catholic, Orthodox, Calvinist, Methodist, and Anglican—embraced these researchers. Unlike Epicurus, Paracelsus, Thomas Hobbes, or Baruch Spinoza, these scientific thinkers mostly kept to their side of the line.

The founders of the Royal Society, having suffered through bloody civil wars, were intent on establishing a domain outside of the warring bands of believers. As their in-house historian Thomas Sprat wrote in 1667, the origins of the Royal Society emerged from the desire "for the satisfaction of breathing a freer air, and of conversing in quiet with one another, without being engaged in the passions, and madness of that dismal Age." The sober and deep study of Nature "invincibly armed" young men against the temptations of spiritual frenzy and enthusiasm, Sprat noted. The price to be paid for this peace was to leave the ethics and the soul to the Church and political life to the king.

Mersenne would have approved. Radically mechanistic explanations of the natural world could freely proceed, for they seemed to require supernatural intervention to fully make sense. If Nature was a machine, then the Heavenly Architect needed to give matter a design. If animals were machines, then God must give them life. And if the human body was a windup toy, then He must wind it up and imbue it with higher powers like reason. No mechanistic science could explain any of that.

In addition, natural science had limited itself in another manner that seemed to call for the intervention of a deity. Premodern views of Nature adopted Aristotle's belief that everything had a number of causes including a final one, which was the purpose it served. Mechanistic philosophies of Nature did not agree. Water did not abhor a vacuum and therefore move away from it. It fell forward blindly, thanks to impersonal forces like gravity. Comets had no destination, no intention. Earthquakes were not meant to cause upheaval. Rather they caused the earth to tremble for geologic reasons that had nothing to do with their final impact.

This antiteleological perspective on Nature countered the tendency to personify acts of Nature and ascribe human or divine intent to such acts. However, as the study of Nature became depersonified, where would that leave the scientific study of persons? By purifying itself of higher-level forces that took action based on intention and purpose, natural science had created a severe limitation. Unlike rocks falling off a cliff, it seemed quite plausible that human beings did act, at times at least, because they *wanted* a goal or outcome. How could a science in which final ends were dismissed, a science based on atoms and passive mechanical motion, take up human desire, thought, will, and intention, much less its disorders? At first, the answer was clear: it could and should not. Quickly, however, this reserve would prove untenable.

THE NEW OCCUPANT of the Oxford Sedleian Chair of Natural Philosophy was an inauspicious choice, a short fellow with a shock of red hair who resembled a pig, or so his friend John Aubrey unkindly

observed. Furthermore, the distinguished new lecturer suffered from
a bad stammer. However, those who knew Thomas Willis understood that he possessed a granite will. After attending Oxford as a
servitor at the age of sixteen, he had joined the Royalist Army and
fought against Cromwell, only then to return to Oxford after King
Charles's defeat. In stark defiance of Puritan rule, he held Anglican services in his rooms, an act that won him undying admiration
from Royalists, who remembered his loyalty when they returned to
power. And if the doctor needed bucking up, he had chosen a wife
even more ferocious in her anti-Puritan convictions than himself.
Along with her sister and mother, she once staged a sit-down strike
against the new regime at Oxford that only ceased when she was
unceremoniously strapped to a board and carted away.

Like Boyle, Thomas Willis's conservative religious beliefs existed
side by side with a desire to study nature. In Willis's case, however,
his chosen area of research would lead him into a dangerous borderland. Fascinated with the brain, Dr. Willis began to study the organ
and cracked open a graveyard worth of skulls. He threw his hands
into that flesh, not the soul of course, but stuff that existed so near
to it.

His training had done little to prepare him for such a Herculean task. Due to the political turmoil in December of 1646, Willis
received a Bachelor of Medicine degree after less than a year of study.
An ignorant, common practitioner, he struggled to make a living,
and rode from village to village in search of patients. He was in
the common parlance a "piss prophet," one of those itinerant medical men who laid great emphasis on the examination of a patient's
urine. The young Willis also employed traditional humoral methods, such as purges, emetics, bleeding, heating, and cooling. Around
1650, Willis's unremarkable diaries record conventional diagnoses in
which he ascribed hysteria to uterine vapors and melancholia to the
humors.

However, as the doctor tried to drum up business, he also began to participate in the Oxford Experimental Philosophical Clubbe, especially a small contingent that met in the rooms of Dr. William Petty. Petty had become a Cartesian while studying medicine in Leiden; he then moved to Paris and conducted dissections with his new friend, Thomas Hobbes. When he arrived in Oxford in 1654, Petty brought with him knowledge of the latest in anatomy and chemistry.

William Petty, Robert Boyle, Thomas Willis, and a group of virtuosi performed chemical studies with the pragmatic goal of finding, if not the elixir of life, at least remedies for illnesses. In the process, Willis began to move from humoral conceptions to more *au courant* chemical theories of the body, disease, and cure. In 1659, he published a book in which he boldly proposed five basic physiological elements, instead of Paracelsus's three. Willis described disease as the result of alterations in these elements. For example, fermentation of the nervous juices caused hypochondria and melancholia. The role of the doctor, Willis suggested, was not far from the vintner, who also monitored fluids and hoped for wine, not vinegar. In this book, this struggling practitioner also followed a disreputable custom; he reported the discovery of a curative compound made of sulphuric and ferrous compounds, but refused to divulge the formula. Drumming up medical business in this cheap manner would later cause embarrassment for the piss-doctor when he metamorphized into an Oxford professor, since such advertisements were routinely denounced by university physicians.

With the Restoration, Willis's place in the medical hierarchy changed overnight. His brother-in-law became university vice-chancellor and Bishop of Oxford, and the doctor's patronage appointment as an Oxford professor was bestowed for life. With the return of Charles II, Willis's credentials were quickly remedied. By royal fiat, he was awarded a doctorate of medicine. And after the departure of the peripatetic William Petty, Willis became the de facto leader of the Experimental Philosophical Clubbe's anatomists.

Willis hoped to reestablish anatomy as the basis for medicine, but which anatomy? Classical Greek anatomical models had been long frozen in place by Christian proscriptions against human dissection. However, in the Renaissance, these strictures had begun to loosen as anatomical theaters cropped up in Padua, Bologna, and elsewhere. Cartographers of the body soon struggled to reconcile the discrepancies they found between classic texts and what they found inside corpses. The biggest challenge to classical teaching came in 1628 when William Harvey, physician to King James I, determined that circulation flowed from arteries to veins and back again due to the pumping of different chambers in the heart. This directly contradicted Galen, who considered the liver to be the source of venous blood.

The newly appointed Sedleian professor had little interest in repeating old views on the body. Willis instead chose to see for himself and focused on nervous life. In 1660, he began working with the talented Christopher Wren (who would later become one of England's greatest architects) and others as they performed anatomical dissections, chemical infusions, animal experiments, and microscopy, studies that would form the basis for his lectures. Willis wrote, "I addicted my self to the opening of Heads especially, and of every kind. . . ." He discovered that much of the brain, as Willis's assistant later informed Robert Boyle, had been erroneously described.

In only a few years, Thomas Willis consolidated a mechanical and chemical view of the brain and nerves. *The Anatomy of the Brain*, published in 1664, was dedicated to the archbishop of Canterbury. Willis made a special effort to proclaim that this study of the "secret places of Man's Mind" would offer no comfort to atheists and heretics. The good doctor had "slain so many Victims, whole Hecatombs almost of all Animals, in the Anatomical Court," so he could lay them at "the most holy Alter of Your Grace."

Willis described awakening from the slumber of received opinion to find a world where much had gone wrong. From now on, the

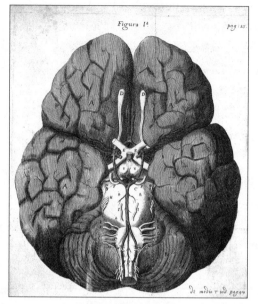

Figure 7. Thomas Willis's *The Anatomy of the Brain*, 1664.

devout Protestant would follow Bacon and trust only observation. Of course, he would not be free from the "calumny" of interpretation and exegesis, since the inward dens of the brain were sealed and the workings of the animal spirits left no traces. He would even dare to launch a "lame" theory. Close examination of the brain and nerves, he proposed, would reveal the functions of the nervous juice and the lower souls.

Willis thus began his pathbreaking work. The empty chambers in the cerebrum, the same ventricles that Descartes believed held animal spirits, were redefined as drains for nervous filth. Like his Dutch predecessor Franciscus Sylvius, Willis insisted that all cerebral functions occurred in the actual brain substance. By severing brain matter and observing the melee that ensued, Willis recognized that the cerebrum controlled motor action. He also discovered that the smaller pair of lobes in the back, the cerebellum, must regulate involuntary automatic acts. Willis carefully tracked the twists and turns of nerves and determined their destinations. This one went to the tongue, that one to the heart. He mapped out the blood sources of the brain, including an otherwise unobserved circle of arteries at the base of the brain that would then bear his name.

In the end, Willis pulled together a model of the brain, much of which would orient researchers far into the future. However in doing so, he could not but stumble over his friend Robert Boyle's red line. Nervous juices, Willis declared, made in the brain and nerves, coursed in and out of different functional areas of the brain, where they animated thought, memory, sensation and motion. Thought, motion, memory? At this point, the archbishop might have wondered just what his humble servant had dared to do. Was the rational soul amid this machinery?

Dr. Willis had not neglected eternity. While anatomical structures implied brain function, Willis proposed one function that required *no* structure. After dissecting dogs, calves, sheep, and other animals, Willis pointed out that countless hours cracking skulls taught him animal and human brains were not so different. Brain differences alone could hardly account for the extraordinary human capacity for thought. Therefore reason and intelligence must be functions with no structure. They existed in the realm of the immaterial soul, which remained the "chief mover of the animal Machine."

The Anatomy of the Brain established a field of study that Willis later labeled "neurology." And the doctor confessed his ambition to go further. The soul, known from antiquity as that which understands all things but itself, would perhaps now be more explicable through a "Doctrine of the Soul" or a "psychologie."

Thanks to the busy pen of the Royal Society's secretary, Henry Oldenburg, news of Thomas Willis's brain studies sped across the Channel. In 1665, *The Anatomy of the Brain* was reviewed in the newly established *Journal des sçavans*. That review noted that Willis's dissections offered up a quite novel, at times extraordinary, view of the stuff inside a head. The reviewer gushed about the brilliant draftsmanship of Willis's partner, Christopher Wren. His engravings were of such precision that critics, like the one in the *Journal des sça-vans*, declared it to be the most reliable and beautiful renderings of the brain ever created.

One naysayer, however, was not so sure. In 1666, the Danish anatomist Nicholas Steno delivered a lecture on the brain, that "marvelous machine," in Paris at the home of Melchisédec Thévenot, one of the founding members of the Academy of Sciences. The speech first took aim at the errors of the Ancients, then those of the Cartesians. He sneered at the idea that the soul was some immaterial stuff. The brain, he simply declared, was certainly the principle organ of our soul. "I don't reproach Descartes for his method," Steno quipped, "but for sinning against it."

He then turned to Thomas Willis, who had claimed the *sensus communis,* that which unites all perceptions into one unified inner experience, was housed in the corpus striatum, and that the imagination dwelt in that rubbery bridge between the brain hemispheres called the corpus callosum. Where was the proof? Steno demanded. Our knowledge of these areas was so paltry that "as long as one has some wits about one, one can say anything you please." He chided those who strayed from what was certain and pointed out that the most common sinners in this regard were doctors and surgeons, who have neither the time nor the luxury to stick only to the anatomical facts. In their zealous pursuit of cures and practical knowledge for patients, these investigators, like Dr. Thomas Willis of Oxford, often were guilty of straying beyond what was knowable.

Steno's words followed those of his guide, the antidogmatic Pierre Gassendi. Both believed that even in the best of all worlds, science could only go so far. It was a question that would resurface repeatedly: When was science on factual ground? And when had it been extended to serve personal, dogmatic, political, or pragmatic ends? In 1669, when Steno's published lecture made its way to London, its cautionary reserve was duly noted in the Royal Society's *Philo-*

sophical Transactions. Little more would be heard from this anatomist, for he soon relinquished his scalpel, converted to Catholicism, and entered the priesthood. While Nicholas Steno vanished, the dangers he described would long persist.

SOON AFTER THE publication of *The Anatomy of the Brain*, the archbishop summoned Thomas Willis to London. While the frolicking court of Charles II had brought pleasure back to the city as dancing, theater, gambling, alehouses, horse races, and bear-baiting resumed along with Christmas and Mayday festivals, the joy proved short-lived. During the early months of 1665, word spread of the plague. The disease was well known to Londoners; it had ravaged them on and off for years. By April, the worst fears were realized. It had returned. On June 7, the memoirist Samuel Pepys noted in his diaries that he had spotted houses marked with red crosses and the desperate words "Lord Have Mercy on Us."

On June 28, the Royal Society suspended its meetings as its members fled to the countryside. Many of the Royal College of Physicians also ran, dramatically illustrating their helplessness before the onslaught. The Court departed as did many parish priests. Edward Cotes, whose dire Bills of Mortality chronicled the staggering toll as it mounted, prefaced one such ledger of death with the plea that "neither the physicians of our souls or bodies may hereafter in such great numbers forsake us."

After thousands of deaths, the London plague abated, but just as the city began to recover, it was devastated again. In 1666, the Great Fire broke out and turned much of the city to ashes. During this apocalypse, prayer and medicine again failed utterly. Many began to waver in their faith in their priests and doctors. Nonconformist theologians of various stripes emerged to comfort the

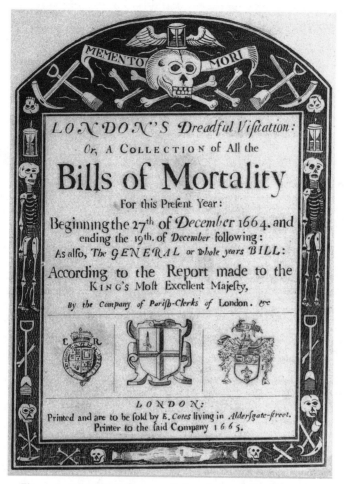

Figure 8. *Bills of Mortality* compiled statistics on the devastating
London plague of 1665.

dying and desperate, and nontraditional healers including astrolo-
gists, magicians, empirics, and charlatans filled some of the need for
care and solace.

The flight of the pastors and the doctors would not be soon forgotten. In London, Galenic medical practitioners, already under a
good deal of suspicion, suffered a further loss of confidence. And
so in 1666, the archbishop requested the presence of the unorthodox doctor Thomas Willis. Dr. Willis came to London and leased a

home on St. Martin's Lane. He did not relinquish his professorship in Oxford, but deputized others to lecture in his place. Quickly he became one of the best-paid doctors in London.

On October 24, 1667, Willis joined the Royal Society, where his sharp tongue was soon heard. The occasion was one of the numerous transfusion experiments that ensued after William Harvey's work on the blood's circulation. One such experiment was performed upon a Mr. Arthur Coga, a maniac whose excitations, his physician reasoned, would be pacified by the blood infused from those most docile creatures, sheep. "Dr. Willis suggested," the record dryly observed, "that this experiment might be proper to make use of upon rotten sheep."

That same year, Dr. Willis extended his studies on the brain to consider its disorders. In traditional humoral medicine, invisible animal spirits constituted an unquantifiable source of the immaterial soul, and formed the critical connections between the body and the spirit world of angels and demons, perhaps even the Holy Spirit itself. But Willis eventually concluded, rather alarmingly, that such spirits were merely flammable liquors. Nervous juices sped through the blood, reached a muscle or nerve ending, then exploded. With that eruption, the body moved. Thousands of tiny chemical fires animated the human corpus.

The *anima*, the sacred source of life, was now reduced to droplets of booze blowing up. These same profane blasts, Willis contended, explained illnesses like convulsive diseases. Here too Willis stepped onto thin ice: epilepsy was often considered the result of demonic possession. Willis cloaked his challenge to religious doctrine with a fawning dedication to the Church, and he reiterated his steadfast belief in the Devil, evil possession, and exorcism. However, the man who once fearlessly defied Cromwell, insisted that many illnesses of the spirit, "the Stupid *Diliriums* of Melanchollicks, the Caninith madness, and others" came from an infirm brain and its sizzling juices, not something supernatural. Violent passions like sudden fear led to eruptions in the nerves and brain that caused hysteria in women and hypochondria in men. Dr. Willis, who once accepted that hysteria resulted from uterine vapors, now rejected that received bit of wisdom. On autopsy, he announced, hysterics had normal wombs, but their nerves were tainted.

Despite his expanding authority, Dr. Willis's claims were confronted by skeptics. In 1670, the Oxford anatomist Dr. Nathaniel Highmore raised his objections before the Royal Society. Where was this so-called nervous juice? How could explosions occur in muscles and nerves without burning up the blood? Despite these unanswerable queries, the most radical element of Willis's thought captured the imaginations of others: animal spirits, once conduits of the immaterial world, might be no more than flammable fluids.

A year later, Thomas Willis's own brain became diseased. His wife Mary died, and the doctor descended into a deep melancholia. Eventually, he forced himself back to work—a remedy he would later recommend. During this period of forced activity, he produced a new book on "psychologie." This study was only meant to account for those higher functions that men shared with animals like monkeys. Published in 1672, *On the Soul of Brutes* would take up these lower functions, while attempting to leave the venerated rational soul to the archbishop.

However, as the reader plunged into Willis's work, such distinctions quickly grew murky. Willis's wily brutes seemed to be endowed with capacities often considered uniquely human. Recognizing this problem, the doctor explained to the Royal Society that while some may find it distressing and paradoxical, he had concluded—in line with the scholastics—that animals possessed a soul. All confusion would clear, if one remembered that man was a "Double-soul'd Animal," who possessed a material soul in addition to an eternal rational soul. Echoing Pierre Gassendi, Thomas Willis argued this material soul was made of brain matter; it performed not just simple sensation, but also the integration and interpretation of these signs, that is, perception.

But how could an animal soul made of corruptible flesh possibly perceive, *how could it think*? Backed into a corner, the Anglican doctor had a reply that others would consider a sign of defeat. Matter was made to think by the "great God, as the only Workman, so also as the First Mover."

Descartes had tried to use skepticism and logic to prove the soul's immateriality, and now Willis used divine intervention to argue for a thinking soul's corporeality! It was a dizzying dance. And while history would soon forget that both Pierre Gassendi and Thomas Willis had called upon God to endow matter with the power to think, this idea would be linked to Willis's most celebrated medical student, John Locke, whose psychology would be forever entwined with this problematic assertion.

Thomas Willis's landmark studies represented the troubles that the new natural philosophy would face as it took up the mysteries of the brain. An Oxford virtuoso and a devout Anglican, Willis worshiped the Book of the Scriptures and devoted himself to the Book of Nature. However, these two worlds seemed to collide in his arena of study—the brain's anatomy, functions, and disorders. For many Royal Society scientists, natural philosophy should steer clear of religion. However, for the students of the brain, this injunction was not easy: they would often land between the two worlds, a wild, unmapped place where brain and soul, spirit and flesh, and Nature and God seemed to touch.

Thomas Willis breached the early modern boundaries for science as he sought to extend naturalistic studies into man's inner being. *On the Soul of Brutes* genuflected to religious authorities, then repeatedly transgressed their dictums. The physician to the Archbishop of Canterbury shockingly asserted that dull matter could think; therefore reason was not wholly immaterial as scholastics and the modern savior of the soul, Descartes, would have it. In fact, diseases of the soul might be illnesses of brain flesh or even more confusing, illnesses of thought itself. Willis himself proposed words that would later mark the split path forward, but he himself found no clarity with his conceptions of "neurologie" and "psychologie." Dr. Willis was torn between his commitments to natural philosophy and his church. He was stranded somewhere between Nature and the Scriptures, between the brain and the soul. Into this undefined domain, an array of physicians and naturalists would soon follow.

3

Witches, Melancholics, and Fanatics

WHEN A COMET was spotted on January 1, 1681, the members of the Republic of Letters lustily attacked the credulous for seeing therein the hand of God. Moderns would busily seek to demystify the natural world, stripping it of spirits and animistic desires. They would deny teleological final purposes and cede the universe to mechanists and mathematicians. However, one line was not to be crossed, the modern border drawn up by Descartes's logic and Gassendi's uncertainty that cordoned off the rational soul. Beyond that line lay human reason, moral law, art, politics, and faith.

If it was possible for astronomers, chemists, and geologists to parade about as Christian virtuosi, the anatomists of the brain faced phenomena that often fell into a complex and politically explosive no-man's-land. However, they were not alone. As the soul's immortality became a source of controversy, an array of disorders thought to straddle body and soul became socially explosive and could not be ignored. At the same time, the trained experts most suited to address these concerns were part of a guild so hidebound by tradition that they had not changed their ways for more than a thousand years.

Late 17th-century physicians were expected to handle questions about where the body ended and the soul began. Traditionally, they distinguished illnesses of one from the other. Doctors had long followed theological dictates which claimed that the rational soul could never sicken: it marked the eternal spirit that survived death. Instead, medical diseases that seemed to affect reason, perception, or thought sprang from two other sources. The faculties of reason could be disturbed by distempers and perturbations, bodily illnesses that crept up from the spleen, liver, or blood. Or the soul could be possessed.

Demonic possession, witches, and Satanic intermediaries were all terrifying occurrences in premodern times. Christian demonology dictated that the rational soul could be commanded by God or Lucifer. In the authoritative 15th-century textbook of witch-hunting, the *Malleus malleficarum*, the authors, two Dominican inquisitors, acknowledged an added wrinkle: sometimes those who seemed to be sorcerers were merely mad. Witch-hunters were implored not to confuse those who made a covenant with the Devil with those whose tales of sorcery were fabrications.

By 1600, traditional demonology also found its critics. The astrologer and occultist Cornelius Agrippa and Paracelsus both claimed a *natural* magic plagued such people. The Devil could manipulate a whole host of hidden poisons and unknown earthly mysteries, so as to take over a human being. Satan employed Nature, but did not possess the power to defy its rule. Hence, if doctors could discover these same occult mysteries, they could combat the Great Deceiver and cure diseases.

This half-step toward a naturalistic view encouraged further critiques of the supernatural. In 1563, Agrippa's student, the Court physician Johann Weyer insisted real witches must be distinguished from mad folks, who simply had a disease. Expecting attacks from theologians, he nonetheless insisted that doctors were required to weigh in on disruptions of reason, bizarre ideas, visions, as well as claims of unusual powers, such as the capacity to speak a foreign language never before encountered, the power to prophesize, or to know another's secrets. He left no doubt that many witches were diseased in their imaginations.

Meanwhile, experts—both physicians and divines—were summoned before the courts to distinguish the possessed from the mad. Naturally, there was some competition between the stewards of the body and those of the soul; however, over the years, accepted criteria were established. It helped that 17th-century physicians, though reputed since Antiquity to be prone to atheism, were almost uniformly devout. Conversely, most Catholic and Anglican clergy accepted medicine for bodily matters, though that was not always so. Some still held to the view most clearly expressed by Pope Innocent III who in 1215 had forbidden physicians from prescribing anything to a sick person that endangered their soul. He warned doctors to call upon physicians of the soul to tend to spiritual health before attending to the needs of the body. But most clergy conceded that some illnesses required more than prayer. And so, doctors and priests worked together to sort out where frenzy ended and evil began. At times, the evaluating doctor and clergyman would be one and the same individual, who moved seamlessly from bleeding cups to prayer.

Gradually in the first half of the 17th century, some medical skeptics began to echo Weyer's concern that witches were often simply crazy. For that reason, in 1625, Dr. John Cotta argued that physicians *must* be consulted in cases of supposed possession or witchcraft. Great doubt should attend common methods of detecting the Devil's work. Tossing a bound witch into water to see if the water would refuse to engulf this unnatural being was a vulgar superstition. Determinations must be made by physicians through proof, such as the presence of a witch's mark, a third nipple that these evildoers used to suckle the Devil or their familiars, their "Imps." Cotta clearly believed that, in many cases, a third nipple would be difficult to locate.

Such consultations were deadly serious, especially as religious wars broke out throughout Western Christendom. Around 1640, as religious strife roiled England, France, the Netherlands, Naples, and

Portugal, heated polemics regarding the authority of competing religious authorities emerged. In this atmosphere, witchcraft became a battleground, part of a broader propaganda war between Catholics and Protestants.

Since the founding of their church, Catholics had held that holy words could effect miraculous change, as in the mystery of the Eucharist service. It followed that, for Catholics, evil spirits in the soul could be rooted out by incantations, following examples from the New Testament. Exorcism by Catholic priests provided a service to the soul-sick and proof of invisible spirits for the rest. However, after Calvin, Protestants denounced such exorcisms as superstitious blasphemy. By 1600, Protestant reformers in England had rid the Anglican Church of such practices. However, the hunger among the populace for miraculous cures did not diminish. While Protestant sects scorned exorcism, a biblical verse from Matthew in which Jesus rid a lunatic of his demon gave them justification for healing through intense prayer and fasting.

In France, the public spectacle of Catholic exorcisms constituted dramatic evidence of that creed's righteousness. More so, hatred for Protestants was stoked when newly extracted demonic spirits at times declared their undying love for Huguenots. Such was the case of Marthe Brossier, whose possession occurred a few days after the Edict of Nantes declared tolerance for French Calvinists. For fifteen months, the young girl was paraded from town to town and publically exorcised. On cue, her demons would be dispatched from inside her and then loudly proclaim their fondness for Protestants. In Paris, the king recognized the danger of this spectacle and called in three trusted physicians to examine the girl. The doctors concluded Marthe Brossier had "nothing from the Devil, much counterfeited, little from disease." The king promptly imprisoned the girl, but somehow she escaped and ended up in Rome, seated beside the Pope. And so, the possessed did not just have the power to terrorize a village; they might also threaten the stability of a nation.

In 1637, the Catholic diplomat, pirate, and founding member of the Royal Society, Kenelm Digby, returned from witnessing a great spectacle. He had traveled to a convent in Loudun in the Loire Valley. Five years earlier, a mass possession had afflicted the nuns there. An offending priest, Urbain Grandier, was accused of witchcraft and duly burnt at the stake; however, the sisters' convulsions and blasphemy did not abate. The Prince of Guémené had asked Digby to evaluate these bizarre events. He was not alone; for some time, gawkers had trekked to Loudun to take in the show.

Digby was skeptical. In his assessment, which he forwarded to Thomas Hobbes, Digby reported that the possessed were "ordered to perform for our satisfaction" and that their affliction was clearly not physical. Thoughts and passions had run riot in them, not least of which was the grandiose pleasure of being the most monstrous of all the Devil's creations. Thus, these sufferers imagined themselves "greater than kings or the Pope himself."

While privately sarcastic, Digby wanted no part of a public controversy. He dutifully declared the events to be supernatural and begged the prince to keep his real views secret, since "I do not want to be on either side of such a disputed issue, in which such zeal and bitterness is displayed." Digby had reason to be careful. Those like Hobbes who promoted naturalist explanations of such events carried the stench of disbelief. Skepticism about the power of evil spirits could easily spread into doubt about the Holy Spirit. Accusations of this sort were easy to hurl and difficult to bat away. In 1584, an English justice of the peace, Reginald Scot, concluded that the spirits inhabiting old crones were mostly the result of "the imagination of the melancholike" and fakery. His book, *The Discoverie of Witchcraft*, was banned by King James I, who personally branded Scot a heretic.

King James understood that if the medical reclassification of the possessed went too far, a critical anchor of his own authority would come loose. The sudden transformation of an old woman into a possessed being was one of very few unassailable proofs of the immaterial soul. It demonstrated that the spirit world existed. And proof of this sort became increasingly important as radicals like Baruch Spinoza and Thomas Hobbes dared to claim the soul was made of matter.

In *Leviathan*, Hobbes was particularly scathing about beliefs of demonic possession. Shockingly, he went further and suggested the only difference between outlawed forms of magic and the Church's sanctioned rites was their legality. "Fear of power invisible, feigned by the mind, or imagined from tales publicly allowed, Religion," he wrote, and those "not allowed, Superstition." Demoniacs who claimed to be possessed, he declared, were simply "madmen or lunatics; or such as had the falling sickness. . . ." As for the performances by which holy men cast out devils with incantations, Hobbes caustically asked, "Can diseases hear?"

This sarcasm did not go unanswered. In 1681, the natural philosopher and Royal Society member Joseph Glanvill rose up to denounce Mr. Hobbes's heresy. *Saducismus Triumphatus*, Glanvill's full-throated defense of demonology, influenced Cotton Mather and provided justification for the Salem Witch Trials. To Glanvill and others, it was quite simple. No spirits, no God. No witches, no miracles. Possession was proof of the power of invisible beings spoken of in the Bible. Hobbes himself believed he had skirted blasphemy by allowing that in the biblical days of the Prophets, possessions and exorcisms may have occurred, but no longer. However, he undercut this claim by insisting that even in the so-called "Age of Miracles," demoniacs were really insane: "That there were many demoniacs in the primitive Church, and few madmen, and other such singular diseases," he wrote, "whereas in these times we hear of, and see many madmen, and few demoniacs, proceeds not from a change of nature, but of names."

The names were indeed changing, and the consequences rippled throughout Christendom. Hobbes and other doubters encouraged the naturalistic study of those who had been called "witches." In

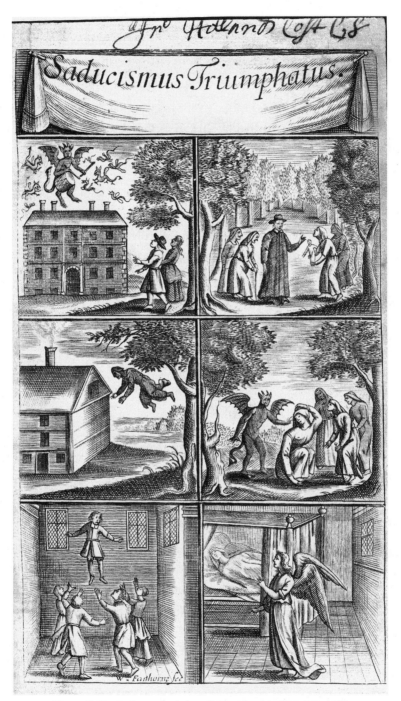

Figure 9. Depictions of witchcraft from Joseph Glanvill's 1681
Saducismus Triumphatus.

1671 while battling accusations of atheism, the doctor John Wagstaffe insisted that there was simply no such thing as a witch; this mass superstition was based on a misreading of the Scriptures, papal trickery, and the limitations of medical knowledge. Diseases of the head allowed men to take their own dreams as magical visions. Physicians and the public were so in the dark about such ills that one day to know these things would be to "discover an unknown world, full of unheard of prodigious monsters."

When such medical materialism crowded too close, as it had during the Renaissance, it threatened those pillars of Christendom based on divine authority. For the vast number of Europeans whose lives were organized around a literal interpretation of the Bible, miracles, exorcisms, and possession were tangible confirmations of the otherwise invisible and unfathomable forces that sanctioned the right of kings and the righteousness of their church. Without these beliefs, what would be the fate of the old order?

DURING THE 17TH century, a far more common phenomenon than witchcraft that straddled body and soul was melancholia. Quite broadly defined, this disease encompassed everything from bizarre intrusions of thought, failures of logic, the loss of voluntary control, love cravings, jealous rage, hypochondria, and a collapse into sadness.

For Hippocrates, melancholia was thought to be due to the burning of yellow bile, which decayed into a black substance that then affected the brain. It created a host of miserable symptoms, including despair, delusions, hallucinations, sleeplessness, anorexia, guilt, and suicidality. Later, Galenic doctors incorporated black bile into their list of naturally occurring fluids; its regulation became the key to avoiding this disease.

However, another ancient tradition could also explain melancholic states. For Socrates and Cicero, for Plutarch and Seneca, cure for a despondent or troubled soul came from philosophy. Practices of *cultura animi* from Hellenistic and Roman Schools sought to guide the lost, enhance reason, and aid the tormented. For Christian healers, a tradition of spiritual counsel also had coalesced from Jewish sages and the ministry of Christ. By the 6th century, Boethius, a thinker influenced by classical sources and his church, could rhetorically ask, "What is the health of the soul, but virtue? And what is sickness but vice?"

And so, alongside the disturbance of essential fluids, causes for melancholia commonly included a wide range of sins and the intervention of the Devil. For that reason, Dante showed little compassion for these sufferers and reserved a special spot in the Inferno for them. The Catholic Church offered confession and sundry healing procedures like the use of relics, holy waters, pilgrimages, and the invocation of saints. After the Reformation, Protestants rejected many of these rites, and filled the vacuum with the power of prayer. To the melancholic Elsa von Canitz, Marin Luther wrote that the Devil had formed her unhappy state of mind. To another who came to Wittenberg for help, Luther declared that her sadness was not a disease for Hippocrates, but would be cured by the Word of God.

Melancholia, this disease of body and soul, preoccupied Shakespeare and his audience. Timothy Bright's *A Treatise of Melancholie*, a 1586 source book for the Bard, provided the clear division between bodily corruption that abused the mind, and the "heavy hande of God" as it weighted upon an afflicted conscience. Countless characters on the Elizabethan stage fell prey to sorrowful, fretful, and melancholic states that followed sin or inner strife. Hamlet suffered from this illness, as did Antigone and King Lear.

In 1621, a monumental compendium of classical views on melancholia appeared. Under the pseudonym Democritus Junior, Robert Burton, the Anglican Vicar of Saint Thomas published *The Anatomy of Melancholy, What It Is, With All the Kinds, Causes, Symptomes, Prognostickes, and Severall Cures of It.* The nom de plume

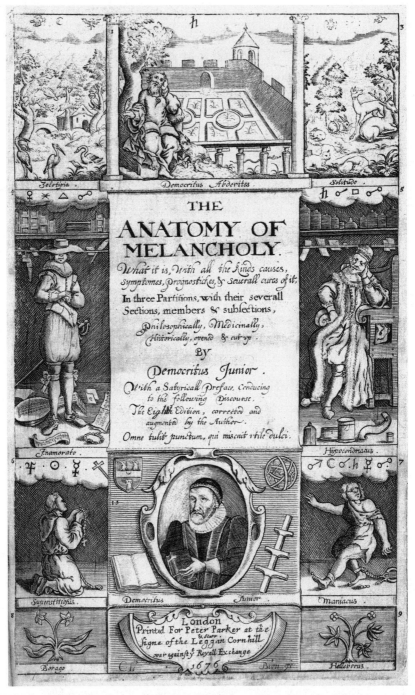

Figure 10. Robert Burton's 1621 work considered a wide variety
of ills to be melancholic.

referred to an anecdote; Hippocrates, it was said, once visited Democritus, whom the townspeople dismissed as crazy. When the father of medicine encountered one of the founders of atomism, he found him under a tree contemplating the carcasses of animals, which were strewn around him. Democritus explained that he had been studying their bodies, in search of the source of melancholia. As he departed, Hippocrates declared that the town's madman was nothing if not wise.

Burton filled his *Anatomy* with knowledge culled not from carcasses, but from books. The result, a gem of English prose, was devoured by the reading public and made the Oxford vicar one of the most popular authors of his time. Sadly, the author did not much enjoy his success. Robert Burton suffered from the disease that was his life's work. He admitted that he was "fatally driven upon this rock of melancholy, and carried away by this by-stream." However, he knew he was not alone. Burton quoted Horace, who wrote, "who is not a fool, melancholy, mad? *Qui nil molitur inepte,* who is not brain-sick?" All the world was mad and who was there to help? Burton acknowledged that some might wonder why a clergyman, not a doctor, purported to illuminate melancholia as well as frenzy, madness, sin, intemperance, dotage, ecstasy, hydrophobia and possession. Democritus Junior was not deterred:

> It is a disease of the soul in which I am to treat, and as much appertaining to a divine as to a physician, and who knows not what agreement there is betwixt these two professions? A good divine either is or ought to be a good physician, a spiritual physician at least, as our Savior calls Himself, and was indeed. They differ but in object, the one of the body, the other of the soul, and use divers medicines to cure: one amends *animam per corpus* [the soul through the body], the other *corpus per animam* [the body through the soul] as our Regius Professor of Physic well informed us in a learned lecture of his not long since. . . .

A divine in this compound mixed malady can do little alone,
a physician in some kinds of melancholy much less, both make
an absolute cure.

A man of the cloth by profession and a doctor by inclination, Burton believed that only such divided men were able to fully comprehend diseases that hovered between sin and humors, love and organ dysfunction, jealous rage and brain deformities. Only a doctor-clergyman could move back and forth between these realms, sorting through the array of disorders, trying to discern whether the source of illness sprang from the soul or the body. Since half of these disorders originated in the body and half in the soul, neither medical men nor clergy could provide a full remedy. The two needed to become one, hence a true soul-doctor.

Burton mixed a vast repertoire of classical adages with Galenic nostrums and Christian theology. Democritus Junior's *Anatomy* identified different varieties of melancholic ills, and moved from jealous lovers to black bile, witches to gassy stomachs, and insomnia to Satan's servants. Melancholy could spring from the intercession of God or the Devil, or forces mediated by magicians and witches. It might also arise from natural sources including astrological constellations, hereditary disease, destructive external influences such as calumnies, imprisonment, and inward influences such as fevers, agues, pox, and a distemper of the brain.

The vicar's therapies included clean air and a moderate diet, the curative powers of the hellebore plant, bleeding, prayer, and exorcism. Soul and body, Nature and Heaven, science and theology were all required. Burton's remedies took aim at consciousness and body, spirit and spleen, but in the end he had a preference. He cautioned sufferers to first pray. They should use medicine only if that failed them. He was not the only divine to emphasize spiritual healing over a bodily one. Thomas Adam's hellfire work, *Mystical Bedlam; or The World of Mad Men*, delineated how the wages of sin was insanity.

Burton similarly worried about immorality and sneered at those who denied the reality of possession. He did not doubt its power.

Among a bounty of classical references, Burton's tome also was sprinkled with astute, personal observations. The soul-sick, he noted, were often blind to their ills. While most sufferers ran to a doctor when their arm was swollen or their stomach churned, the one faculty whose disorder could not be perceived was precisely the one that allowed a person to perceive the world. The intellect managed to not know its own troubles and could not heal itself. Sadly, this would prove true for Burton himself. This erudite, witty, and elegant scholar of melancholy, according to John Aubrey, lost his battle and hung himself in Christ Church.

Burton wrote as the classical divisions between soul afflictions and humoral illness had begun to break down. In addition, magical and astrological medicine were waning. In the future, Anglicans would continue to acknowledge supernatural causes for melancholia, but deny rationales that came from the stars, such as those put forward by the Reverend Richard Napier. Napier was an orthodox Anglican clergyman, whose medical studies were anything but orthodox. Apprenticed to the infamous astrologer Simon Forman, he spent the rest of his life looking to the sky for guidance. He believed that planetary movements were macrocosms that mirrored the microcosm of a human being.

At the time of his death in 1641, sixty volumes of Napier's case records were preserved by Aubrey and others, who scoured them for Gnostic secrets and magical elixirs. They found that Dr. Napier moved back and forth between bleeding plasters and leeches, chemicals, and ritualized prayer. His practice included many lunatics, 40 percent of whom were either melancholic or what he called "mopish." During his career, over 513 patients claimed to be enchanted or haunted, but Napier, who frequently consulted with angels himself, was quite skeptical. He diagnosed over half of these as mad. Despite his heretical practice, which included prognostications based on readings of the moon as well as direct advice from spirits, Napier managed to avoid condemnation by the Church. His good fortune likely had to do with his zealous devotion, which prompted him to pray incessantly, so much so that "his knees were horny with frequent Praying." It was said he died while bowed down in reverence.

And so, in the decades before the Restoration these priest-doctors offered prayer and bleedings, and openly considered a wide array of in-between illnesses lumped under melancholia that could easily be framed as either natural or theological in origin. *The Anatomy of Melancholy* would be reprinted eight times until 1671, when Burton's work suddenly stopped being read. Burton's veneration of the classical past would go out of fashion and his soul-body thinking on melancholia would lose ground. In the modern world of mechanists, chemists, and empiricists, this illness would be more fully pulled into medicine. Anatomies of such things, no matter how erudite, required the study of carcasses. Take no man's word for it.

⁓

IN PROTESTANT COUNTRIES, the most explosive trouble that forced a reexamination of the line between soul and body was called enthusiasm. Enthusiasts were men and women who believed that they had been directly spoken to or touched by the Lord. Thus, they often claimed divine power, and insisted their followers live by the commandments they received, not rules handed down from a prince or king. Enthusiasts, it was feared, might ignite a rebellion.

Once, enthusiasts were considered the chosen and the gifted. For early Christians, these were the "inspired," the lucky few who had inhaled God's breath. After the Reformation in Switzerland, German lands, and especially England, a proliferation of radical dissenting Protestant sects, unchecked by any priestly caste, claimed to commune directly with the Lord. They spawned a new generation of prophets, seers, and apocalyptic messengers, visionaries who entranced or terrified their neighbors. "Enthusiasts" and "fanatiques" engendered chaos, it was feared, and not without reason, for claims of revelation spawned sects that helped to stoke war across Europe. What once was a blessing had transformed into a bloodstained curse. Physicians soon offered a new framework by which to view these self-proclaimed saviors: they suffered from a madness called religious enthusiasm.

The 16th-century Anabaptists were an early, favorite example of enthusiasm. This sect denied the efficacy of infant baptism and, based on that, called for whole-scale revolt. Originally from Switzerland, Germany, and Holland, their radical movement spread. These believers considered themselves graced with prophetic instruction through divine voices and visions and hence refused to recognize any king's laws. He could not compel them to go against the dictates of Heaven.

The term Anabaptist soon became shorthand, a smear against a host of often tiny, obscure sects that privileged private revelation over received authority. Loyal members of the Church of England were confronted with an array of such soapbox visionaries. The Anglican Church denounced these Dissenters and insisted the Biblical Age of Miracles was over. Those who said otherwise were Satanic. To Anglicans, religious enthusiasm was a devilish contagion that swept up whole villages and led to civil strife.

Declaring that no physician had yet addressed this epidemic, Robert Burton took it up. He called those who "seem to be inspired by the Holy Ghost" victims of religious melancholy, a variant of love melancholy in which the object was not Anne or John, but rather the Redeemer. The numbers of afflicted were vast: "Give me but a little leave, and I will set before your eyes in brief a stipend, vast infinite ocean of incredible madness and folly," Burton wrote. He considered anyone throughout the world whose worship was misdirected to be mad in this manner. Mahommedans, Jews, heretics, enthusiasts, diviners, prophets, and schismatics were all enthusiasts. Superstition affected their brains, hearts; understanding, their souls.

And the cause of this widespread plague was the Devil, who "rangeth abroad like a roaring lion."

Over the next decades, this disease spread in Burton's homeland. Radical sects announced their prophecies across England, Ireland, and Scotland. The beheading of Charles I by Oliver Cromwell and his forces led to the collapse of the Anglican, Royalist order and victory for the Dissenters. With no central religious authority, visionary splinter groups sprouted up. Among the Parliamentarian rulers of England, these movements could not be easily dismissed, for hadn't the new rulers fought for the right to follow one's individual conscience? And so, aided by the collapse of censorship, new sects spread their message with an outpouring of pamphlets, tracts, ballads, and sermons, which told of miracles, visions, and prophecies. Britain became a country of prophets. Anabaptists were joined by Levellers, Diggers, members of the Family of Love, Grindletonians, Muggletonians, Roundheads, Brownians, Methodists, Seekers, Antinomians, and Separatists. Village squares filled with self-avowed messengers from God who told of their communion with Heaven and Hell. In the British Isles, it seemed, the Age of Miracles had returned.

The Ranters were one group whose questionable existence did not prevent them from inciting panic. Established sometime around 1649, the group never had a recognized leader or an organization, but they were said to share a disdain for traditional morality. Christ was within all, they preached, and hence believers, by definition, were blameless. Confident of their own purity, Ranters were said to grant themselves orgiastic sexual license and were known to allow blasphemous language, hence their name.

If the Ranters were in part a collective fantasy, as some historians now believe, the social problems engendered by those who privately communed with God gained prominence with the emergence of the Society of Friends, or Quakers. The founder of this dissenting group, George Fox, was a Puritan who believed his people were not pure enough. Disillusioned with the slack morals of his elders, he fell into

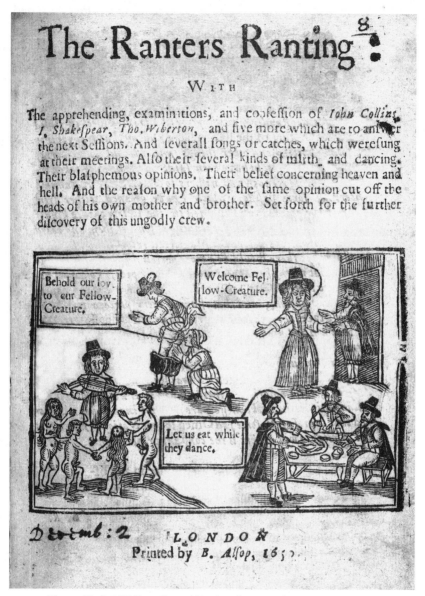

Figure 11. A 1650 Royalist publication showing the Ranters engaged in wanton sex, naked dancing, and gluttony.

despair, then had a revelation. In 1647, Fox heard a voice that marked his path forward; he began to preach that each individual should follow his own divine Inner Light, the presence of the God in his own soul. Biblical times were no less miraculous than these, Fox preached. He himself engaged in miraculous healings, exorcisms, and prophetic judgments, and believed any and all could minister to others, if they had been touched by the Holy Spirit.

Oliver Cromwell and the Parliamentarians were in a bind. Nonconformists themselves, they could not discount individual revelation, and yet sects like the Quakers scorned the rule of law. George Fox and his Friends were repeatedly imprisoned for fear that their doctrine would spread civil disorder. It became increasingly critical for moderate Nonconformists in England to find a legitimate way to support an individual's private conscience while at the same time discounting the potentially revolutionary claims of radical prophets and visionaries. The need for such a dividing line was made clear in the notorious trial of James Nayler.

In 1651, this one-time cavalry quartermaster fell under the sway of Fox's teachings; he sold his farm, left his wife and family, and roamed the land as a Quaker evangelist. His plainspoken eloquence and his supposed resemblance to Jesus led a group of devoted women to much admire his Inner Light. They declared that he was, in fact, God's Son. On October 24, 1656, in Bristol, Nayler and his worshipers staged a Palm Sunday reenactment, in which he rode a horse. At his side, female disciples kept up an ecstatic chant of "Holy! Holy! Holy!"

This self-proclaimed King of Israel was quickly arrested. At his trial before the House of Commons, Nayler would not deny that he was Jesus Christ, and so he was pilloried, publicly whipped, and branded on his forehead with "B" for blasphemer. Then, as if that were not enough, Nayler had a hot iron plunged through his tongue. The extraordinary brutality of his punishment reveals something of the time. After all, there had been other frauds and fools who claimed to be the Messiah, people like William Franklin and Arise Evans: they had been treated far more leniently. However, this new Christ, if he was believed, had a potential movement behind him: if the Quakers aligned with him, he would represent a threat to the regime.

In a Commonwealth filled with dissenting religious groups that prized personal revelation, what were the Parliamentarians to do? On what grounds could they denounce one sect and embrace another? In Paris, a then-exiled Thomas Hobbes thought he knew the answer. He viewed claims of divine inspiration through the dark lens of decades of brutal warfare that roiled Europe. Again and again, one sect had declared itself to be in possession of the Truth and the other to be Satanic. Such beliefs were a quicksand that could sink a nation. Hobbes believed the authority of private revelation must be strictly contained, but to do so required more than the torture of some misguided false Jesus. It required a new view of the state.

Concern over religious enthusiasm was critical to Hobbes's famous reformulation of the standing political order. Thus, the reader of *Leviathan* found rather strangely that this political treatise quickly veered off to discuss the problems of madness and this common form of disease. Hobbes insisted that enthusiasts were religious terrorists who needed to be compelled to follow the monarch. Thus, he elevated the state above any church. Only a dominant, secular authority could provide longstanding political stability. Then, religious enthusiasm would be a matter for police, jurists, and doctors.

Hobbes was ignored and the problem grew. In 1655, Méric Casaubon published the first full-length work on the problem of enthusiasm. The son of a French Calvinist persecuted by Jesuits, he found asylum in England and became an Anglican clergyman. In *A Treatise Concerning Enthusiasme*, Casaubon allowed that divine inspiration might exist, but only rarely. He took up his pen in disgust after reading a French nun's account of her own revelations, which had been authorized by Catholic bishops and scholastics. To Casaubon, the woman's tale was one of madness. Insane enthusiasm had spread to Turkish dervishes, prophetic rabbis, Catholic nuns in ecstasy, German maids with fits, Spanish Alumbrados or Illuminati, and even saints. In the second edition of his work, Casaubon added another mad tribe, the Quakers. This English sect were, he suggested, a new

edition of the Alumbrados, as "if the Devil, in such times of libertie
. . . play the same pranks in England." "Let others admire Witches
and Magicians . . . I honour and admire a good Physician much
more, who can (as God's instrument) by the knowledge of nature,
bring a man to his right wits again, when he hath lost them: and I
tremble . . . when I think that one Madman is enough to infect a
whole Province."

Many trembled by his side. In the free-for-all that was interregnum England, the diagnosis of religious enthusiasm was embraced
by moderate Protestants to mark the difference between divine grace
and grave disease. For Anglican proponents of the status quo, however, enthusiasm was a disease of all Nonconformists, not just James
Nayler. In 1656, the Cambridge Platonist Henry More, in his *Enthusiasmus Triumphatus*, declared enthusiasm always to be a matter for
doctors, for it was nothing more than "mad or Melancholy men,
who have confidently affirmed that they have met with the Devil, or
conversed with Angels, when it has been nothing but an encounter
with their own fancie." Intoxicated and distempered, they dreamt
with their eyes open. The return of Charles II in 1660 reinforced this
broader view. As the Anglicans returned to power, many embraced
"rational religion," the view that all of God's acts should be fully
accessible to reason. In 1674, John Owen proclaimed that the Lord
did not work by inspiration, but through the God-given faculty of
thought. The rest was insanity.

Charles II cracked down on Dissenters, who were imprisoned
and routed. A new law forbade any non-Anglican religious meetings
from hosting more than five people at one time. For Royalists, Oliver Cromwell himself became an example of a dangerous enthusiast,
a man for whom "every crime becomes Lawful, and every Design,
that turns up in his Head, is a divine Impulse." At the Royal Society,
discussions of politics were themselves deemed signs of enthusiasm
and were strictly forbidden. Enthusiasts promulgated bloodshed, regicide, and war.

In Catholic countries like France, Austria, Spain, and Italy, the Pope and his robed emissaries still stood between each believer and his or her God. This hierarchy possessed the power to curtail and marginalize any religious enthusiasm that it deemed not in its interest. However, in Protestant countries, especially in Restoration England, where no such barrier was in place, the elite increasingly began to proclaim that many who were supposedly inspired in their souls were touched in the head. And so they turned to doctors. Physicians expanded their role in the interstices of their splintering society, so as to ensure the safety of the status quo from *I heard it from God* insurrectionists. Anglican clergymen, jurists, and landed gentry joined moderate Calvinists and reiterated that the Age of Miracles was over. Those who saw God's face or heard His voice had not been touched in their souls, but were actually medically ill—in a word, mad.

A Crisis of Conscience

THE 17TH-CENTURY discourses on witchcraft, melancholia, and enthusiasm manifested a shift in the old divisions between the soul and the body. These phenomena, once clearly defined theologically, now had become controversies that existed in the nebulous border region between religion and medicine. While Robert Boyle confidently pursued natural science and reserved the realm of spirits for his faith, early modern physicians entered a murky borderland where the claims for the soul were in direct conflict, not just with a mechanized or chemical natural world, but also with social and political demands.

This medicalization of some soul phenomena was not simply a collective turn to reason. Rather a crisis had settled over Western Christendom as heterodoxy undermined claims of authority based on divine knowledge. The sacred miracles of one community were decried as the Devil's work by other sects. If, for some, the Pope was a holy, revered figure, for others, he was a possessed Antichrist. Hence, the debates of a few philosophers—who argued over the realm of the soul and the material claims of the brain, the body, and Nature—became implicated in the religious wars of the many. Was a witch truly possessed, or melancholic? Was George Fox a prophet or a terrorist twisted by enthusiasm? In the face of these volatile questions, a growing number turned to answers from earthly sources.

To confront these disruptive problems, a few doctors began to suggest that the faculty of reason, that defining function of the rational soul, itself could become sick. Medical explanations expanded to take up the soul's perturbations. Even devout citizens were eager to accept the notion that claims for possession or commands at insurrection heard from God were not real, but rather madness. Exhausted from decades of bloodshed, the authority of the competing Christian churches lost sway and such secular conceptions inched forward.

However, these often theatrical and explosive controversies like that of James Nayler or the nuns of Loudun were but the most visible demonstrations of a deeper and more ubiquitous problem that troubled the feudal order. The rise of Christian heterodoxy and the simultaneous ascent of scientific materialism undercut the very basis for ethical conduct.

During the Classical Age, moral life was predicated on a balance between the passions and reason. Plato considered reason powerful enough to control these desires. The Stoics agreed. Passions, they believed, were simply false judgments that reason could correct. During the late 16th century and early 17th century, a revival of Stoicism emerged in France and the Netherlands led by thinkers like Justus Lipsius and Guillaume du Vair. In their own way, each highlighted the famous Delphic injunction, "Know Thyself," for they insisted that rational insight could serve as a regulator of behavior and work as a moral compass.

Aristotle was never persuaded of reason's power, and a long line of theologians from St. Augustine to Thomas Aquinas agreed. Passions were not errors, but rather fixed parts of human nature. These urges could be managed, but never vanquished. In the Thomist view, unruly passions were common to all beasts, including mankind. However in humans, these cravings traveled to the stately home of reason where they were subdued. When passions overtook the rational soul, illness and vice ensued. Aristotle counseled men to reign in these inner forces, while Stoics sought their elimination. Throughout Christianity, this was an organizing drama of daily existence. Passion-driven sins and temptations must be controlled, but thanks to the God-given soul, humans were up to the task.

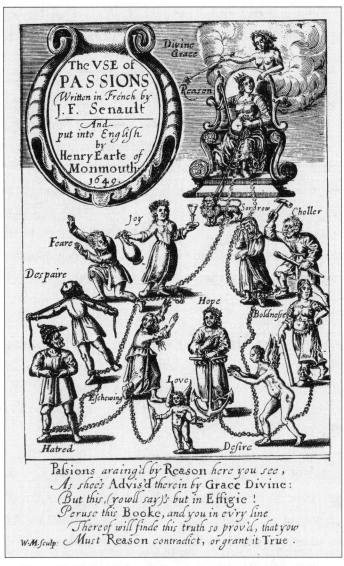

Figure 12. This 1641 frontispiece shows reason as a divine grace that chained the passions.

As Protestant sects grew, the importance of the individual conscience expanded. Without a priest to offer confession and absolu-
tion, each man was left alone to judge his own inner world and guess
his everlasting fate. After his conversion to Calvinism, Cromwell
himself fell into despair, tormented by the worry that he was not one
of the Elect destined for Heaven. In 1678, John Bunyan wrote: "How
can you tell if you are elected? . . . My thoughts were like masterless
hell-hounds; my soul like a broken vessel, driven into the winds, and
tossed sometimes headlong into despair." With the stakes being no
less than eternal torture, the reliability of one's conscience became
central to Protestants.

However, by the late 17th century, early modern thinkers like
Descartes, Gassendi, and Boyle had sought to alter these old views.
The passions would be renamed: those who considered them the
result of inner motion spoke of "emotions." As a mechanical and
chemical human body assumed the functions of the sensitive souls,
only an immaterial spirit stood in the way. For modernists, the battle
for salvation now seemed to pit a clanking machine against something
holy. In 1681, Andrew Marvell in his poem "A Dialogue Between
the Soul and the Body," captured this weird mix of metal and spirit:

> Oh who shall, from this dungeon, raise
> A soul enslaved so many ways?
> With bolts of bones, that fettered stands
> In feet, and manacles in hands. . . .
> A soul hung up, as 'twere, in chains
> Of nerves, and arteries, and veins. . . .

Could pumps of flesh be contained by a spirit? How was it even
possible for matter and its opposite to intersect? Some quickly recognized the profundity of this challenge to the divided world of science
and faith that the moderns had fashioned; one of them was the philosopher most responsible for that division, René Descartes.

GALENIC MEDICINE WAS primarily a closed system in which alterations
in the body's fluids caused disease. However, Galen and his followers
did allow for six environmental disturbances that might disrupt these
inner workings. These "non-naturals" remained a part of medical
logic until at least 1800. For Robert Burton, the list included diet, air
quality, exercise, sleep patterns, bodily intake and evacuation, and,
lastly, excess passion. With this last of the nonnaturals, Galenic medicine held a small place for illness that might be considered moral.

In ancient Greece, intense passion played a critical role in theories of madness. Influenced by the Stoics, Galen considered unruly
feeling to be an assault on the body. It shook one by the shoulders,
sent fumes flying about, and rattled the soul. The heart—which he
believed to be the seat of all passions—when disrupted, made nox-
ious vapors that traveled through secret channels to the brain, where
the result was melancholia or frenzy. Never at a loss for support from
the classical canon, Robert Burton supported this logic with lines
from Horace, who wrote:

> By yesterday's excesses still oppressed,
> The body suffers not the mind to rest.

Most doctors agreed that excess passion caused disease, but the
descriptions of those passions varied widely. Burton himself employed
old terminology that divided feelings into the "irascible," which
were complex and powerful, and the simpler "concupiscible," which
were desirous. Some classical authorities believed the four wheels on
the human chariot were love, hope, hate, and fear. Others substituted
joy for love, or added desire and sorrow to the inventory. Aquinas
was not satisfied until he distinguished eleven passions. And it did
not stop there, as other authors sought to construct complex entities

out of simpler ones and thereby account for shame, envy, malice, vengeance, ambition, and covetousness.

And so, this single nonnatural cause opened the floodgates for Galenic doctors to imagine emotionally based illness and consider ways to reign these in. Primitive forms of psychotherapy focused on Stoical philosophy. Galenic doctors counseled patients to avoid long and extreme feelings of grief or anger or jealousy. Such admonishments pervaded Elizabethan theater, such as Shakespeare's *All's Well That Ends Well*, where a girl mourning her father was counseled to snap out of it, before excessive grief unhinged her.

Furthermore, such perturbations might not just make one mad; they also might undo a whole people. In 1601, the English author Thomas Wright opened his extensive work on the passions by observing their importance for the body, the soul, and the nation. First, passions altered the humors. Second, they "trouble wonderfully the soule" for good Christians; they induced vice, corrupted judgment, and seduced the will. When out of control, individuals, then communities, become frenzied. Wright told of a "Christian Orator" who could "effectuate strange matters in the minds of his Auditors." This preacher could twist his audience into tears, then turn them to laughter. He had the power to make his listeners lose their senses and run riot.

Thanks to his Jesuitical convictions, Wright was repeatedly imprisoned and finally banished from England. He dedicated *The Passions of the Minde in Generall* to Shakespeare's patron, the Earl of Southampton, in the hopes that his famously pugnacious lord would be delivered from his own fervors. However, the moralist in Wright insisted on a broader point. The passions were naughty servants who tried to defy their master. Bathed in corporeality, they could not defeat the ethereal ruler on her throne. The almighty soul was to govern the body and guide the passions as "subjects and vassals." As God reigned over man, and a king ruled his subjects, so did the soul control the passions. Passions could rebel against reason; similarly, a nation could be caught up by revolts or general sedition and be torn apart by its wild-eyed members. Perturbations of the soul led to madness, vice, and warfare.

Like many tracts on the passions that began to appear during this tumultuous time, Wright sought to keep his feet planted firmly in the Old World: for him, Nature, Christian ethics, and monarchist politics were three pillars of the same civilization. *A Treatise of the Passions and Faculties of the Soul of Man* written in 1640 by Edward Reynolds held the same assumptions. The prince was the "soul of the Commonwealth." In the same way that the body politic could send its passions and false reports to the prince, the body machine could misdirect the soul. Those called good or evil were made so by their passions. For the disturbed and tormented, Reynolds recommended moderation along with Christian repentance. Faith, education, and good habits strengthened the rational soul against its sometimes frenzied invaders.

Reynolds's *A Treatise of the Passions* was dedicated to Princess Elisabeth, daughter of the Queen of Bohemia, a reader eager to consider such matters. Around that time, however, the brilliant, multilingual, dark-haired beauty, so astute that she was nicknamed the "Grecian" by her siblings, had fallen under the sway of another counselor. In 1643, she had commenced an intense correspondence with Descartes, in which she pressed this thinker to more fully address the problems *he* had created, the same problems René had disdained when his nemesis, Pierre Gassendi, had raised them.

Cartesian metaphysics always suffered from a grave difficulty. Challengers asked how two different substances, one immaterial and the other material, could affect each other? Among the growing band of Cartesians, "occasionalists," most famously the ingenius Nicolas Malebranche, rose up to defend the belief that no such interactions took place, thereby further segregating the immortal Christian soul from the body. This, however, only raised more questions and prompted endless metaphysical duels.

Descartes had little patience for all this. However, the pressing queries from the princess were different. In May of 1643, she asked, if the mind had no extension, how could it propel the body? Under her persistent queries, the philosopher confessed that he had no idea. He called for a new "Human Science" to solve this problem, but he didn't just drop the subject. For Elisabeth's questions were not merely academic; the princess suffered from severe melancholia. And so the intense devotion between the Frenchman and the free-thinking Princess steered away from loftier considerations to discuss her passions and the burden they placed on her. After 1643, in these intimate exchanges, Descartes worked out the details of a new theory, which he put into practice. Elisabeth dubbed him the best doctor for her soul.

In 1649, Descartes's last work, *The Passions of the Soul*, was published with a dedication to the princess. In it, the author distinguished himself from those of his followers that denied consciousness and the body ever mixed. During his years immersed in animal dissections, Descartes had told Mersenne that he hoped to locate imagination and memory somewhere in the flesh of the brain. "I doubt whether there is any doctor who has made such detailed observations as I," he declared. During these studies, he stumbled upon a small olive-sized structure at the center of the brain known as the pineal gland. In his unpublished "Treatise on Man," written in 1637, Descartes had constructed a theory in which that little protuberance held enormous significance. It was the precise place where the immaterial Cogito attached to the body. We see only one image with two eyes, hear one sound through two ears. Therefore, the soul must unify our senses. The pineal gland might be, no it *was* the center of that unification. Thereafter, it also became the precise location of the rational soul.

A dozen years later, Descartes further developed this idea. The pineal gland was the meeting place between the soul and the mechanical disruptions that came from memories, sensory information, pas-

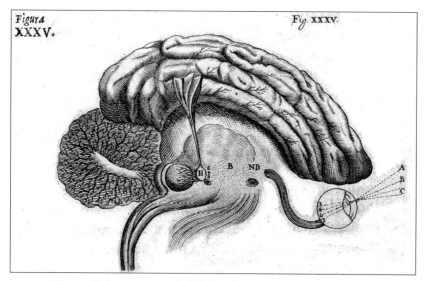

Figure 13. Descartes concluded that the pineal gland (labeled "H")
was the seat of the soul.

sions, appetites, and bodily forces. Passions did not originate in the
heart and work through their way to the head through vapors. Passions were forces in the brain communicated to the Cogito through
this little gland. Descartes imagined that the pineal gland must
vibrate back and forth to convey desire. For example, the impulse to
run would spur the little gland into rotary action. The soul, in turn,
sought to push and pull the pineal gland as it saw fit. The struggles
of conscience, the dark night of the soul now seemed to have been
reduced to the swirling of a little bulb in the brain.

This model had important medical applications. In 1645, the
princess wrote Descartes to complain of a fever and cough. He
promptly informed her that this was due to sadness. He advised
her that great souls do not abandon themselves to their passions;
their reason must subdue such affects. Elisabeth thanked him for
this advice. Encouraged, Descartes elaborated further. Imagine a
man who constantly immersed himself in pitiful tragedies, and
another who despite his share of misfortune, directed his imagina-

tion toward things that could furnish him with contentment and joy. This exact psychic treatment was the one he had imposed upon himself, when after his mother died days after his birth, his own weak constitution and lingering ills often made others think he was not long for this earth.

This Stoical cure was echoed in *The Passions of the Soul.* The soul must hold on during great commotions. Weak souls fail to resist and become prey to hatred, desire, sadness, and love; they become enslaved and unhappy. For while positive passions fortify good thoughts and feelings, negative passions harm us by prolonging bad ideas and feelings. One's pineal gland was groomed in "our earliest years," but it could be reeducated and linked to new thoughts and new capacities, much like an animal can be trained. The goal was to have an "absolute empire over all the passions."

Descartes's theory meshed with traditional Christian ethics. While passions could drive the will of a man as in the case of melancholic desperation, human beings possessed the capacity to control these feelings. Virtue and happiness were predicated on the soul's management of the mechanical disruptions from the body-machine. However, Descartes's call for a human science perched between the soul and the body-machine was novel. In his attempts to bridge inner experience and bodily input, his efforts were no longer traditionally Christian, but something stranger.

Descartes's *The Passions of the Soul* was widely debated. Its most lasting innovation was to relocate passions from the heart to the nervous system. All Descartes needed to make his neural machine mesh with thought and rise into being, was that pineal nub in the center of the brain. News of the Frenchman's claims regarding that pineal gland spread. While welcomed by dedicated Cartesians like Regius, this discovery proved to be a disaster. While Henry More attacked this notion as nothing more than speculation, Nicholas Steno's 1666 lecture in Paris, which questioned some of Thomas Willis's assertions about the brain, saved special contempt for Descartes's pineal gland theory. Steno's criticism made its way to Huygens and the Academy of Sciences and raised doubt with French anatomists. However, the most lethal rejoinder came from Thomas Willis. In his *The Anatomy of the Brain*, Willis let it be known that animals of all sorts, including the most cruel and brutish, had supremely well-endowed pineal glands. The celestial soul of humans did not reside there. By the 1670s, according to Spinoza, such theories provoked only ridicule and disgust.

WHILE DELIVERING A crushing blow to Descartes's theory of soul-brain interaction, Thomas Willis did not have a better solution. Like the Frenchman, he had done much to naturalize much of the Thomist vegetative and sensitive souls, while carefully preserving an immaterial place for reason and the rational soul. Nonetheless, if the pineal gland was an absurd suggestion, Willis had no better one for how an immaterial soul could interface with nervous matter and contain the passions.

As the basis for ethical conduct was debated, civic strife reigned. After the Restoration of Charles II, Anglicans and moderate Dissenters both longed for a way to preserve social stability, by creating individuals whose liberty of conscience could be protected, because their passions were in check. With that goal in mind, Thomas Hobbes proposed a radical solution.

In *Leviathan*, Hobbes was remorselessly, single-mindedly materialistic. He argued that Heaven and Earth, as well as God and the soul, were made of matter. This stance was in part the result of "the disorder of the present time," phenomena like the Thirty Years War, decades of religious extremism, and sanctified terrorism, in which competing spiritual groups ravaged the body politic. Only through a dry-eyed analysis of individual conduct could one comprehend this "madness in the multitude."

Passion and reason, for Hobbes, were both matter in motion. However, the frenetic movement inspired by lust or joy or hate led Hobbes to conclude that reason provided a rather weak restraint. Given the dominance of animal feeling, individuals were doomed to be the playthings of their passions, easily provoked by their own selfish desires and in constant conflict with each other. Their dearest pleasure—power—drove them. Reason and ethics were slaves to this tyrant. Things that were vehemently desired always seemed to be ratified as noble. That which was despised just as easily was rationalized as vicious. Men never could peacefully coexist, for their natural state was selfishness, all versus all, a life, in his famous phrase, "solitary, poor, nasty, brutish and short."

Passion made men not just rapacious, but also crazy. Vainglorious or dejected feelings led to insanity, as was clearly evident from religious enthusiasts, whose folly of believing themselves inspired allowed them to rage against the laws of the nation and pursue their own selfish ends. Troubled minds of this sort were far from rare; Catholics who accepted transubstantiation and the Pope's infallibility were lunatics. So were many criminals, possessed demoniacs, and an array of modern Protestant prophets. These disturbed individuals created and sustained superstitions:

> From the ignorance of how to distinguish dreams, and other strong fancies from vision and sense, did arise the greatest part of the religion of the Gentiles in time past, that worshipped satyrs, fawns, nymphs and the like, and now-a-days the opinion that rude people have of fairies, ghosts, and goblins, and of the power of witches.

Liberty of conscience meant such unhinged believers could freely declare that their folly was inspired. In a society where everyone was a prophet, no one was safe. To live in peace within such a dangerous, deluded tribe, Hobbes could see only one choice: individuals must give up some personal liberty and hand it over to an absolute monarch. What others might call a tyrant, Hobbes called a sovereign whose job was to regulate a population filled with brutes and fanatics.

Unlike those early moderns who placed their faith in the power of the rational soul, Hobbes considered that faculty to be a machine quite prone to error. All around as he surveyed his brethren, he found false beliefs, bad logic, and imaginings taken as reality. In this, he mirrored the conclusions of Sir Thomas Browne, whose 1646 *Pseudodoxia epidemica, or Vulgar Errors* detailed volumes of absurdities that reasonable folk accepted, from belief in griffins, phoenixes, unicorns, and mermaids, to myths about biblical times. For Hobbes, reason was frail and fallible. The sole assurance that we did not exist in a dream came from our senses, our brains, and our minds. And thought disorders—not just passions overrunning reason—but illnesses in the rational faculty itself, must be "rightly numbered amongst the many sorts of madness."

If the intellect could be ill, it was also our only hope. A nominalist who leaned heavily on the universal meaning of words, Hobbes placed great weight on "mental discourse," the natural processes by which the perceptual, naming, logical, and imaginative functions churned together to make for human understanding. Names linked into general affirmations, then syllogisms, to make up thought. Such was the process that men called being conscious. Reasoning for Hobbes was computation, a kind of logical accretion and subtraction of meaning. By this account, one could discern which kinds of mental discourse added up, and which ones veered off into lunacy. Therefore, the claims of conscience were analyzable. It was not the word of God written in men's hearts, but another mental operation, that could be evaluated. Logical grounds existed to declare some acts of conscience legitimate and others folly.

Anticipating a storm of criticism, the author of *Leviathan* ruthlessly critiqued defenders of ethics who based their analysis on the rational soul. What, he asked, could a Cartesian phrase like "immaterial substance," or "free will" or "free subject" possibly mean? Any examination revealed nothing more than a descent into meaningless self-contradiction. Wills and subjects were by definition not free. Substances were material.

Hobbes dared to go further and explain how functions previously attributed to the soul operated. The inner world began as an empty warehouse. Outward turbulence provoked nerve activity from the senses that was then formulated by our imagination. Information was strung together and unified into what he called "associations." These secretly connected thoughts "run over all things, holy, profane, clean, obscene, grave and light, without shame or blame. . . ." When supercharged with passion, associations transform into zealous beliefs. For those who heard voices from the other world, the passions had been victorious.

Safely ensconced in Paris, Thomas Hobbes watched as war ripped at his homeland. Without the soul, without a unified Church, the tutor of the future King of England believed there was only one solution. The monarch must protect the general Commonwealth from waking dreamers, ranting zealots, and the rabble. In a world of matter and motion, where passion so easily took hold of reason, where warring religions justified ethical injunctions to kill, social order would need to rest with the state. An absolute monarch could act as ethical reason for the body politic, reigning in its wild desires. There was no other way, or so Thomas Hobbes concluded.

THE BREAKDOWN OF scholasticism and the religious wars in Europe led to grave concern about a linchpin of the Old World, the human soul. By the second half of the 17th century, philosophers such as Descartes, Hobbes, and Gassendi sought to find a place for this human essence in a mechanical world. Scientists and anatomists pushed the boundaries by exploring the brain and searching for that impossible space, a home for reason and eternal consciousness. As competing claims to absolute truth polarized and in part undermined religious authority, doctors and clerics renegotiated the boundaries of the natural and the supernatural, madness and soul sickness, when considering diseases that traditionally resided between body and soul, such as enthusiasm. Some worried about the nature of ethics in an increasingly natural world, one where nothing divine held back a man's animal cravings, a fallen world where the rewards of Heaven and the pains of Hell did not backstop law and order.

All this meant that between 1650 and 1700, a torrent of writings appeared focused on the anatomy of the soul and the brain, the perturbations caused by the passions of inner life, novel models of consolation for the tormented and disturbed, articulations of politics, rhetoric, and logic that analyzed and situated the intellect anew, and medical works on madness that took stock of an array of disturbances once considered soul disorders.

To be sure, much of this work was apologetic in nature. Many authors wrote with the hope that they would keep the Old World from breaking apart. A growing minority, however, took steps toward the profane idea that the rational soul and its highest functions might be material, prone to illness and errors, and not divinely endowed. No one went as far as Thomas Hobbes in making these claims. However, the strained refutations and partial calls for reform would lead to a break and a new theory for human reason that would be of monumental consequence.

PART II

THE ENGLISH MIND

My mynd to me
a kingdome is.

—EDWARD DYER

"Myself in a Storm"

O N OCTOBER 25, 1656, a twenty-four-year-old Oxford medical student traveled to London, where Cromwell's second
Parliament had recently cracked down on dissent and purged itself of
nearly a third of its members. Unlike many Anglican virtuosi such as
Boyle and Willis, this man was of strict Calvinist stock, though his
convictions had been softened during years at the elite Westminster
School, then at Oxford. Nonetheless, his trip to the capital, where
men of his creed now held power, brought only consternation. The
city had gone crazy.

His letters home describe how the most radical of the Dissenters,
the Quakers, refused to don hats, an eccentricity well founded, he
quipped, since a hot head was "dangerous for mad folks." He then
detailed the debacle created by that symbol of enthusiasm, the new
Christ, James Nayler, and his singing Mary Magdelenes. Finding his
way to the chamber where Nayler had retired after his examination before Parliament, the young man found quite a scene: female
worshipers wore white gloves, some hid their heads in white bags
and hummed continually, while one sang "Holy! Holy! Holy!" Disgusted with the never-ending fragmentations of Protestantism and
the chaos it had engendered, the doctor who would one day reshape
modernity went home convinced he was a denizen of "great Bedlam

England." A few years later, he wrote of the unceasing confusion that surrounded him: "I no sooner perceived myself in the *world* but I found myself in a storm. . . ."

Back at Oxford, John Locke threw himself into his medical studies and his research with the experimental philosophers. He befriended luminaries of the Invisible College like Robert Hooke and Robert

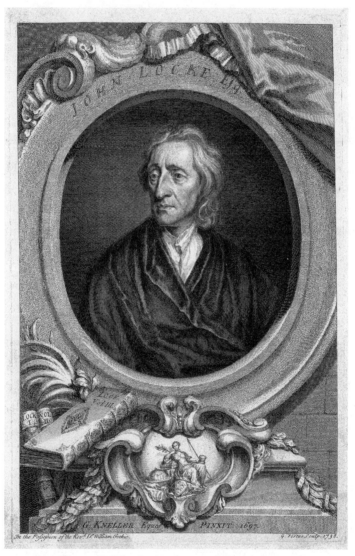

Figure 14. John Locke, doctor, philosopher, spy.

Boyle, who became a mentor. Along with Anglicans and many Calvinists eager for stability, he rejoiced when Charles II returned: he
could now be counted as a full-fledged monarchist. Meanwhile, he
soaked up novel medical theories that broke from Galen and took
close notes on the lectures of the newly appointed Sedleian Professor
of Natural Philosophy, Thomas Willis. His student notes carefully
track Willis as he mixed chemical and mechanical theories of disease
and offered nervous explanations for hysteria and epilepsy.

Willis's Oxford lectures also set out central ideas that later
would be attributed to this pupil. The Sedleian Professor spoke of
sensations registering on an otherwise clean mental slate, a "tabula
rasa." Like Gassendi, Willis insisted brain matter could perform
cognitive functions. God, Willis lectured, had endowed humans
with "thinking matter." This paradoxical phrase circumvented the
problem of how matter could, in a mechanical or chemical manner,
emerge with higher powers of reason, such as free will. This finesse
would be adopted by Locke, who would incur decades of derision
for what would be considered an absurdity. Yet, this solution—half
natural and half religious, a paradox that could all too easily be
dismissed—would prove critical for the younger man as he began
to do what was otherwise unthinkable: redefine the soul so that it
no longer had any dominion over cognition, reflection, free will,
or personal identity.

⌒

AS A YOUNG man, Locke's commitment to medicine was deep. Through
his formative years, he traveled to medical Meccas like Montpellier
in France, befriended local doctors, and dutifully recorded recipes
for cures for everything from pimples to gonorrhea. Such matters
dominated not only due to Locke's chosen profession, but also to his
own constant health worries, which included asthma. The doctor's
movements around Europe, ostensibly for his own well-being, may

also have been motivated by more clandestine pursuits, for while at Oxford he had plunged into a murky world of espionage.

A serendipitous encounter led to his turn to political intrigue. In 1666, Anthony Ashley Cooper, the first Baron Ashley, traveled to Oxford to visit his son and take the medicinal waters. To aid in this, he had written to a Dr. Thomas, who, being out of town, called upon the younger Locke to stand in his stead. The doctor and Lord Ashley hit it off. In 1667, Ashley asked the thirty-five-year-old to come to London and treat victims of the plague. Soon, however, Ashley developed dire troubles of his own. He had contracted a mysterious ailment, likely a liver abscess, which was a potentially lethal matter. A conference of doctors recommended surgery, which when performed unleashed a torrent of pus. Passionate medical arguments ensued over what to do next; some thought a candle should be inserted to stop up the wound. Thanks to Locke and others, instead a silversmith was summoned to craft a tube, which was inserted into the Lord's stomach to drain his suppurating wound. Each day, attendants flushed the tube out with wine to keep it clean.

The patient survived to become the Lord High Chancellor of England and the Earl of Shaftesbury, and he never would forget his debt to the young physician who helped see him through this near-death experience. In gratitude, Lord Ashley got the king to write Oxford authorities to secure Locke's position. Ashley never discarded the silver drain, which became a symbol of his survival and a focus for the mockery of his many political opponents. John Dryden had a ghost in one of his plays proclaim: "Bid Lord Shaftesbury have a care of his spigot; if he is tapt all the plot will run out." Dryden's concerns about Shaftesbury's behind-the-scenes conspiracies were not far off: over the next decade, the earl would be involved in secret negotiations and backroom deals that held England in the balance.

John Locke became Ashley's confidant, secret courier, and doctor; he also became a devoted follower of Dr. Thomas Sydenham. One of the most prominent physicians in Restoration London, this fervent Calvinist had taken that creed's antitraditionalism and commitment to personal experience and applied it to his profession. Too much of medicine, he concluded, was empty theory, grand mansions of vanity. Sydenham preached observation by the bedside and, following Francis Bacon, the accretion of reliable facts, not grand symphonic notions. He positioned himself against the Galenists with their bloodletting, and natural philosophers whose mechanical and chemical presumptions cured no one.

Sydenham sought pragmatic remedies. He was one of the first to advocate the cooling of feverish patients, rather than the traditional strategy of keeping them warm. He was renowned for creative, often improvised, therapies. In one case, he set a melancholic man out on an expedition to find an imaginary doctor who never existed: the trip itself, Dr. Sydenham happily reported, gave the man purpose and shook him out of his torpor. In 1668, it had been Sydenham who advised Locke not to stop up Ashley's wound, but rather to construct the celebrated drainage pipe. John Locke became this renowned doctor's sidekick, coauthor, and collaborator; he trailed Sydenham on his rounds and began a book with this "Great Genius of Physik," a never-completed compendium of clinical medicine.

Locke also remained in conversation with the natural philosophers and virtuosi whose perspectives he shared. Like them, he was highly skeptical of superstitious occurences, such as the famous mass possession of French nuns in Loudum; in his medical notebooks, he jotted down that it "all was a cheat," a case of fraud. In 1668, Locke was elected to the Royal Society and appointed to the committee for considering and directing experiments. However, he preferred smaller settings for discussion, such as his own rooms at Exeter House. There he met with intellectual friends like Sydenham, Ashley, and James Tyrell, and during one such gathering during the frigid winter of 1671, Locke and his friends fell into deep discussion.

The question they debated was one that both Thomas Sydenham and Robert Boyle had addressed themselves. What were the powers and limits of the human intellect? Where did our rational capacities end, and where did faith in biblical revelation begin? The argument inspired Locke; he jotted down a page of ideas the next day and thought that would be it. Instead, the question haunted him. His subsequent quest for answers took many years, and his proposed solution eventually ballooned to nearly 1,000 pages.

Though his ideas were initially hatched in 1671, Locke's time to write was repeatedly overrun by politics and the roller-coaster ride that was Lord Shaftesbury's fortunes. In 1672, Shaftesbury was appointed Lord Chancellor to head the government; his loyal advisor Locke gave up his medical practice to assume a government post. A year later, Shaftesbury fell from favor, and Locke was sent by his lord to Montpellier, the home of a great medical faculty, but also the center of power for the dissident French Huguenots. In 1679, Lord Shaftesbury reconciled himself with the Court and asked Locke to return to London and serve again. Finally in 1681, Lord Shaftesbury, convinced a Papist plot to overtake England was in the works, conspired to overthrow the king, whom he deemed to be treasonous. By then Charles II's behavior had alienated many; the whoring and boozing of his court led some commentators like Samuel Pepys to conclude that hedonism seemed to be their sole purpose.

Wary of Shaftesbury's machinations, Charles sent spies to carefully watch the lord and his emissaries, among them Dr. Locke. Shaftesbury was arrested for high treason and locked away in the Tower of London. Though he was eventually released, the message was clear for opponents of the regime. In 1682, after one of his aides was hung, Shaftesbury dressed up as a Presbyterian minister and escaped to Holland. Locke knew what would come if he didn't act quickly. He too fled England.

However, the battles over religion were only becoming more intense on the Continent as well, as Charles's cousin, Louis XIV, revoked the Edict of Nantes in 1685 and attempted to cleanse the country of Huguenots. Acts of brutal repression, torture, and imprisonment preceded an exodus of Protestants from France. Huguenot intellectuals, like Pierre Bayle, became deeply embittered. A Protestant from Foix who converted to Catholicism, Bayle had come back to his father's faith in time to be forced from his home. In Holland, his journal, the *Nouvelles de la République des Lettres*, took up the battle against religious orthodoxy and absolutism. In his zeal against the dictates of Catholicism, Bayle was accused of being not just another follower of Calvin, but rather a Socinian. This 16th-century heresy argued that belief could only be demanded when textual claims from the Scriptures survived the test of reason. Given that criterion, little in their view survived. Bayle himself declared that he would reject the Holy Book, Moses, and the Apostles, rather than disbelieve "the clear and definite conclusions" of his intellect. He made it especially clear that this reliance on reason over belief should take precedence in the domain of ethics.

As these refugees of religious absolutism made their way to the countries bordering France, John Locke settled in Holland and sought to avoid the public eye. In exile between 1683 and 1689, Locke steered clear of controversy and devoted himself to his ever-expanding manuscript on the boundaries of human knowledge. First called *De intellectu humano* and then *An Essay Concerning Human Understanding*, this tome went through numerous drafts. Back in 1679, the author had eagerly declared the book to be finished, only to reconsider. In Holland, he substantially revised and expanded his arguments. Finally, in 1688, *An Essay Concerning Human Understanding* appeared; strangely, this central work of the British Enlightenment first was published in an abridged French translation.

The book did not appear in toto until December of 1689, after Locke sailed back across the Channel to a radically altered political landscape. His treatise itself advocated for changes in the traditional views of the soul and proposed new frameworks for metaphysics, medicine, natural philosophy, ethics, and politics. At the center of these changes was a new conception attached to an old term: the mind.

LOCKE WAS NOT the only one trying to synthesize the last decades of debate over the soul and formulate a new framework for inner life. After initially landing in Rotterdam, Locke had moved to Amsterdam, the home of a Jewish lens grinder who had died six years earlier and bequeathed to the world a treatise that almost magically made sense of soul and mind, passion and reason, God and nature. The renegade Baruch Spinoza had been shunned in life; after his death, in his writings, Benedictus de Spinoza would continue to be ostracized, but he could not be ignored.

The son of successful Portuguese Jews who took refuge in Amsterdam, the young Spinoza became captivated by Descartes and the power of geometry, which seemed to possess the power to rewrite the soul and the world. By attempting to do exactly that, Spinoza was expelled from his synagogue in 1656. He gave up the family business, a renunciation made easier by the fact that it was failing. Instead, this determined Cartesian wrote. At the same time, his remarkable talent for optics put him in touch with the great scientists of the time, including Huygens in France and Boyle in London. While making lenses for their viewing devices, Spinoza had hoped to prepare the way for his own masterwork with a preliminary work, an anonymously published natural history of religion, which sought to debunk superstition and argue for secular rule, free inquiry, and toleration. Published in 1670, that work caused such a scandal that Spinoza felt his life was in danger. He completed but held back his grand synthesis, which was only published after his death in 1677.

This daring analysis, simply called *Ethics*, sought to dismantle Cartesian dualism and collapse its distinctions between the supernatural and the natural, thought and substances with extensions, the Cogito and the mechanics of the universe. The soul was natural,

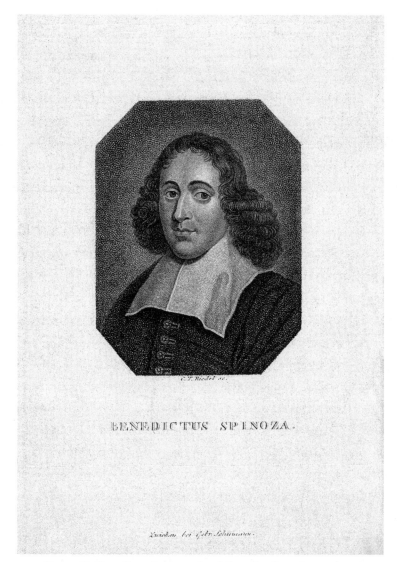

Figure 15. Benedictus Spinoza, the philosopher from Amsterdam.

Spinoza announced, and Nature itself possessed a soul. If God was in Nature, then Nature was animated. Nature could not be divided into thoughts and things, God and matter. For any thought was also a material thing, and any material thing was a thought. The mind *was* a thinking thing but so too was all of the natural world, which was made up of infinite, eternal susbtance.

These formulas made Spinoza's name a swearword for believers, and important reading for radical thinkers. For some, his theory was pagan, another pantheistic heresy, however it was particularly suited to resolve impasses about the soul and the body, thought and the human machine. While dismantling Descartes's central distinctions, Spinoza also proposed an especially compelling model for the roles of passion and reason. "Affects," as he called them, were not qualitatively different from thoughts, but were inadequately known ideas. Reason and passion were not distinctive things, but they presented themselves to consciousness differently. Passions were dim ideas that required clarity for their control. Once understood, affects could be tamed by reason. Understanding could control man's unruly passions. Knowledge became the force for morality as well as spirituality. For if Spinoza was correct, through understanding Nature, one could touch God. The intellect became supremely empowered, for thought could make God's designs apparent.

The foundation of virtue rested on the striving of the mind for understanding; God had nothing to do with it. For Spinoza, God was not a force for human good. Rather, goodness came from acts freely guided by man's reason, and human bondage was the result of our being controlled by blind affects. In this way, Spinoza's ethics did not enter into the tortured debates over how or where the corporeal and the immaterial interacted. He dismissed Descartes's attempt to marry his incorporeal *cogito* to the pineal gland as "a hypothesis more occult than any occult quality of the Scholastics."

Spinoza's writings began to penetrate the British Isles and English debates over the soul in the 1670s. In 1676, Henry More wrote Robert Boyle to report that he had been "informed out of Holland, from a learned hand there, that a considerable company of men appeared there, mere scoffers at religion and atheistical" and one was "Spinosa, a Jew first, then a Cartesian, and now an atheist." Spinoza and Boyle were particularly poised to clash, since the former dismissed belief in the Devil, possession, and miracles, all matters the Englishman cherished. Spinoza's demystifying zeal linked him more to Hobbes, despite their crucial differences. Hobbes considered the passions wild and uncontrollable and thereby rationalized the need for absolute monarchy. Since Spinoza believed reason could control inner urges and freedom of thought ensured morality, he insisted that the most sound political structure was a democratic republic.

While in Holland, Locke likely encountered Spinoza's followers; he had that innovative radical's works in his library. However, John Locke was no Spinoza. Unlike his Dutch counterpart, whose Euclidean notions rose high above the hurly-burly of the everyday, Locke was a man of affairs, a medical clinician, and a political operative, who always seemed to have an eye on the pragmatic effects of his writings. Locke similarly kept his distance from Thomas Hobbes, though the young Locke clearly cribbed from *Leviathan* in his earliest unpublished writings. He cited the much-maligned Englishman rarely and ignored the older man's influence, even when it was blatant. Pierre Gassendi's neo-Epicurean hedonism also influenced Locke, but that too would go mostly unacknowledged. Used to keeping secrets, this spy did not readily give up his sources during this dangerous mission. All his diplomatic skills would be required if he was not to be tarred as an atheist.

On the run, through a landscape dotted with competing divine claims to truth, Locke began to create a natural model for functions generally attributed to the rational soul. In that way, a man's knowledge and understanding could be fully susceptible to rational analysis; one might distinguish claims that were true from those that were false, mark boundaries between supportable fact and belief, and create a new language for the ills of reason and unreason. Like many virtuosi, Locke saw delusion and superstition as the darkest cloud that lingered over humanity. In 1681, he wrote in his journal: "The three great things that govern mankind are reason, passion, and superstition. The first governs a few, the two last share the bulk of mankind and possess them in their turns. But superstition most powerfully produces the greatest mischief."

And so, in the service of analyzing the subjective processes that undermine reason, Locke's *Understanding* contained something shocking. Locke stripped the rational soul of its greatest attributes, forcefully repositioned the faculties of thought, memory, and consciousness into a natural faculty, and thereby hoped to distinguish passion-ruled and superstitious fanatics from rational gentlemen who freely differed about matters that were beyond human understanding.

Not content with Descartes's Cogito or Gassendi's and Willis's partial preservation of the rational soul, Locke sought to create a new vocabulary for the intellect and its world. He adopted his teacher Thomas Willis's notion of thinking matter, in order to effectively contain if not resolve the soul-body problem. When challenged as to how freedom could emerge from an animal-machine, how the greatest of human capacities could be produced by flesh, he happily replied that an omnipotent God made it so. The Lord could "superadd" active forces like thought to matter, should He please. To those who would cry that he had made the immortal soul into a fleshy substance, Locke replied that understanding could not judge whether the soul was material or immaterial. Locke never wavered from his belief in Heaven and Hell. There was an immortal soul, as his religion made clear; however, this superadded thinking thing was not part of the soul, and should be studied through natural philosophy.

Without access to the private daybooks in which Locke explicitly made his logic clear, Gottfried Leibniz read this new philosophy based on matter that could think and concluded that he had stumbled across a new extrapolator of Pierre Gassendi's thought. And through his work in Oxford and the Royal Society, as well as his long stays in France with Gassendi supporters like Gilles de Launay, his studies in Montpellier with the colleagues of Gassendi's physician, Dr. Bernier, and his reading of that physician's collation of Gassendi's work, Locke's anti-Cartesian positions were likely honed by the study of this modern Epicurean. However, the *Essay* was not just a synthesis of preexisting positions. Locke created a new anatomy of inner life, relying heavily on neologisms like "self," a word he concocted, and others with long histories like "idea," "person," and most critically, "mind."

In Old English, *gemynd* and *mynde* first referred to memory alone. During the Elizabethan period, the words were widely employed to denote inner experience. Poets and writers had many a notion in mynd and were of a mynd to act on them. A smattering of phrases employed this meaning—to remind, keep in mind, bear or have in mind, or come to mind. Another connotation also existed. From the earliest days of Chaucer, Englishmen could have another in mind, speak their mind, or set their mind on a task. Thus, personhood might be abstractly associated with this word. William Shakespeare, in one of his famous sonnets, referred to "the marriage of true minds."

A century before Locke, the meanings of this word began to migrate. Having in mind, having to mind, and needing to remind grew to imply the concept of an inner possession, first synonymous with the soul, but gradually different. The Bard anticipated this usage when he refered to the mind as an inner organ: love saw not through the senses, but through the mind's eye. The alchemist and diplomat Sir Edward Dyer composed his poem on the mind as his personal kingdom, man's greatest treasure. And if the mind was a possession, it was something that could also be lost. From at least the 14th century forward, men were said to lose their minds, go out of their minds, or not be in their right minds. Shakespeare wrote of a "mind troubled by deep melancholy" and of futile attempts to "minister to a mind diseased."

However in these cases, the mind was still a working synonym for the rational soul. There was no hint of trespassing on holy ground, no apparent contradiction yet between that mind and the soul. However, along with Thomas Hobbes, Thomas Willis, and Gassendi's expositor Walter Charleton, a few intrepid English thinkers had begun to develop concepts and theories of the mind that tilted away from Platonic and Cartesian souls, and headed toward the dangerous belief in the mind as an object of Nature, a thinking *thing*. In 1645, the Catholic Kenelm Digby, from his exile in Paris, alongside Mersenne and Hobbes, published his *Two Treatises*. Sensation, memory, and imagination were material, the result of matter in motion. Lower forms of reason were also bodily, such as the fox's behavior as it stalked a hen. Digby still considered higher forms of thinking to be in the domain of the immaterial, but anyone who considered his example closely would need to wonder.

Another early expositor who moved toward a natural mind was the English doctor trained in Leiden, Richard Burthogge. He shared many of Locke's political concerns and wrote his 1674 *Organum vetus et novum, or a Discourse of Reason and Truth*, to forward the belief that the mind clothed its sensations with subjective "notions." Anticipating Immanuel Kant, Burthogge concluded that reality itself was not knowable, and claims of absolute knowledge simply demonstrated a diseased mind, one filled with prejudice. Sanity consisted of a freedom from the delusions manifested by philosophical enthusiasts like Paracelsus or theological ones like some Dissenters. Later, Burthogge would propose the Platonic idea that pure mind was God, but the doctor would also argue that in humans the mind was a thing impure, one merged with matter.

These were some of the gestures taken toward the notion of a brain-based mind, one that obeyed the laws of matter and somehow also had active powers to think and will. However, no English writer of great influence had dared to explicitly oppose the mind to the rational soul. Locke did that. He took the sundry meanings of the word "mind" and transformed them into a full theory of a bodily thinking object inside us. He offered a systematic, exahaustive account of the operations of the mind, which now became the theater of subjective experience. In this reworking, the ontological and metaphysical concerns of Descartes's "I think, therefore I am" became transformed. I think and I am, Locke might have said, because I possess a mind. More than anyone before him, John Locke reified the mind, made it a thing.

Ideas populated Locke's mind; they were its natural inhabitants. If the word "idea" had deep roots in Platonic thought, it also had long been commonly used in English as a reference for a notion or conception or image. However, those meanings were not so clear in France, where some of Descartes's followers took the contents of the ethereal Cogito on a supernatural path. Nicolas Malebranche argued that our ideas must exist outside of us to be real. Therefore, they existed in God's mind, and the study of ideas must by necessity be the study of the Lord.

John Locke's *Essay Concerning Human Understanding* opens with a blast in these battles. Against those who believed ideas were deposited in us by the Deity, Locke announced that the mind was an empty tabula rasa at birth. What we know, how we think, and how we process reason and passion all derive from natural sensations and reflection. Abstract, mathematical, and moral ideas were not innate. Faith, justice, God, and reason itself were not given but acquired, as demonstrated by the fact that whole nations differed over those matters. If there were no innate ideas, it followed that the immortal and universal soul of man could not be endowed with . . . well anything mental. Locke wrote:

> I know it is an opinion, that the soul always thinks, and that it
> has the actual perception of ideas in itself constantly, as long as
> it exists; and that actual thinking is as inseparable from the soul
> as actual extension is from the body; which if true, to inquire
> after the beginning of man's ideas is the same as to inquire after
> the beginning of his soul.

However, he argued, we still have our souls while we sleep, don't we? And yet, while asleep, we do not think. The soul existed, but it must be divorced from this newly conceived of object, no longer the same as the soul, but critically different, the fallible and mortal mind.

For Locke, anything that was the object of understanding—pain, inner meditation, and perception—came from ideas. Locke catalogued simple and complex ideas and different modes of thought—sensation, contemplation, and remembrance. In addition, modes of pleasure and pain—passions—were also ideas gained from sensation or reflection. Like Spinoza, Locke rejected the traditional distinction between animal passions and supernatural reason. For him, this ancient battle was now a contest between two different kinds of ideas. In this fight, reason could be relied upon to be the source of the moral truths prescribed by natural law and God.

While reason could rule, Locke's mind was also prone to error, breakage, and decay. If the rational soul was never ill or mistaken, Locke's meaty mind was vulnerable in all these earthly ways. If predecessors ranging from Robert Burton to Thomas Willis to Descartes, blamed cognitive miscues and delusions on the bad influence of bodily passions and humors, following Hobbes, Locke inaugurated the possibility of minds that were fallible not due to other aspects of the body, but to themselves.

An Essay Concerning Human Understanding came out in English at the end of 1689, but Locke could not stop working on it. In letters with correspondents, especially William Molyneux, Locke pushed his conception of the mind further, so that it housed not just the play of ideas, but something whole and stable, something that would stand alongside the soul or the *Cogito*. In the second edition of Locke's work, published in 1694, he added a chapter on identity, the foundations of which were built upon "consciousness."

If the mind was the structure by which we think and have ideas, consciousness was the inner apprehension of that thing. Consciousness made up one's individual identity and self. It linked memories and unified the me from yesterday with the me of tomorrow. The soul did no such thing: at death, it flew from us and could inhabit others. Hence, it could hardly be said to make up individual identity. Consciousness consolidated experiences and actions, so as to give unity to the same person. The "self" was a complex idea attributable to consciousness.

This framework offered new vistas. Instead of possessed souls, one might now consider false ideas, disturbed or fragmented states of consciousness, and troubled or defective selves. Morality, as well, could be considered not a matter for metaphysics, but the natural science of inner life. A madman who was not aware of his own acts, Locke asserted, must be thought of as two people, and could not be justly punished for the acts of his sick self. No longer based on sin, belief, and the state of one's soul, individual identity became a construct predicated on conscious experience in the mind. Hence, the self was continually a work in progress; it could grow, split, falter, take small or large false turns, even disintegrate. Traditional physicians of the soul, under Locke's conception, would need to make room for new diseases. Physicians would be challenged to consider idea-sicknesses and pathologies of self and consciousness that were not the simple result of fevers, vibrations, chemical fires, or humoral imbalances.

Locke himself explored how the mind could spin off into chaos. In the first edition of the *Essay*, he declared that while simple ideas were never wrong, human confusion arose with mixed ideas. Fantastical ideas were based on correct simple ideas passively taken in then combined in a jumbled-up manner, in a way "really never united, never found together in any substance."

Early on as a doctor, Locke had considered madness the result of the false connection of ideas. In 1678, his medical notebooks record his thoughts; "query whether mania be not putting together wrong ideas and so making wrong propositions from them, notwithstanding the reason be right? But madness is a fault in the faculty of reasoning. . . ." Then: "Query whether madness be not the wrong application of mad ideas to things that exist, but are neither having of wrong ideas nor wrong reasoning, and then so that it seems to exist wholly in proposition into simple ideas or syllogisms, as for example made in phantasy him to be either king or candle." And: "Madnesse seems to be noething but a disorder in the imagination, and not in the discursive faculty; for one shall find amongst the distract, those who phansy them selves kings, &c., who discourse and reason right enough upon the suppositions and wrong phansys they have taken."

In the fourth edition of the *Essay,* published in 1700, the one-time doctor would elaborate on these mistaken associations. Madness and the more minor delusions "sprang from the very same root, and depend on the very same cause we are here speaking of. This consideration of the things itself (madness), at a time when I thought not the least on the subject which I am not treating of, suggested it to me." In that 1700 edition, Locke also added his celebrated chapter "Of Association of Ideas," which startlingly acknowledged no predecessors. In his correspondence, this student of Hobbes's writings appeared to be blissfully unaware of his elder's precedent.

While Hobbes saw passion bullying associations into odd tangles, Locke declared that without any excess passion, "in the steady calm course of his life," a man's thought could weave itself into bizarre knots. Calm delusions, not marked by frenzy or furor, were widespread. False education and strange cultures could make whole peoples insane. Once an impression was made on an innocent child, it could structure her moral actions, passions, and reason. When a foolish maid shared the idea of goblins hopping about in the night with a child, such superstitious fears might easily plague her former charge deep into adulthood. Locke turned to his medical experience to hammer home this point. A patient had been "perfectly cured of madness by a very harsh and offensive operation." While deeply grateful for the cure, the man's associations nonetheless made him shudder when he saw the doctor. Such glued-together associations, if learned, could be prevented or perhaps, with difficulty, unlearned. If the mind was made of old experience, it could be fixed by new experiences.

The widespread madness that truly concerned Locke had nothing to do with goblins or melancholics, but rather religious fanatics. In the last section of the second book, he declared that wrong combinations of ideas were often the source of the irreconcilable opposition found between various sects. Nurtured in small subcultures where the same false connections were reinforced, these throught-disordered partisans "applaud themselves as zealous champions for truth." This kind of thought disorder, he wrote tellingly, "is the foundation of the greatest, I had almost said of all the errors of the world; or if it does not reach so far, it is at least the most dangerous one."

In case Locke's meaning remained unclear, in 1700 he affixed a new chapter to the *Essay* entitled "Of Enthusiasm." Based on "ungrounded fancies of a man's own brain," these sick men, some melancholic, others grandiose, "flattered themselves with a persuasion of an immediate intercourse with the Deity." No sane man can set up "fancy for our supreme and sole guide." Rather, he declared, *"Reason must be our last judge and guide in everything."* It must check passions, fancies, and persuasions, including those related to religion.

And so, this son of Puritans redefined what his parents had meant by private conscience. That inner experience of the Lord had expanded to a much broader thing—consciousness—the core of subjectivity or individual selfhood. And that domain was no longer private, spiritual, and therefore unassailable; it could also be mad. Such quiet insanity might not manifest itself openly, but in the privacy of their own chambers, minds easily fell into disorder and became dedicated to delusions. By this analysis, the once-sacrosanct private conscience of Quakers, Levellers, and Diggers was no longer beyond inquiry and reproach. Such claims were now open to a rational anal-

ysis and could become a matter for judges and doctors. For visionaries who flouted the state might be simply mentally ill.

⌒

BEFORE LOCKE, NO one other than the hated Thomas Hobbes and
Baruch Spinoza had dared to give such a systematic and naturalistic
account of the mind as a natural object. And unlike those thinkers, John Locke's mind proved less offensive and more persuasive to
a multitude of believers. A sincerely devout man, Locke laced the
Essay with affirmations of God's presence, the reality of spirits, and
the everlasting soul. Instead of undercutting the rational soul, Locke
amputated much of it, cutting away mental life, while reiterating that
eternity still awaited the good and virtuous.

As Locke completed his masterpiece, political events led to his triumphant return from exile. In 1688, King James II, the openly Catholic monarch, was overthrown by William of Orange and Queen
Mary. A parliamentary democracy was established, and a year later,
a Bill of Rights was enacted. The Glorious Revolution launched
Locke into a pantheon of British heroes: he was the emissary of the
now-vindicated Shaftesbury. After the English publication of his
Essay, John Locke became a figure of national pride. A naturalistic
conception of reason and consciousness, though still controversial,
would ride Locke's fame into English society.

The *Essay* was acclaimed as a work of genius. In 1694, John Aubrey
pronounced this work "the best Booke that was writt by *one* man."
Over the next half-century, the prestige of this treatise grew despite
a storm of opposition. Sermons and popular lectures denounced
Locke and his mind philosophy. Endless arguments ensued over the
nature of matter, the notion of extension, the essence of substance,
the definitions of bodies, volition, the soul's immateriality, as well
as the dangers of atheism, freethinkers, and other heresies. Divines
recognized the threat posed by the crafty Locke: he had breached the

boundaries between science and religion that had been so carefully constructed by Mersenne and Descartes. Mr. Locke bowed down before his God, while he proposed that human reason was natural and based in matter. Unlike Spinoza and Hobbes, however, this was no fire-breathing materialist, but someone more restrained. This diplomat was a vexing opponent, more difficult to demonize.

A series of thinkers tried nonetheless. These included, rather appropriately, more than one of the Robert Boyle Lecturers, who had been chosen to further Christian belief in an honorary forum endowed by the great chemist. In 1705, Samuel Clarke's popular sermon railed mostly against Hobbes and Spinoza, but then added a third to make an unholy trinity. Without going so far as to name the illustrious Locke, he launched the soon-repeated charge that thought superadded to matter was absurd, an act of "Violence on Reason," for it meant the soul was corruptible and could not be immortal. However, Locke's followers could rightly retort that their hero was an agnostic on such issues, and only believed that human understanding could never answer questions regarding the soul's survival of the body.

One anonymous pamphlet concluded that Locke's trickery meant God was just a metaphor, a position that was "in all probability the last great Effort of the Devil against Christianity." Others argued that Locke slipped into absurdity when he gave passive matter an active force like thought, an argument that weakened substantially after the emergence of Isaac Newton's theory of gravitation. Newton's findings were taken to suggest, contra the physicist himself, that the force of attraction resided in matter, which might also therefore contain active processes such as thought. Others rose up to claim Newton's law of inertia meant some immaterial mover was needed to set the universe in motion, and therefore Locke's thinking matter was impossible.

Locke himself engaged in some of these quarrels, but over the next decades he relied on a band of admirers who defended him.

Anthony Collins refused to let Samuel Clarke's charges go unanswered. In their well-publicized debate, Collins took up the Boyle Lecturer's sundry accusations, including the charge that Locke had become an animist who had endowed everything including rocks and trees with thought. Collins replied that Nature contained more or less complex forms of life. Hence, it was quite logical to think that not all matter possessed thought. The brain alone came together in a way that created this new quality.

Mersenne would have rolled over in his grave. For if Collins was correct, the temple of Nature did not require an architect. Without the notion of the sensitive and rational souls, it had become deeply problematic to account for the qualitative shift between the dead and the living, life forms that were still and those that moved, and, finally, unthinking beings and those that could reason. The three-tiered soul once accounted for the emergence of each of these new qualities; each added a new level of complexity. Descartes mechanized the vegetative and sensitive souls, and now Locke and his followers naturalized much of what was left in the rational soul. If matter, with God's help, might organize itself into a higher-order system with utterly new qualities such as the capacity to think and act, then who was to say that matter might not add up to something larger and more creative in the universe, such as God?

Since Locke argued that God could be discovered by reason, *The Spectator*'s Eustace Budgell—who urged fellow Englishmen to consider atheists excellent balls to be shot out of cannons—embraced Locke and counted him among the nation's great protectors of the faith. Pious himself, Locke deftly skirted a number of thorny theological questions and—no doubt for himself as much as his readers—preserved the eternal, God-given soul. At the same time, he insisted on a natural model of inner life that was rule-based and systematic. Borrowing his teacher Thomas Willis's sleight of hand—matter superadded with active thought—he leapt from passive flesh to a mind animated by consciousness and motivated action. While thinking matter raised a flurry of questions, Locke refused to be deterred, leaving the finer points of that assumption to others.

Perhaps the most astute response to Locke came from a French visitor to England, François-Marie Arouet, known after 1718 as Voltaire. For him, the political contrast between Great Britain and nearby France was stark. As individual liberty expanded across the Channel, King Louis tightened his grip, dismissed all notions of religious tolerance, and tamped down on dissent. Voltaire had been forced to flee to this haven, which he grew to love. His *Philosophical Letters*, expanded from his *Letters Concerning the English Nation*, extolled the genius who authored the *Essay*. While Descartes discovered the errors of antiquity, he and his followers only substituted new errors for old ones, Voltaire believed. Locke was different:

> Such a multitude of reasoners having written the romance of the soul, a sage at last arose, who gave, with an air of the greatest modesty, the history of it. Mr. Locke has displayed the human soul, in the same manner as an excellent anatomist explains the springs of the human body.

Voltaire mocked scholastic arguments in which the soul was endowed in the womb with ideas of God, space, and abstract metaphysics. Experiences and sensations were the stuff of the mind. The rest was nonsense. I am a body, he had declared, and I think. Locke's thinking matter was perhaps a contradiction, but it was *our* contradiction.

While the Frenchman's chosen metaphor of the soul—a clock with a spring of unknown materials—did not make him friends among the clergy, Voltaire grasped the essential point. Even if Locke's suggestion was philosophically assailable as nothing more than an oxymoron, all other options were worse. With thinking matter, Locke managed to contain the dichotomies forced upon him by his in-between culture. With decades of debate over the soul behind him, he danced around numerous theological landmines and scientific roadblocks, and in the space made by paradox, freed reason from the soul.

And so, Locke's thinking matter was not mere wordplay. Through this forced union of opposites, first inaugurated by Gassendi, then adopted by Thomas Willis, John Locke united inner experience with the rest of Nature. Unlike Descartes and his followers, Locke bridged thought and nature by insisting on this paradox. Neither Willis nor Gassendi went this far; for them, the rational soul still took over for the highest-level processes. After John Locke, however, it was possible to imagine humans differently. Thinking matter meant that one might bow before God's power, for it was He who superadded thought to flesh, and at the same time employ empirical and experimental tools to understand *all* of inner life.

On this ground, shaky as it might be, Locke built a new city. Brain matter and inner experience jointly presided inside us. Locke called the brain "the mind's presence room." Meanwhile his mind was a shape-shifter: it could be passive machine from one angle and inner agent from another. Filled with working parts—sensation, ideas, associations, reflections—it was rooted in matter, as well as a powerful higher-level function directed by a conscious self. While the machine churned on, Lockean consciousness utilized the power of reason to act. Thanks to the powers of consciousness, man was morally responsible for himself. Hence, it was now possible to imagine a new culture in which self-definition, ethics, knowledge, and political authority could be further divested from theology and souls, and predicated on secular knowledge of conscious selves, beings with minds.

The Sagacious Locke

A FTER HIS TRIUMPHANT return to London, John Locke's
theory of the mind gradually spread, as did his views on the
processes of thought, consciousness, delusion, and the capacity of
reason to control man's passions. Along with Francis Bacon and Isaac
Newton, Locke became synonymous with the progressive advances
of English culture.

Throughout Western Europe, Locke's thought moved quickly
throughout literary and philosophical circles, where its political
implications were not missed. A swarm of French refugees, often
trained in Protestant seminaries to reject divine right and employ
private conscience, embraced Locke's model of consciousness with its
justification of inner difference. The French Huguenot exile Pierre
Coste became Locke's interpreter and French translator, and through
Coste's efforts the *Essay* spread throughout the continent.

Locke's theories of the mind would become part of the curricula of universities, often finding a home among those who taught
and studied logic. It also would be enshrined in those warehouses
of learning, the Enlightenment dictionary and encyclopedia. In his
seminal *Historical and Critical Dictionary*, the exiled Huguenot Pierre
Bayle traced a line of thought from Thomas Willis's animal soul to
Locke's thinking matter to an anonymous freethinker who consid-

ered humans to be no different than brutes. The 1747 *Biographia bri-tannica* lavished seventeen pages of small type on the "celebrated" philosopher's life and thought. Denis Diderot and Jean d'Alembert in their great *Encyclopedia* included a lengthy section on Locke, as did Johann Zedler's German *Universal-Lexicon*. And in his famed *Dictionary*, Samuel Johnson turned to Locke's authority 138 times. Johnson's definition of madness as a disorderly jumble of ideas neatly followed Locke's.

As this naturalized notion of the mind began to spread, some sought to push aside the paradoxes of God-given thinking matter and map out a fully natural model. In 1729, Ephraim Chambers's *Cyclopaedia* defined psychology as "a Discourse Concerning the Soul" which was not a part of theology, but anthropology. In 1740, the Scotsman George Turnbull announced that he would study the human mind precisely as he studied the human body. When the *Encyclopaedia Britannica* emerged from Edinburgh, though it defined the mind as akin to spirit, the opposite of matter, it also allowed that the mind was now explored in the science of logic and morals, natu-ralistic inquiries that owed much to Locke.

The spread of Locke's notions on the mind was greatly aided by his general celebrity. To many in England, he was a political hero. Magazines like *The Spectator* and *The Tatler*, created in the first years of the 18th century for an educated, middle-class audience, frequently referred to this great man as well as his model of reason. So assumed was it that a gentleman should have read Locke, that *The Spectator* found it amusing to contemplate the hilarity of men in the kitchen making cheesecakes, and ladies in the parlor reading Locke. In 1712, Joseph Addison assumed his readers were acquainted with the "great modern discovery, which is at present universally acknowledged by all the inquirers into natural philosophy" regarding the ideational nature of perception. For those shamefully in the dark, he cited chap-ter and verse from the *Essay*.

As Locke's philosophy began to be assumed knowledge for the literate, his name and notions would be dropped in essays and poems. Christopher Smart's poem "The Furniture of a Beau's Mind" poked fun at the empty-headed lover, who resembled a Lockean child:

> *When infants are born, by experience we find,*
> *   With ideas so few they're supply'd,*
> *That Locke has most justly resembled their mind,*
> *   To a cabinet empty and void.*

Among coffeehouse chatterers and those men and women of leisure, Locke's theory would encourage interest in the minute, the private, and the fleeting, the most ephemeral moments of an individual's consciousness. For according to John Locke, we become these experiences; they populate us and fill an inner void. Hence, Locke contributed to the explosive growth of autobiography. While precocious examples of the written examination of inner life predate this period—consider St. Augustine's spiritual awakening in the *Confessions*, Renaissance writings like Benvenuto Cellini's *Autobiography*, and the essays of Michel de Montaigne—this form of self-scrutiny truly emerged as a robust English tradition after 1650 and especially took off in the later part of that century.

The earliest of these 17th-century autobiographies often fell into two genres: a legalistic brief based on complaints of being wronged or victimized, or come-to-Jesus spiritual conversions. The later narratives centered on God and the dramatic action took place around the soul's private state of crisis and eventual rebirth. Examples include works authored by Dissenters such as John Bunyan in his 1666 *Grace Abounding to the Chief of Sinners* and by Quakers like George Fox. Often, when the spirit of the Lord spoke to a man, he wrote it down. In 1648, Gerrard Winstanley, one of the legendary Diggers, went further and proclaimed that all of biblical history existed within:

therefore every man's story included that of fallen Adam, Cain, and Moses all the way to the savior Christ. He urged his fellow men to discover this by taking an inward journey.

Before Locke, few of these accounts took up the classical demands of narrative in which the self must rationally weigh dilemmas and sort out its fate. One precocious exception was by Margaret Cavendish of Newcastle, the second wife of Hobbes's patron. In 1656, this poet and natural philosopher published *A True Relation of My Birth, Breeding, and Life*, a work that prefigured Rousseau's *Confessions*. Cavendish's self-portrait included a searching meditation on her crippling fear of social groups and her extreme bashfulness. It was a brave attempt to burrow into her inner world and make sense of her differences, qualities that made her individual.

Locke's sensationalism encouraged reflection on the inner world as it was constructed through bits of daily experience. And so, side by side with these older narratives, there began to be a number of detailed, everyday stories of a person's feelings and thoughts. Early autobiographers mixed the emergence of sin and reborn faith with the rise of worldly knowledge. For example, Samuel Johnson's journals contained meticulous records of his gross sluggishness, dissipation, excess, and negligence. He noted his idleness and pressing need to approach the Lord with a clean heart, not today but tomorrow. His list of resolutions included worshiping more diligently and keeping a journal.

The most famed practitioner of quotidian self-scrutiny was Samuel Pepys. If the London functionary and member of the Royal Society conducted no laboratory experiments, he may be said to have conducted a running dissection of his own mind. Pepys catalogued the events of his day as they impacted his thoughts and feelings; without blushing, he recorded the socially shocking alongside the conventional. As an elaborate record of his misdeeds grew, he increasingly became concerned with the state of his soul. His many illicit amours would be attended by the hopeful phrase "may God

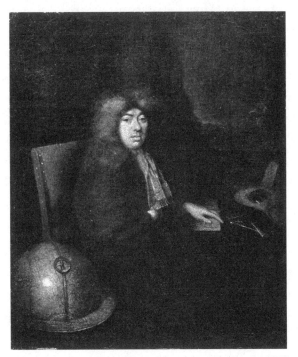

Figure 16. Samuel Pepys began his celebrated diary in 1660.

forgive me." While God might be so generous, Pepys's chronicle cast him as everyman, struggling under the sway of his gluttonous desires. There was no redemption in this story, no renunciation, only moments of pained self-recognition and an attempt to give coherence and meaning to the frayed strands of sensation and reflection that made up his days.

Pepys's writings came before a flood of English autobiographies. Men and women like the young James Boswell kept, and sometimes published, revealing records, attempts to find meaning in more secular lives not so tightly bound to religious narratives. In addition, writers like Daniel Defoe, Henry Fielding, Samuel Richardson, and the doctor-turned-Grub-Street-hack Tobias Smollett, took to the novel to trace the formation of character, not through Christian allegory, but through the shifting impact of secular life and social environment. These two forms of self-exploration, memoir and fiction, merged at times as in Defoe's masterful 1719 fictional autobiography, *Robinson Crusoe.*

By 1751, Samuel Johnson could write that England was passing through the Age of Authors, as men and women delved into the birth and growth of their own consciousness. By that time, Lockean verities were so widespread that they had become ripe for parody. In his farcical masterpiece *The Life and Opinions of Tristam Shandy,* Laurence Sterne's hero related the sad story of his conception, a most unfortunate event in which his mother at the moment of sexual climax asked his father whether he had forgotten to wind the clock. From this "unhappy association of ideas which have no connection in nature," his mother could never again hear a clock wound up without "thinking of something else," and vice versa. It was a little bit of madness, the author agreed, a strange mix of ideas that "the sagacious Locke, who certainly understood the nature of these things better than most men, affirms to have produced more wry actions than all other sources of prejudice whatsoever."

DURING THE FIRST decades of the 18th century, England built new legal and political structures. After 1688, when William of Orange took the throne, absolute monarchy died. With Anglicans and Dissenters mingling with Papists and Deists, a period of openness ensued in which rules for social and political conduct were in play. The demise of the Licensing Act, which had established laws of censorship in 1643, led to an explosion of publications and robust debates in print, as Grub Street became synonymous with a battalion of writers who churned out tabloids and pamphlets. Ever-expanding London became the central stage for debates over the emergence of a new kind of culture and a new kind of morality, one that placed more emphasis on reason and individual rights, and less on the fate of one's soul.

The growing force of secular reason rattled the robed men behind their altars as well as those on their thrones. In every state save for England, the Netherlands, and Poland, princes and monarchs ruled, secure in the belief that they were divinely licensed to do so. It had once been a crime in England to argue against the divine source of royal authority, for if this power was stripped of its supernatural source and seen to stem from earthly reason alone, then these rulers would be naked. And John Locke knew it. A year after the Glorious Revolution, he released a series of essays that sought to finish off the old order.

Locke's *Two Treatises of Government* appeared in December of 1689. It began with a full-throated refutation of the hereditary, divine right of kings, and a scathing dismissal of Scriptural justifications for such power, such as claims by kings to be descended from Adam. The second essay outlined a civil society in which all men were created equal. This cohered with Locke's theory of selfhood and the mind. What could all those blank slates be but equal at birth? Nearly simultaneously, he sent out his letter on toleration, that divisive subject that had long simmered in Western religious and legal circles. Hiding behind anonymity, Locke argued that civil interests included life, liberty, health, and possessions, but not the salvation of souls. Since belief emerged from the full persuasion of the mind, error could be challenged by reason only. Force was useless. Dissenters, Locke proposed, should be treated like odd fellows who did their hair up in a silly manner.

This too followed from Locke's psychology. In an absolute world where the soul was saved or damned, it made sense to torture the possessed so as to rid them of evil, then convert and save their souls. However, if reason was in charge, with its quirky faults and little delusions, such absolute authority over others had no basis. Locke, who once denounced the Quakers as mad, now insisted state policy toward such religious dissidents be one of acceptance. The care of the soul should be left to "every man's self," he wrote. This little phrase signaled a stunning reversal: for over a millennium, the soul was the guardian of the self. Locke now would have the thinking and judging self be responsible for the soul.

Locke's *Letter Concerning Toleration* engendered scalding rebuttals. Jonas Proast, an Anglican clergyman, was incensed. Reason, he reminded his readers, could not alone battle Satan. Since the Church of England possessed the Truth, its members should not tolerate all the misguided and dangerous works of the Great Deceiver. Under the pseudonym "Philanthropus," Locke quickly published a rejoinder: since absolute truth in Rome differed from absolute truth in Geneva, which differed from absolute truth in London, magistrates of all three places should get their noses out of such matters. They could secure the state by generally protecting individual rights and restraining those who were deemed to be mad.

Proast was falling out of step with the times. Decades of murderous religious warfare had done their work. So too had Baconian natural philosophy and the broad effect of skepticism toward the claims of scholastics. For nearly half a century, natural philosophers had been turning away from those old dogmas. And that meant that political and legal power would have to change shape as well. Absolute knowledge meant absolute power. Truth from supernaturally empowered monarchs and clerics compelled action and brooked no dissent.

However, if the monarch was but a man, then reason was his sole source of authority. And after John Locke, the mind that furnished a leader with intellect was often seen as filled with potential error, wrong conclusions, even cracked delusions. If the mind could so easily wander off, then it could not command unquestioning obedience from others.

In England over the late 17th century, a number of thinkers began to separate different kinds of knowledge claims and the kinds of certainty they commanded. If God's knowledge was absolute and infallible, man's was neither. By 1700, a consensus emerged in

England regarding the hierarchy of human knowledge. Mathematical proofs and some metaphysical logic held universal truths that must be accepted by all reasonable gentlemen, while sensory observation and introspection offered perhaps a modicum of certainty that generally left room for error and debate. History, religious belief, and conclusions from everyday life were close to sheer opinion; this knowledge was at best probable and could not compel assent from others.

In this shifting landscape, years of attempts to increase toleration for religious difference were increasingly successful. The Toleration Act of 1689 suspended penalties against Nonconformists, though it did not mention Catholics, Deists, or non-Christians. Over the next twenty years, over 2,500 places of public worship for Nonconformists sprang up. Joseph Addison in *The Spectator* was delighted to espouse Locke's notion that God was a complex Idea, which of course meant it would be necessarily different for varied people. Religious truth became a matter of different possible truths. Fallible minds armed with probable knowledge would necessarily need to accept disagreement. Of course, there were limits to such tolerance. For Locke, the line was clear. Enthusiasts and maniacs were not just of another opinion. Any religious group that espoused the eating of babies, for example, would be prosecuted. Any that reached such a "degree of madness" as to push for attacks on the foundations of society would also be intolerable.

As the eternal soul ceded more ground to the fallible mind, conceptions of everyday morality also began to shift. Before 1700, moral philosophy was simply a branch of theology, but increasingly that was no longer so. While French Cartesians living under their absolute monarch rejected the naturalization of reason, in England morality began to be thought of as a more mundane affair, a conflict between passion and reason in which the Prime Mover moved nothing. Like Democritus, the Epicureans, Hobbes, and Gassendi, Locke believed the dynamics of pleasure and pain motivated humankind. But he also followed Plato's insistence that reason could still rule supreme. By taking this stand, Locke and his followers faced quandaries about how a loom of ideas could actively choose, want, or desire. At one point, Locke considered adding another component to his theory of the mind to reinforce reason and give it power: the will. But Locke remained suspicious of the scholastic tendency to explain phenomena by inventing new faculties. He dismissed this strategy and followed Hobbes, pointing out that the very term "free will" was oxymoronic. By definition, will was *unfree*; it was what made the blood pulse.

While motivated by their own desire, humans gradually learned which impulses must be resisted. In this way, they found freedom. Liberty came from the mind's capacity to consider its urges and then freely choose how to act. Those who believed freedom meant orgiastic license lived in a misbegotten world where "madmen and fools are the only freemen." Only the blind hedonist embraced intense moments of pleasure that resulted in long-standing remorse and pain, and only the cowardly refused to accept some pain now for long-lasting happiness. The ethics of pleasure-seeking were not the same as childish desire, and stemmed not from godly devotion and sanctity, but rather from a capacity to choose that which secured one's sanity.

Could the social order stand on such a rickety foundation? Many shuddered at the thought. However, in placing so much weight on the power of reason to manage and guide our desires, Locke was not alone. The emergence of ethics predicated on the workings of reason mirrored the rise of rational religion among freethinkers who sought to silence enthusiasm's loud party. Called Deists, they insisted God's works could be known by logic and inquiry. No priest, rabbi, or pastor was required. No dogmas, creeds, or rituals, either. True understanding emerged from the discovery of immanent principles in Nature, which were the inscription of God's moral law. Early forms of Deism relied on "right reason" to unveil God's moral order. For many, Isaac Newton's laws of universal order were crowning achievements of this movement.

John Locke didn't quite fit the Deist mold, for he fully believed in miracles and biblical revelation. Furthermore, while Deists argued that the rational soul with its heavenly heritage could unveil God's work, Locke's mind had no such power. Worse, his rejection of innate ideas actually undermined Deism. For if the mind was a net of imperfect associations, prone to prejudice, superstition, and delusion, then it was hardly dominated by a universally endowed right reason, but rather pedestrian, often wrong, reason. Nonetheless, Locke's ethics echoed some Deist views and attracted its advocates, since he also believed God's desire was encoded in His design and could be found in natural law.

Among the most prominent of Deists was the Irishman John Toland. In 1696, he penned his *Christianity Not Mysterious*, a book deeply indebted to Locke's *Essay on Human Understanding*. Reason, though deeply vulnerable to deception, was still the only grounds for certitude. Matters of faith should always be rational. Even biblical commandments must stand up to logic before becoming law. Hauled before a grand jury, Toland became notorious. Shunned as a pariah, he ended up homeless and destitute. Thirty years later, incensed believers, still bitter, assaulted his idea that God was an analogy.

In 1707, Locke's pupil Anthony Collins dared to publish *An Essay Concerning the Use of Reason*, which denied religious mysteries and revelations, and argued that all morality rested on logic. Another Lockean, John Trenchard, used the master to debunk superstitions, noting how easily the mind could be fooled to worship shadows and clouds as gods. The deistic Matthew Tindal wielded Locke like a whip to demand that reason test all Christian beliefs.

These freethinkers were members of a tiny vanguard. During the early 18th century, British Deists were routinely chased down and prosecuted. Their books were dumped in bonfires. In French and Dutch periodicals, scandalized opponents breathlessly covered these developments, quick to denounce atheists and materialists. An "impious Sadducee who denies any immaterial substance," snarled one journal, as it announced Locke's death. Even Pierre Bayle, in his influential *Dictionary*, worried about the perilous implications of Locke's thought, merely one step away from turning men and women into beasts.

However, decades of bitter warfare in which the absolute moral claims of Catholicism crossed swords with the absolute moral claims of Protestants, led a growing number of European thinkers to conclude this: either God was on everybody's side or He was on no one's. Disgusted by the waste of human life, a stream of dissidents dared to consider heretical alternatives like Deism. And a few went even further. After Louis XIV revoked the Edict of Nantes and the rights of Huguenots in 1685, a disgusted Pierre Bayle dared to ask an almost unthinkable question: could a society be moral *without* religion? Could a society of atheists be safely governed by reason alone? From his exile in the Netherlands, Bayle brazenly answered yes. With Locke as their guide, others now considered a path in which the "thou shalt nots" of an individual's conscience could be transformed into rational operations guided by the mind.

LOCKE BELIEVED ETHICS were the "proper Science and Business of Mankind in general." His theory of the mind underwrote a form of secular morality that he believed could ensure virtue, as well as public safety and order. In his last years, this venerated figure searched for ways to ensure the growth of a more tolerant, liberal society. In 1693, he published a book on education that claimed parents, not God or the church, created the inner regulations of reward and punishment that resulted in reason, conscience, and good or bad character. Conscience, Locke contended, was the residue of parental instruction, not matters of the soul. This parenting book went through twenty-five English and sixteen French editions by 1800.

At his death, Locke also left behind *Of the Conduct of the Understanding*, a work that promoted skepticism as a new ideal of mental health, one that did not get ensnared in that "disease of the mind as hard to be cured as any," delusion. Madness settled in when "sandy and loose foundations become infallible principles" and became reinforced by habit. The cure for false beliefs was not more indoctrination of a contrary type, but rather the fostering of mental liberty. Children must be encouraged to question themselves, down to the roots of their own thought, a capacity often squashed by overbearing teachers. Those who possessed this reflective ability corrected the fallacies and fantastic constructs of their minds by themselves.

Moral conduct depended on such self-scrutiny in which the mind exerted mastery over itself. Of course, a man might also lose his head; passions might take control. Love, anger, grief, or fear all had the power to enchant, confuse, and provoke a "perfect madness." Reason could also create delusion, by rushing off like a river, never pausing to consider its course. Finally, Locke spoke of spontaneous, bizarre experiences like hallucinations. All three of these were threats to one's sanity and in large groups could imperil the moral order.

And so, morality and sanity both were rooted in mental freedom. In a heterodox world, the soul with its verities must yield to an autonomous, reflective self whose capacity to question, consider, and judge became the surest bulwark for a stable and just society. After centuries of absolutism, this claim struck many as bizarre. Virtue was dependent on self-questioning? The Anglican cleric and geologist Thomas Burnet was alarmed by the absence of any universal morality in Locke. But the Englishman refused to budge; education was the best we could do to create moral men. The payoff from this seemingly flimsy model was immense: no universal moral code meant no wars over absolute moral claims. Rome and Geneva and London each could have their own moral codes, as could natives of the New World, Asia, and Africa.

Still a number of Locke's followers were discomforted by this ethical relativism. They dreamed of securing Locke's theories by transforming them into universal laws, not unlike the law of gravity. However, these attempts to follow Newton faced problems, one of which was the howls of protest from Sir Isaac himself.

In 1693, Locke received an enraged letter from Britain's genius. It had been six years since Newton published his masterpiece, *Philosophiae naturalis principia Mathematica*, which demolished what remained of Aristotelian teleology and codified mechanistic science for the coming century. Newton and Locke were acquaintances, but long ago the physicist had demurred when asked to venture into Dr. Locke's domain, saying discussions on the soul and mind were "too hard a knot for me to untie." "I can calculate the motion of Heavenly Bodies," Newton had added, "but not the madness of people."

After reading Locke's *Essay Concerning Human Understanding*, however, Newton became furious. He accused Locke of destroying morality, being an atheist, and trying to embroil the mathematician in unseemingly sexual affairs. The last accusation was a tip-off that all was not well. Later, Newton apologized: "I beg your pardon . . . for representing that you struck at the root of morality in a principle you laid down in your book of Ideas. . . . I took you for a Hobbist." Locke pressed Newton to further explain his strange and harsh censure. On October 15, 1693, the man who possessed perhaps the greatest mind of his age revealed that he had fallen victim to a mad delirium, and could not recall a single word of his own outburst.

Likely poisoned by alchemical experiments, Newton recovered his senses but did not change his view of Locke's *Essay*. And this was not merely one dissenting voice. As honor surrounded him, Newton assumed the leadership of the Royal Society, where he exerted great influence over its agendas and exercised a good deal of vindictiveness toward his enemies. In these latter years, Sir Isaac dedicated himself to prophetic treatises and esoteric theological study, in which he would beat back the notion of materialism and fill the mechanical world with spirits of absolute morality and divine reason. There was no place for Locke's mind in that.

And so as Locke's psychology spread through the corridors of culture, most early modern natural philosophers like Newton refused to accept thinking matter, or a society dislocated from its religious commitments. And why should they? The kinds of evidence offered in Locke's *Essay* were not experimental proofs or mathematical calculations. For the natural philosophers, logic could not compel assent. Demands to know the mind by ocular observation and experiment created an impasse, since the mind, though immediately knowable to itself, remained hidden to others. As Locke and his followers sought to establish a natural philosophy for inner life, they would find themselves cast out from the Church and denied entry into science.

A century after his death, Mersenne's words were still mouthed by others. The Scottish Presbyterian clergyman Andrew Baxter, wrote that mechanics required the presence of a Prime Mover. Were Locke and his supporters ready to believe that the spontaneous movement of an elephant was but the "dull and dead" earth? "Our Moderns forget," he wrote, "that he who believes that dead matter can produce the effects of life and reason, is . . . credulous."

There seemed to be no way to adjudicate the disagreements between these new disputants, the soul and the mind. Locke's *Essay* fell between the borders of mechanistic science and theology. However, unlike the work of Spinoza or Hobbes, Locke's writings took root in that no-man's-land. While undermining the rational soul, Locke's mind made room for belief. And if Locke's mind could not be proven in equations or experiments before the Royal Society, nor could it be falsified. A naturalistic conception that seemed to make sense of aspects of inner experience neatly mirrored scientific theories of knowledge. The inductive and empirical method required a mind that constructed its understanding of the world based on sensation and experience. According to Locke, Bacon's rules were simply natural to the mind. Other perspectives became wrongheaded.

THE MOST POWERFUL rejoinder to Locke's moral relativism did not come from horrified representatives of the Church or Royal Society stalwarts. Rather embarrassingly, his most vitriolic critic was a gentleman who knew Locke's pedagogy better than anyone alive. Delivered into this world by John Locke, Anthony Ashley Cooper, who would become the third Earl of Shaftesbury, was educated for the first eleven years of life by his grandfather's trusted physician, since his own father was deemed mentally unfit. Locke had been given dominion over the boy's family: he had chosen Shaftesbury's mother for his father and had absolute control over the education of the seven progeny that resulted from this union. Anthony, the least robust of the children, grew deeply attached to his tutor and referred to him as his foster father. Ultimately, however, this student would pay his teacher back with bitterness and ridicule. Mr. John Locke, he declared for the world to know, was a prig whose rejection of universal morality was absurd.

As Cooper revealed, being raised as a tabula rasa, a Lockean child, whose every experience might alter his identity, was intolerable. As he sailed off to Europe, the young man wrote to Locke and confessed that he needed to make the greatest efforts to be an honest man and a friend. Later, he would conclude that thinking of his own goodness in such contingent terms only fostered intense anxiety. It made it seem as if one "prostituted thy self and committed thy Mind to Chance and the next comer . . . as if there were nothing that rul'd within, and had the least control."

That conclusion, however, only dawned on Cooper after years of discomfort and dislocation. In 1689 with the Glorious Revolution, Anthony, now the grandson of a national hero, returned home to take up politics. It didn't suit him. Asthma and bad health prompted him to abandon London's foul air for the Netherlands, where he surrounded himself with Locke's enlightened friends like Pierre Coste and Jean Le Clerc, and turned his energies to writing. In 1708, Shaftesbury published his "Letter Concerning Enthusiasm." Like Locke, he argued that hostile and punitive responses to crazed Dissenters only worsened their madness. The surest antidote for such fanaticism was satire, raillery, and laughter. Zealots should be ceaselessly lampooned, as should their grim, melancholic adversaries, a bit of advice that delighted and inspired Jonathan Swift.

In 1704, Locke died, and a few years after his death, Shaftesbury began to privately voice skepticism regarding the philosophy that his tutor espoused. "'Twas Mr. Lock that struck at all Fundamentals, threw all Order and Virtue out of the World, and made the Very Ideas of these . . . unnatural and without foundation in our Minds," he wrote on June 3, 1709. In 1711, he published *Characteristics of Men, Manners, Opinions, Times,* which argued that humans possessed a universal, inborn ethical core, one not based on any theology. God was not necessary for ethics, since priests could be terrorists and heretics might be loving and Christ-like. Wise men of different cultures differed in their gods, yet many found the same path to goodness.

Therefore, humanity did not require any creed or any particular form of education to be ethical. Morality was everywhere. Just as we recognize beauty without being schooled in aesthetics, women and men have no trouble distinguishing virtue from vice for a natural moral sense resides in all. These moral antennae were as intrinsic to human beings as eyes and ears. And while others considered the control of the passions a key to moral behavior, Shaftesbury reversed things. Thanks to our inner moral sensor, virtuous acts feel good, and vice makes us pained. Hobbes was wrong: we don't cynically categorize everything we like as good, but rather instinctively recognize what is moral and naturally like it.

This new spin on a secular theory of ethics shared Locke's emphasis on tolerance. Pleasure from virtue and pain from vice was not a matter for Christians, Jews, or Muslims. A universal conscience, possessed by all, established harmony between the self and society, whether one was a priest, a heathen, or an animist. Amused skeptics congratulated Shaftesbury for his great discovery: humans had a "moral nose"! They wondered how this astonishing protuberance had been ignored for so long. Others rolled their eyes and reminded their readers that according to Shaftesbury, we lived in a blissfully good, kind, and peaceful world. Cooper's celebration of universal moral goodness was echoed by the poet Alexander Pope:

> *All Nature is but Art, unknown to thee;*
> *All Chance, Direction, which thou canst not see;*
> *All Discord, Harmony not understood;*
> *All partial Evil, universal Good:*
> *And spite of Pride, in erring Reason's spite,*
> *One truth is clear, WHATEVER IS, IS RIGHT."*

Decades later, Voltaire in *Candide, or The Optimist* lampooned such views through the character of Dr. Pangloss, who after each rape or disembowelment, proclaimed this to be the most perfect of all possible worlds.

In this growing debate over the nature of morality, another voice rose up to scoff at such optimism. A Dutch émigré to England, Dr. Bernard de Mandeville agreed that ethics could not be taught. That was because what pedagogues like John Locke called virtue was actually vice. Born in 1670, Mandeville studied medicine in Leiden and developed a practice that first focused on hysteria and hypochondriasis. He traveled to London and took to writing fables, following Jean de La Fontaine. In 1705, he published *The Grumbling Hive, or Knaves Turned Honest*, a twenty-six-page poem that garnered little notice. In 1711, Mandeville's *Treatise of the Hypochondriack and Hysterick Passions* included a scathing indictment of his own profession, which previewed his views on morality. Doctors? They were hypocrites whose high-minded ideals hid a covetousness lust for money and vanity. Galen? A liar, who must have known his remedies did nothing. Thomas Willis made up discoveries to win fame. Speculation in medicine was nothing more than a ruse.

Shaftesbury's ethics exasperated Dr. Mandeville. And so he expanded and republished his poem and gave it a more provocative title: *The Fable of the Bees; or, Private Vices, Publick Benefits*. There was no inborn moral sense. In fact, what do-gooders called virtue and vice were like wine in the morning and breakfast at night, all upside down.

This theme of moral insincerity and hypocrisy was of course not new. On the Elizabethan stage, for example, portrayals of scoundrels who wrapped themselves in high-minded ideals were commonplace. Mandeville himself took inspiration from a different source: a group of 17th-century French satirists who had upended Christian and Stoical adages of "la Morale." At the center of this circle of writers was an aristocratic Royalist, François de La Rochefoucauld, who in the 1660s began to toss out amusing aphorisms that mocked his society's ethical dictums as screens for vanity and *amour-propre*. Stoical claims for superhuman self-restraint were just lies. Passionate self-love lurked beneath saintly acts of sacrifice. "Our virtues are, most often," he wrote, "only vices in disguise." French readers swarmed to La Rochefoucauld's delicious turns of phrase, and some took up their own pens, such as Marin Cureau de La Chambre and Jean de La Bruyère.

With them, Mandeville concluded that Christian culture labeled self-interest as immoral, when it was in fact unavoidable and necessary. Therefore, the most upstanding men and women of a community were mostly pretentious frauds. But there was hope. While many honestly tried to resist their selfish passions, most failed. And that was a good thing. If too many succeeded, it would result in catastrophe for the community. For the "vice" of selfishness was critical to the maintenance of the hive. Without it, no society would survive. Mandeville's paradox was that public well-being came about indirectly from private selfishness. Greed was good.

Reason, Mandeville also assumed, was acquired as per "Mr. Lock"; the child was a carte blanche that was filled with ideas. However, this doctor had a less hopeful view of education: it taught children to conceal their passions, not conquer them. It fed them shame and falsehoods. Higher morals were elaborate fictions used to control others, for without self-love, humans would be suicidal. As for the soul's immortality, that was a farce that simply flattered the species.

In 1723, Dr. Mandeville added a new attack onto his *Fable.* It focused on a certain deluded "Noble Writer." Only a gentleman born into luxury and indolence and educated "under a great Philosopher, a mild and good-natured as well as able tutor," only such a

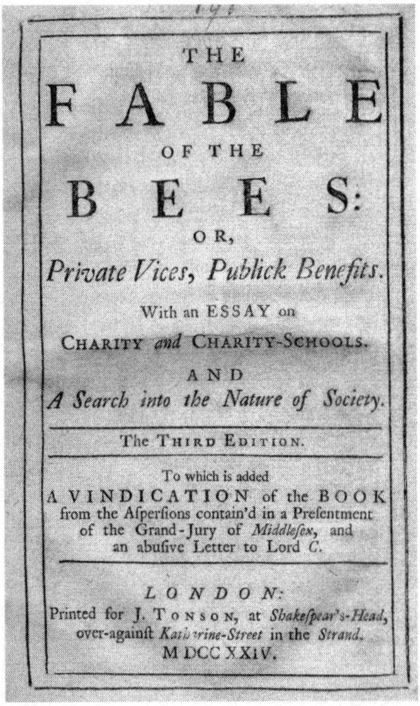

THE

FABLE

OF THE

BEES:

OR,

Private Vices, Publick Benefits.

With an ESSAY on

CHARITY *and* CHARITY-SCHOOLS.

AND

A Search into the Nature of Society.

The THIRD EDITION.

To which is added

A VINDICATION of the BOOK from the Afperfions contain'd in a Prefentment of the Grand-Jury of *Middlefex*, and an abufive Letter to Lord *C.*

LONDON:

Printed for J. TONSON, at *Shakefpear's-Head*, over-againft *Katharine-Street* in the *Strand.* MDCCXXIV.

Figure 17. Bernard de Mandeville claimed that Christian vices were often natural and healthy.

fool might be tricked into believing in universal goodness. For those who could not see through the thin veil, the index at the end of the poem explicitly referenced "Shaftesbury." There, the indexer acidly defined him as an optimistic believer in Goodness who was "refuted by his own Character."

In England, Mandeville provoked outrage. Twice summoned before judge and jury, he did not shrink from denouncing philanthropic activites such as the supposedly opulent conditions wasted on the poor in hospitals. He rejected schooling and other forms of aid for the impoverished.

And so, in addition to the older models of Thomas Hobbes and John Locke, Shaftesbury and Mandeville constructed their own brands of secular ethics. If morality once referred to religious rules of conduct, in England by 1730, this assumption was increasingly challenged by competing theories based on man's relationship not to God, but rather to Nature. These views varied from asserting man's innate righteousness to his inborn selfishness. In 1743, a professor named David Fordyce articulated this new approach: "*Moral philosophy* has this in common with *Natural philosophy*, that it appeals to *Nature* or *Fact*; depends on Observation, and Builds its Reasonings on plain uncontroverted Experiments, or upon the fullest Induction of Particulars of which the Subject will admit." A modern mind and self had begun to vie for prominence with traditional notions of the soul as the new foundation for ethics, behavior, and social life. However, as the debates between Locke, Shaftesbury, and Mandeville demonstrated, the conclusions varied so far and wide as to call the whole endeavor into doubt.

AT THE HEART of the debates over secular ethics was a problem Shaftesbury knew well. Locke had made the mind radically contingent. If every impression and experience could twist a man

toward insanity or evil, then every moment, every day, was filled
with uncertainty and dread, for events and environments molded
humans like clay. Shaftesbury and Mandeville both disputed this,
arguing for inborn forces that rooted human identity in something
transhistorical. Shaftesbury mocked Lockists who required "schools
of Venus" to teach lovers to do what they did, and assumed in
some sober nation that the race of man might otherwise perish.
Over the next centuries, some would line up for the forces of the
environment and "Nurture" in the creation of human interiority,
while others would take the side of inborn essences, instincts, and
"Nature." Did goodness stem from caring and hospitable surroundings, or was it inherent? The personal and political implications of
each view would be vast.

As fascination with English progressive thought swept Europe,
the competing secular proposals for morality and the mind filtered
into an underground network of pamphleteers, freethinkers, lapsed
abbés, natural philosophers, Huguenots, Quakers, and French *philosophes*. For by 1700, among those who dared to know, it was obvious
that the jumble of absolute God-given truths in Christendom could
not *all* be true. More thinkers began to share the goal expressed by
philosophers like Hobbes and Locke: moral life, human conduct, and
political order could not securely rest on belief and claims of divine
knowledge.

While the English were enshrining individual liberties in a Bill
of Rights, the publication of works by John Locke and Isaac Newton made it clear that whole new vistas now existed in the British
Isles. Visitors began to come from Italy, Switzerland, and France,
for it seemed that in merry England, Descartes's theory of planetary
motion and his theory of the soul had been simultaneously exploded.
Foreigners returned home and then spread the word, but there was
an impediment. Few on the Continent read English. This was especially problematic for Locke's achievement, a good deal of which
came through the creation of a new working vocabulary distinct

from the discourses on the soul. Even worse, many of his terms had no obvious equivalent in translation.

Most centrally, there was no French or German cognate for "mind." And so, Locke's theory crossed linguistic borders in disguise: his mind was translated into words that meant "spirit" or "soul." "Consciousness" presented another headache for Locke's translators. Of course, these ambiguities could be a tactical strength. While Spinoza and Hobbes were vigorously condemned across Europe, Locke's mind, filled with consciousness, did not elicit the same response. In French and German, his bold proposals were couched in familiar words—conscience, spirit, and soul—that created confusion which proved useful when confronted by censors and defenders of the faith.

And so, while natural philosophers at the English Royal Society or the French Academy of Sciences restricted their research to empirical demonstrations, mechanics, and mathematics, belief in a naturalized mind and secular ethics began to grow. The Christian Church's dominion over moral life, long challenged from within by different sects, now faced a new challenge. Breathtakingly, the great John Locke had proposed that all of moral life could be subsumed in mental life. Ethical conduct could be created or destroyed, understood or mistaken, based on mental functions. If so, a new cadre of experts would be needed to focus on this modern mind and its capacity for good and evil.

Bedlam in Britannia

AROUND CONTINENTAL EUROPE, the skeptical sons and daughters of Galileo and Descartes had consolidated their authority over Nature, while the priests retained their unchallenged positions as physicians of the soul and guides to salvation. Mechanistic science did not pretend it could explain higher-order human functions like reason, and in many branches of Christianity, theologians relinquished older views of the natural world, and hunkered down to defend the immaterial soul from animists and other atheists.

The emergence of a reified mind, an object that was a natural source of reason, no longer a synonym for the soul, but in critical ways its opposite, disrupted those clean divisions and created new possibilities and anxieties. The old dichotomies of body and soul now became a three-way contest between body, soul, and mind, with the last term existing somewhere between scientific discourse with its prerequisites of materialism, mechanization, and quantification, and the metaphysical credos of an immaterial human essence.

These abstract controversies became concrete for a growing array of citizens, whose troubles once were of the soul and now could be thought of as mental. Long involved with bilious forms of madness, 18th-century doctors were gradually forced to confront this competing mental paradigm. And as with the prior century's scares over

witchcraft and religious enthusiasm, after 1700 the need for such sorting of reason and its ills took on broader political importance. In the
self-proclaimed Age of Reason, the not-so-hidden secret was that no
one could be secure of their own mental powers. If John Locke was
correct, then that faculty was dependent on an easily influenced, fragile thinking thing in which minor forms of madness afflicted many.

In rapidly changing Great Britain, it was imperative to be able to
be sure as to who had a trusty mind and who was delusional, as well
as who had the capacity for moral judgment. Hopes of a social order
based on individual liberty, voluntary self-restraint, and the pursuit
of individual happiness seemed to depend on mental competence.

After the Glorious Revolution, England increasingly allowed a
clamor of opinions and the polis needed to be safeguarded, ironically,
by securely defining the limits of such openness. Locke, Shaftesbury,
and other moral philosophers agreed that on the other side of the line
lay madness, those who acted under false beliefs generated not by a
divergent theology, but rather the fumes of fever, bad bile, tangled
ideas, and wild passions. Locke explicitly excluded "Ideots and Madmen" from either civil toleration or criminal punishment. These
were not true Dissenters or outlaws; they were ill and should not
be accepted as merely different. Persuasion might cure them, Locke
argued, but imprisonment and torture would not. Even Locke's
opponents relented on this point; mad "heretics" should not be punished. They knew not what they did.

And so, in 18th-century Britain, the political experiment of toleration went hand in hand with an increased scrutiny of the sanity of
citizens. An impetus emerged to recognize and define certain forms
of difference as not just divergent opinions from varied creeds and
cultures, but rather madness that resided outside the bounds of liberal
freedoms and rational debate. New forms of madness—often said to
be exclusively English—began to proliferate alongside the expanding
liberties of that society.

At the same time, older notions of soul trouble lost credence. If in the 1680s the Royal Society's Joseph Glanvill still fiercely denounced anyone who denied evil spirits as a heretic who also denied God and the soul, a few decades later witchcraft had become a laughing-stock. In 1714, the inaugural issue of *Gentleman's Magazine* shared as common knowledge the belief that "apparitions, genii, demons, hobgoblins, sorcerers, and magicians, are now reckon'd idle stories." By 1736, every witchcraft statute in England had been repealed. By then, support for these claims had long waned. No witch had been convicted for over twenty years.

This retreating tide of supernaturalism occurred alongside a steep decline in Galenic theories of madness. In 1689, Thomas Tryon, a self-styled "physick" in London, attacked Galen's wisdom as nothing more than hot air. Tryon declared, rather charitably, that bloodletting did nothing. "The truth is," he wrote, "Madness and Phrensie do generally, and for the most part . . . arise and proceed from various Passions and extreme Inclinations, such as Love, Hate, Grief, Covetousness, Despair." Humoral theories, he pointed out, could not account for mass delusions. Enthusiasts, Tryon noted, could infect an entire town, provoke a congregation, and make an entire country go insane simply with ideas. A crazed notion could leave one man's mouth, enter another's ear, and somehow spread. Ideas, not just passions, upset minds, and a model of disrupted humors could offer no explanation for such a thing. However, Dr. Locke's mind did rather well on these counts. Jonathan Swift, who followed Shaftes-bury's advice and mercilessly derided both enthusiasts *and* mechanis-tic virtuosi as equally insane, also found Locke's mental framework convincing. Madness, he concluded, could not be from bodily vapors alone, for what of the epidemic of religious madness in which one man's fancy became that of a whole army?

And so as the 18th century commenced, the stage seemed to be set in England for mentalist views to sweep away the old and estab-lish themselves as the new paradigm for reason and its disorders, thus helping to contain concerns about fanatics and deluded members of this more open society. However, surprisingly for the first half of the 18th century, the impact of Locke on doctors continued to be small, for the drawbacks of this view remained imposing.

As Locke's well-read contemporaries knew, Lucretius had famously argued that illnesses of thought proved the soul itself was mortal. In 1702, William Coward in *Second Thoughts Concerning Human Soul* dared to insist that the soul died with the body. Evidence for that came from cases of madness and more so, its cure by medical means. Coward engendered a wave of rejoinders from theologians and doctors like Nicholas Robinson, who in defending the immaterial soul, also felt obliged to dismiss the mind. Locke would have been quite astonished, for by segregating thinking and ideas from the everlasting biblical soul, he had hoped to undercut Lucretius's logic and establish a limited, natural domain for the intellect. Madness, for him, had no impact on the eternal soul, which now stood outside reason. Arguments pro and con filled many pages and turned many ways, but in the early decades of the 18th century, defenders of the faith still hesistated before Locke's mind.

Furthermore, for those interested in law and order, Locke was vexing. For him, the line between madness and sanity was not clear. To be a touch mad like Tristam Shandy's mother was supposedly common. Most labored under strange associations. Locke blurred the difference between sanity and madness, and made it difficult to categorically distinguish the truly crazed from the merely harebrained. If reason was to determine who would and would not be tolerated in the political order and who would be held responsible before the law, it was a minefield.

Meanwhile, the ascension of King George I in 1714 consolidated the Whigs' progressive, rationalist vision. This new order was heralded when the new king abolished the Royal touch. For over four centuries in England and in France, it was widely believed that the king or queen could cure scrofula through a miraculous laying on of hands. Along with ideas of divine right, this procession of sufferers who patiently waited for their political leader to cure the King's Evil, reinforced notions that the monarch was God's emissary. Upon ascension to the throne, kings took up the responsibility of curing this affliction; hence, they endured lines of desperate tubercular patients, including in 1712, the two-year-old Samuel Johnson. While this tradition continued in France, the new king from Hanover, George, put an immediate end to it.

In Georgian England, ameliorative philanthropic efforts for the poor and troubled also began in more earnest. In London, concerned wealthy individuals began to concern themselves with not just the salvation of souls; they funded the construction of schools and hospitals, including asylums for the mentally ill. In 1719, Westminster General Infirmary was established, and six years later, a wealthy bookseller established Guy's Hospital, which included four hundred beds and a wing for the insane.

The creation of these new large spaces to house, care for, restrain, and study the mad would be transformative. Prior to that, the mad in England were mostly cared for by their families, or when necessary, they were placed in small madhouses, privately owned businesses in which a proprietor, rarely a doctor, agreed to house a few mentally ill for a fee. These businesses advertised kindness and care, but often delivered little. In 1702, Dr. Gideon Harvey decried the bleeding by "pretended Masters of mad-houses." Their purges, vomits and bloodletting sought to throw off putrid particles from the brain, but the treatments disturbed many who turned to gentler remedies, like moderate diets, gentle purging, and opiates. Such kinder treatments, Harvey announced, allowed him to cure a whole hospital-worth of the mad.

The exception to the rule of small private madhouses was London's fabled St. Mary of Bethlehem Hospital variously known as Bethlehem Hospital, Bethlem Hospital, or "Bedlam." Founded in the 14th century, this structure years later at its entrance held two sculptures of human agony, Raving Madness and Melancholy Madness. In 1600, the hospital housed thirty ragged, chained patients. However, as soul sickness began to be reframed as a natural illness and as possession and enthusiasm began to be redefined as delusion, melancholia, mania, and delirium, the numbers of the mad grew. In 1675, the hospital moved into a new building created by one of the Oxford virtuosi, Thomas Willis's assistant, Robert Hooke. Bedlam became a symbol and a spectacle, in which Londoners lined up to gaze at the insane; in 1707 alone, some 96,000 visitors toured the facility and its few dozen inmates. If this was hardly a Great Confinement of rabble and deviants, it was a fascination for Londoners who paid for the privilege of viewing what it meant to lose one's mind. They came to witness a slew of 18th-century James Naylers, who claimed to be Jesus, Mary, or some prophet. No longer branded or revered by chanting worshipers, they were hospitalized and placed on display as exemplars of everything a reasoned man was not.

Over the course of the next decades, the terror of madness would begin to compete with the religious terror of damnation. Johnson wrote: "Of the uncertainties of our present state, the most dreadful and alarming is the uncertain continuance of reason." If reason and the sentiments ruled, then it was horrifying to consider the fact that understanding may "make its appearance and depart, that it may blaze and expire." In Scotland, the moral philosopher Adam Smith agreed: "Of all the calamities to which the condition of mortality exposes mankind, the loss of reason appears, to those who have the least spark of humanity, by far the most dreadful and they behold that last stage of human wretchedness with deeper commiseration than any other."

However, if reason was so fallible, who was to judge between different claims to rationality? Was it merely one man's word against another? The dramatist Nathaniel Lee bemoaned his fate after he was locked away in Bedlam. "I asserted that the world was mad, and the world said that I was mad, and confound them, they outvoted me," he wrote.

Daunted by his uncle's descent into dementia, Jonathan Swift also feared madness. While strolling in an orange and yellow forest that was shedding its foliage, he predicted to a friend, "I shall be like that tree; I shall die first at the top." A governor of Bedlam in 1714, Swift put much of his wealth into founding St. Patrick's Hospital in Dublin, the first lunatic asylum in Ireland. Three years before it opened, he was declared incompetent, for his sad premonition had come true.

Still even as John Locke became synonymous with English progress, before 1750 the great majority of doctors in England rejected his theory of the mind and its ills. Though Georgian society offered them an opportunity to expand their power, expertise, and practice, most early 18th-century physicians largely refused to enter the traditional province of the Church. Jeered at and often treated with mockery, humoral theory still remained central to their practice, for it provided them with ready-made answers for everything from a headache to a fever. Widely satirized and lampooned, physicans nonetheless stuck to it. Christopher Smart wrote a sketch on the Old Mock Doctors, who from behind hypocritical masks seldom cure and more generally kill the poor. Derided yet depended on, Galenic medicine staggered about like a bullet-ridden man who had not yet fallen.

During periods of strong monarchist control, the traditional English medical elite remained propped up by the authorities, but after the Glorious Revolution that changed. Eighteenth-century British medicine became an open and frequently deluged marketplace. Apothecaries and chemical doctors rushed forward, as did eccentric clergymen, midwives, and alternative healers who employed astrology, folk herbal methods, faith healing, and secret potions to tend to the ill. Empirics, mountebanks, surgeons, and sundry oddballs also offered up their services, mostly to the poor who—in one of the very rare examples of poverty's advantages—could not afford the bleedings prescribed by expensive academic physicians. Pamphlets,

broadsides, and books advertised miraculous herbal or chemical concoctions, and thereby put the professionals on the defensive. Grub
Street churned out claims for new discoveries. One best-seller promised relief from Cephalick Purging Pills, Emetick Powder, and the
Nerve Fotus for frenzy and madness.

A prominent purveyor of chemical cures was Dr. Robert James,
whose patented Fever Powder, a mix of antimony and mercury, found
its way to the heated brows of Thomas Gray, Horace Walpole, Oliver
Goldsmith, numerous lords and ladies, and King George III himself.
James extended the uses of this powder to nervous and mental disorders. Christopher Smart dedicated a poem to James and his potion,
predicting: "Millions yet unborn will celebrate the man." The poet,
a grateful patient himself, took time out from his laudation to decry
cutthroat competition from other retailers, who were "mercenary
and mean enough" to attack poor Dr. James.

In this freewheeling setting, established physicians were more
concerned with protecting their traditional patient base than with
entering into controversies over the soul and the nature of thought.
Those who sought to abandon humoral theory often turned to a
mechanical system of physiology and pathology. Medical mechanists,
who first emerged in the 17th century, insisted the body was a contraption. The jaws were pincers, the stomach a container, veins were
water mains, the heart a piston, the lungs a bellows, the liver a filter,
and the corner of the eye a pulley. Reason had no place among these
chains and gears.

In Leiden, the Calvinist doctor Herman Boerhaave stood out as
the leader of the medical mechanists. Considered one of the greatest
physicians on the continent, he first took a Cartesian stance in which
immaterial reason could conquer the passions, but over time his famed
medical system sank back into a purely theological one: mental peace,
he contended, came from the teachings of Jesus Christ. This mix of
mechanistic medicine and Christian devotion was echoed in Rome
by Giovanni Borelli and Giorgio Baglivi and in Pietist dominated

Halle, by Friedrich Hoffmann, a physician to the King of Prussia.
Writing in more repressive environments than London, these doctors pushed for Newtonian materialism and beat back accusations of
atheism by steering clear of the soul. Hoffman's intellectual adversary
in Halle, the radical Pietist Georg Ernst Stahl, went even further. He
sought to rewin the body for God's dominion. Passive matter could
not explain life, he argued, which must be due to an "anima," a vital
life force. Reversing over a century in which more and more of the
natural world and the body was ceded to mechanics, Stahl argued
that the soul in fact controlled mental and bodily functions. Sickness,
as the Bible taught, came from sin.

Stahl's animism quickly became a source of ridicule, but for doctors who did not want to return to that premodern model, there were
no easy choices. Writing about the soul and body was a dangerous
game in which outward devotion was no insurance against censure.
For the flimsiest of reasons, the deeply religious Dr. Boerhaave was
accused of atheism, a frightening charge that could bring ruination.
Most doctors stayed on their side of the soul/body line; in Holland
and England, the freest of places, the early 18th-century doctor
crossed over this demarcation only with great trepidation. Most had
no interest in the rancor they would then face. The denunciations
would not just come from outside of medicine; in 1702, the English
doctors Gideon Harvey and John Purcell condemned the offensive
suggestion that madness was anything other than either a humoral
disruption or a soul–sickness.

And so, the philosophical debates Locke instigated over the
mind, madness, and moral psychology initially spread to educated
readers, but made little headway with English doctors, who kept
mum about thinking matter. Threatened on one side by unlicensed
competition, they were also pressed on the other by natural philosophers of the Royal Society. Sir Isaac Newton had championed
mathematical knowledge and natural science in a way that undercut
the pragmatic, clinical rationales of physicians like Thomas Syden-

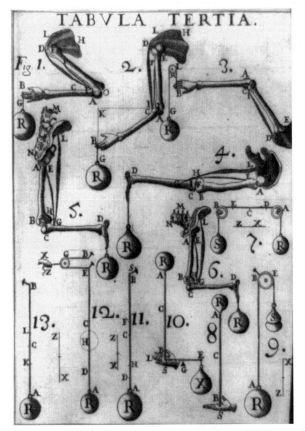

Figure 18. Giovanni Borelli, an early advocate for mechanical theories of the body, and his study of the arm, 1685.

ham. While Locke's indefatigable support for Sydenham led to the doctor's empirical method making some headway in the Royal College of Physicians, Newtonian physicians emerged as his competitors. Advances in medicine, they argued, must be linked to new knowledge in math and physical science. Fashionable models of flesh pulleys and bony rods took hold in London. Many doctors embraced Newton and pursued the hydraulics of the flesh. Nicholas Robinson even sought to apply Newton's theory of ether to the soul's actions on the body.

Archibald Pitcairne, a Scottish friend of Sir Isaac, was perhaps the most prominent Newtonian physician in Britain. After the Glorious

Revolution, this Edinburgh doctor went to Leiden and helped found a medicine based on action and motion. In this way, he proposed to free medicine from any philosopher's "tyranny," any philosophy, that is, save his own. Pitcairne attracted a group of pupils that included George Cheyne, a larger-than-life figure who vehemently opposed Locke and emerged as a conservative spokesman for the nervous troubles of Georgian England.

A Scotsman, Cheyne began his medical career alongside Pitcairne, but his teacher's boozy nights drinking, gorging on food, and carousing through London brought the younger doctor to his knees. In 1705, after one too many vomit-drenched evenings, Dr. Cheyne retreated to his native Edinburgh; he now weighed 450 pounds. During his retreat from London's high life, the obese doctor had a spiritual awakening. He settled in the fashionable town of Bath, a place known for harlots and hot springs. A steady stream of patients with nervous ills came to take the waters. Soon they also came for Bath's new doctor.

George Cheyne's medical thought was predicated on a machine-like carcass and a mystical soul. He dismissed Locke's mind and maintained the old Cartesian divisions. However, times had changed, and unlike his medical predecessors, Cheyne ended up mixing moral and medical matters in a way that embodied the creeping secularism of English life. For him, sick livers and spleens were not just mechanical diseases, they were ethical failures. In his popular book *The English Malady; or, A Treatise of Nervous Diseases of All Kinds*, he made the case that a host of behaviors, traditionally considered moral lapses, had led to rampant nervous illness in the most modern of nations. Fully one-third of all the illnesses in tolerant, rich England, he declared, were of the nervous sort. The country that *illuminati* from the continent looked to for guidance was actually in the corner twitching uncontrollably and throwing up.

Intemperance was the root cause of these ills, but Cheyne did not bother to develop medical theses about why some lost control. He simply blamed moral weakness for the unending feast of spices, fats, and spirits, and the pandemonium of sensual pleasure. Immorality made fat, lazy, whoring, lying, and gambling England develop tics. However, while the putative cause seemed moral, the Lord did not play a large role in Dr. Cheyne's prescriptions.

In fact, a contemporary, Edward Strother, pointed out that Cheyne meddled in moral matters without a priest's sanctity. For all his religiosity, Cheyne gave the soul little room in his account of groaning, rumbling, and stinking bodies. An exception was full-blown madness. There, Dr. Cheyne let it be known that only He who calms the tempests could quell this storm. And the author of *The English Malady* admitted his appeal would touch only those like himself who were pained by their own excesses. Others would ignore him. For them, he promised not the wrath of the Fallen Angel, but rather fatigue and flatulence.

Cheyne's autobiography, published in *The English Malady*, was a cautionary tale. However, unlike Bunyan's *Pilgrim's Progress*, Cheyne did not directly invoke religion to chastise London's revelers, but rather portrayed himself as a brother-sufferer who had learned his lesson. For him, the body was an indisputable benchmark for immoral excess. While some accused him of being an enthusiast and Puritan zealot, Cheyne steered past these criticisms. In his large hands, nervous illness was Nature's way of saying you have sinned.

And so, while the Witchcraft Acts were passed by Parliament, and madness began to be viewed less in supernatural terms, it could still be conceived of as a moral failing. These wild beings may not be possessed by demons, but they had succumbed to their passions, and come undone. In *Bedlam*, Thomas Fitzgerald warned his readers:

And hence this just, this useful Lesson learn:
If strong Desires thy reasoning Pow'rs control;
If arbitrary Passions sway the soul,
If Pride, Envy, if the Lust of Gain,

If wild ambition in thy Bosom reign,
Alas! Thou vaunt'st thy sober Sense in vain.
In these poor Bedlamites thy Self survey,
Thy Self, less innocently mad than They.

Robert Burton's book on melancholia reached out to the
conscience-stricken in Puritan England, but George Cheyne's *English
Malady* addressed different anxieties that emerged alongside the newly
won freedoms of liberal, well-to-do Georgian England. Would a less
religious society based on hedonistic morals lead to crazed licentious-
ness? Printed in 1735, William Hogarth's paintings, *A Rake's Progress*,
warned of such a fate. Tom Rakewell, a wealthy young man indulged
himself in fox hunting, music, and finery, which then led to orgies
with syphilitic prostitutes, gambling, debtor's prison, and in the end,

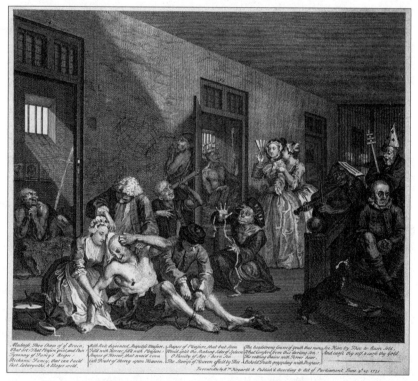

Figure 19. William Hogarth's *A Rake's Progress* (1732–1733) chronicled
the descent of Tom Rakewell into madness.

saucer-eyed madness. Hogarth's last painting depicted a broken, mad Tom, stared at by finely dressed women who have traveled to Bedlam to take in the show.

In Georgian England, the embrace of increased liberty and the fear and confusion it engendered were also dramatized in Daniel Defoe's 1722 novel *Moll Flanders*. No simple figure, Moll was a whore and a mother, a liar and a sweetheart, an impoverished criminal and an eager capitalist, a selfish rogue and a virtuous heroine. Unlike *A Rake's Progress*, in this and other accounts such as George Lillo's 1731 play *The London Merchant*, Christian categories of good and evil became scrambled. Restraint did not always equal virtue, and freedom was not an absolute good for it could veer out of control.

Increasingly, traditional moral failures—such as gluttony, wantonness, and drunkeness—began to be seen as illnesses. In 1736, a number of authors argued that the urban poor—interestingly, not others—were out of control with drunkenness, which would spoil not their souls, but their brains and nerves. Similarly, in 1737, an anonymous tract on masturbation called *Onania* became a huge bestseller. It revealed that the damage from this sin was not spiritual but rather physical. The masturbator should expect enervation and anxiety, and dead or puny offspring. As a treatment, the author still advised repentance; furthermore, one should carry a picture in one's pocket of the most flawless beauty penciled over by "rotten teeth, bleary eyes, and no nose at all" to help dampen one's ardor. This mix of Christian morality and medicine also informed the writings of John Wesley, the founder of Methodism and author of the popular primer *Primitive Physick*. Wesley enthusiastically endorsed Cheyne's views on dietary and physical immoderation as moral failings that led not to Hell, but terrible decay.

Perhaps the most extreme example of English medicine expanding into moral matters can be found in discussions of suicide. Prior to the 17th century, suicide was a heinous sacrilege, a crime against God, king, and man. Despite their difficulty testifying, the dead were put on trial and, if convicted of self-murder, denied a Christian burial. In England, their properties would be confiscated, and their bodies would be dumped at a crossroads, in some cases with a stake driven through them. As in the cases of witchcraft, physicians were called in to these trials to determine the criminal's state of mind. If the self-murderer was found to be an idiot or mad, he was acquitted of any crime and his properties would remain with his family. Between 1550 and 1660, such acquittals were quite rare. Over 95 percent of suicides tried before the King's Bench were found to be sane and worthy of punishment. Popular broadside ballads reflected this same belief; suicides were not insane, but rather spurned, pregnant, or betrayed lovers like, for instance, "Fair Philis": "For with her fatal dagger, she/ Stab'd to the heart, set sorrow free." These lovers succumbed to passions and ended their lives not out of madness, but often as a final testament to their wounded sincerity. No matter for physicians, these suicides would be found guilty as charged.

However, by 1720, the number of self-murder cases deemed *non compos mentis*—not of sound mind—had ballooned to over 40 percent. Part of the impetus for this change was no doubt economic; the rise of a middle class made the property of suicides worth the fight. More families went to great lengths to avoid the penalties imposed on a relative who had killed him or herself. Still, such redefinition was only possible because of a shift from the sins of religion to the mad acts understood by medicine.

In this atmosphere, some doctors went even further. That libertarian enemy of social intervention, Bernard de Mandeville, claimed suicide was neither wicked nor mad, but rather a rational choice in which one hoped to avoid pains worse than death. The philosopher David Hume shocked many with his defense of suicide, a view seconded by the writer Joseph Addison. In 1737, when Eustace Budgell took his own life, he left behind a defiant note that read: "What Cato did, and Addison approved Cannot be wrong."

These views, in which a heinous crime against God was now

normalized, convinced few and frightened many. England, it began to be said, suffered from an epidemic. In addition to its many nervous ills, its gloomy, liberty-loving people were quick to end their lives. Self-murder, 18th-century visitors from France and elsewhere reported back home, had become an epidemic; it had become the "English disease." The most progressive, modern, and free country in the world, it seemed, was also eager to destroy itself.

Sympathy, Idea, Nerve

I N S C O T L A N D, a quite contrary set of views on the mind and morality emerged. Opposition of this sort was not surprising. In 1707, the Scots had formed the union with England to create Great Britain. Long treated with contempt by their cousins and consciously resistant to their hegemony, the Scottish, over the next decades, established a vigorous intellectual tradition that rivaled any other in the world.

A loosening of Scottish religious authority allowed for such ferment. By the early 18th century, the strict Calvinism that once dominated Scotland was countered by the increasingly influential Moderate Party, which despised enthusiasm, touted rational religion, and helped shape a bustling, economic, philosophical, literary, and scientific life. Novel perspectives on politics, economics, medicine, and philosophy found fertile ground.

A leader of this intellectual community was Francis Hutcheson. A progressive Scottish Presbyterian, Hutcheson became chair of moral philosophy at Glasgow University and, instead of focusing on the Great Book, pressed forward with efforts to create a science of morality and behavior. To do so, Hutcheson sought to synthesize Locke's views with those of his rebellious pupil, Shaftesbury. In this way, he hoped to account for internal cognition and swat away beliefs that morality was a serendipitous affair. For his effort to bear fruit, the Ten Commandments and Epicurean hedonism would both need to be supplanted by a fuller account of virtuous and vicious behavior.

Hutcheson accepted Locke's argument that sensations created ideas which then furnished the mind, but he also believed with Shaftesbury that an innate moral sense was the primary motivation for humans, and the source of their emotions. Sentiments arose from that moral barometer—joy from acts of charity and remorse from deceit. Through this moral sense, we experienced another's emotional state deeply and directly. Ethics and social stability rested, not on the Good Book, but on this natural state of shared compassion, what he called a "sympathy" between human beings. Like muscles in the body, this shared emotion balanced private desires and yielded both personal and social harmony.

While John Locke naturalized the mind, named it, made it an object, and split it off from the rational soul, Francis Hutcheson propelled forward a line of thought in which minds interacted not just as individual rational agents, but also as connected, feeling ones. Elaborating on Shaftesbury, Hutcheson began to envision groups who maintained feelings of commonality through shared sympathies. When telescopically expanded, all people could be thought of as linked in an immense system of interacting, looping, and reinforcing affective exchanges. Sympathy was the glue of society, Hutcheson argued, and disruptions of this bond led to immorality, criminality, and social fragmentation.

Hutcheson's student David Hume took up some of the same questions as he sought to establish himself as the long-awaited Newton of moral science. After suffering a nervous breakdown, this humble and patient scholar published *A Treatise of Human Nature* in 1739. Hume made the frailty of reason central, and the solidity of knowledge, even of reality and the self, were subjected to grave doubt. Humans make associations, he argued following Locke, not based on reality but simply contiguity. Things that happened in a sequence were glued together and understood to be causally related, whether they were so or not. Our unified knowledge of the world was thus born of mere accidents in time and space. Hume dismissed an inborn moral sense, but he also did not believe reason accounted for morality. The mutual sympathy described by Hutcheson and healthy self-love allowed for virtue and happiness.

Professor Hutcheson fostered another illustrious student who initially set out on the same intellectual path. Before his name became linked with economics, Adam Smith took up the task of building a theory of behavior based on shared feelings. As a Glasgow professor of moral philosophy, he published *The Theory of Moral Sentiments* in 1759. Dismissing Mandeville as a sophist and rejecting Locke's excessive emphasis on reason, Adam Smith followed his teachers, Hutcheson and Hume. Self-love must be balanced by an inner sympathy for others, he argued. Social bonding and morality were based on this capacity for feeling. Famously, Smith later extended this notion to his theory that an "invisible hand" guided free-market economies and created a happy hive. If unimpeded, economies would self-regulate, thanks to shared, natural sentiments.

By 1750, these Scottish models of mind, morality, and behavior offered a stark alternative to those found in England. These efforts were thoroughly modern: they did not advocate a return to souls in Heaven and Hell, but rather sought a path forward by conceptualizing the mind as a feeling, interactive entity. When James Boswell left Scotland, he professed to comprehend himself thanks to the moral and psychological dictums learned from his professors, like Adam Smith. To aid in his self-knowledge, he had a compass: "A man cannot know himself better than by attending to the feelings of his heart and to his external actions, from which he may with tolerable certainty judge 'what manner of person he is.' I have therefore determined to keep a daily journal in which I shall set down my various sentiments and my various conduct," he wrote. For Boswell, he was not defined by his apprehension of reality or acts of reason, but rather by his *feelings* and the behaviors they engendered. Consequently, his journal detailed his lusts, anxieties, and aspirations, the waxing and waning of his pride, his guilt, dejection, and anger, all building blocks that he believed made up his inner being.

Scottish moral psychologies also touched on the sources of immorality, but much of that was left to the physicians. Hutcheson believed those without a moral sense were sadly deformed, like a man without ears. Vice was simply disability, an inborn illness. Acts of cruelty and evil were not due to possession or sin, nor were they the result of crazed thoughts. These were innate and pathological.

Hutcheson invited local doctors to consider illnesses of sympathy and the sentiments, but at first he found little interest. When founded in 1726, the Edinburgh Medical School was staffed with stalwart medical mechanists like Archibald Pitcairne, who had no interest in mental or moral pathologies. However, the next generation of Edinburgh doctors turned away from levers and pulleys and started to develop a medicine founded on the self and sympathy, sentiments, and the nerves.

Dr. Robert Whytt led this new generation. Born in 1714, he attended medical school at Edinburgh before taking a medical tour to London, Paris, and Leiden. By 1738, he returned home to commence medical practice; in 1747, he became professor of theoretical medicine at the Edinburgh University, a position he held until his death. With his university appointment secured, Whytt turned his efforts to research and made a startling discovery. The spinal cord, he showed, was critical to what would later be called reflex action. It was not just human beings who responded sympathetically to each other, but also different parts of the body. Whytt brought the concept of sympathy from philosophy into the body, and it helped him conceive of the automatic interactions of what became known as the "sympathetic" nervous system.

In his research, this doctor also turned to face the complications that mechanists confronted with biological problems. While the vegetative soul once established the difference between the living and the dead, mechanists with their pumps and pulleys could offer no explanation for life itself. Nor could they explain actions once attributed to the sensitive soul like voluntary and involuntary movement. For Robert Whytt, life and thought were both due to a "sentient principle," a force that charged nervous matter. The doctor did not intend this force to be supernatural, and he ridiculed Dr. Stahl's soul-dominated body. Nonetheless, Whytt would find himself mocked as a mystic who believed that some animistic force infused all of Nature.

Armed with his new model of sympathetic nervous and mental action, Whytt sought to reconceptualize nervous illness. Morbid cases arose from failed sympathies in the nerves, spinal marrow, or brain. The sentient power might be too sensitive, or deficient. None of these dysfunctions were due to souls or animal spirits, Newtonian ether, electricity, or chemical fluids. They were disruptions of an interconnected neural system. Sympathetic interactions of nerves and the brain coordinated and unified a body into a beating, breathing, acting, and thinking whole. More strangely, the same sympathies linked individuals into a social unit. There was a "wonderful sympathy between nervous systems of different persons, whence various motions and morbid symptoms are transferred from one to the other." When one man yawned, Whytt noted, yawns erupted all around. Hysterical fits could be similarly contagious.

Scottish medical theories on shared sentiments and sympathies in the nervous system sharply contrasted with reigning views in London and Leiden. In Edinburgh, morality, mental health and illness, were the result of an integrated web of feelings. When William Cullen took over Whytt's professorship in 1766, he furthered this perspective. A friend of Adam Smith and David Hume, Dr. Cullen believed illness was often due to an excess or depletion of sensibility that led to nervous irritability or torpor. And he considered the mind a critical domain for the treatment of illness. The doctor, he concluded, "must on occasion be the Moral Philosopher also, and he will sometimes practice with little success unless he can apply himself to the Mind."

SCOTTISH DOCTRINES OF sympathy sought to synthesize some of the contradictions facing those who would consider body and consciousness, medicine and morals. However, their proposed solutions—post-Lockean hybrids of mind and body—were poorly received in England. When Boswell arrived in the great capital, he was flattered to befriend Samuel Johnson, who quickly informed him that Hume was a vain fool, and that both morals and sympathy were obviously acquired through Locke's model of reason. Johnson applauded his young devotee, however, when he found Boswell lugging about the thick volumes of the genius who had rightly merged mind with matter, Dr. David Hartley.

Born in 1705, Hartley was heading for the Anglican clergy, but after studying at Cambridge, he turned to medicine. In 1731, he published a pamphlet in favor of variola inoculation against smallpox, which won him accolades. Five years later, he moved to London and swiftly established himself as the personal doctor to the Cavendish family, a regular member of the Royal Society, and an expert on "the Stone," bladder calculi from which the author himself greatly suffered.

Hartley turned his attention to psychology after reading a refutation of the Scottish moralists by Reverend John Gay. Gay cast doubt on any innate moral sense, and strove to show that ethical behavior easily could be accounted for through the interweaving of ideas. Hartley entered this fray, if very hesitantly. After seventeen years of endless revision, he published *Observations on Man, His Frame, His Duty, and His Expectations*. Initially a moral treatise, by the time of publication, his essay had ballooned into a multivolume work with

soaring ambitions. To make sense of man's moral life, Hartley took
up the body and the mind, as well as the spiritual hereafter. The
chemist Joseph Priestley became his acolyte, and Samuel Johnson, his
proselytizer. The poet Samuel Coleridge named his son Hartley, and
the founder of psychiatry in America, Benjamin Rush, commended
Hartley to Thomas Jefferson and John Adams. David Hartley, they
believed, had succeeded where other modern thinkers had failed: he
had stitched man, Nature, and God into one seamless whole. Despite
his explicit rejection of the unfashionable term "system-builder," Dr.
Hartley was precisely that.

Hartley tried to synthesize Newtonian physics, Lockean mental life, and his own peculiar brand of Christianity. First, he dove
into the paradox of "thinking matter." John Locke contended that
outer stimuli resulted in mental experiences, but he never dared to
explain that transformation. He never spelled out how, for example,
we came to see primary qualities of red or feel secondary qualities
like heat. After studying Newton, Hartley believed he had a solution. Vibrations in ether stimulated nerves and created traces in the
brain he called "vibratiuncles." Vibratiuncles were ideas that massed
into associative nets, which accounted for complex mental processes.
And while physical gyrations traveled up nerves and resulted in ideas,
ideas could create vibrations and thereby stimulate activity. Thus, the
mind could regulate the body and take charge of actions, including
moral choices.

This was what many of the moderns had been hoping for: a biological model that allowed for mental causation, a model of consciousness that was placed within a deterministic universe and still
allowed for free will. Hartley also solved a theological problem that
had long troubled him. He refused to accept the belief that God, the
benevolent source of all that was Good, the Cause of all Causes, was
behind Original Sin, Hell, and eternal damnation. If God set everything in motion, then all motion was godly and good. This theological position, known as Necessitarianism, framed Hartley's view that a

mind, even if driven by mechanical forces and the pursuit of pleasure, still pointed itself toward Heaven. The doctrine of original sin was wrong. Mankind was not destined to suffer, but rather to gradually reach greater states of beneficence and perfection, culminating after death, in an eternal merging with the pure love and divine body of Jesus Christ.

Dr. Hartley's views were long in the making. In anguished prayers written as a young man, he spoke of being "afflicted in body, mind and estate," tormented by his sensual passions until a spiritual awakening called him toward the Light. At the same time, he wrote a friend to report that he had proven "we must from the Law of Association at last become benevolent." Mistaken associations could be reworked, a conscience could grow closer to God. A sinner could be saved, a child enlightened, a criminal reformed, and a deluded madman set straight. Christian morals thus transformed into a therapeutic ethic that focused on correcting the errors of the mind.

Hartley was disturbed, however, by an alternative view. While readers were assured in the preface of his book that the author had not eliminated free will, later in the text, he seemed to do just that. The sight of a flame led to an automatic set of mental connections that made a man dart back. Conscious motivation took a backseat to this "train of internal sensations." In the end, Hartley tried to finesse the problem of a mind that was free and mechanical by distinguishing what he called practical free will (we have it) from a philosophical free will (we don't). Still, he couldn't fully convince himself. In a moment of defeat, he privately confessed, "I am mechanical."

Readers were left scratching their heads. Hartley's correspondent the Reverend John Lister recoiled from Hartley's suggestion that free will was no different from vomiting, an analogy he considered very objectionable. Hartley's own editor, after going through his many manuscripts, wearily concluded the author allowed for no transcendental soul, a point Hartley was known to sometimes concede.

Strange Dr. Hartley—vegetarian, Lockean, Newtonian, moralist,

and mystic—in trying to bridge the newly open divide between matter and mind, landed in a netherworld. While some were delighted
by his unification of energy and ideas, enemies appeared on all sides.
Anti-Lockean opponents like the Scottish academics scoffed. He was
met by incomprehension by the majority of doctors looking for practical methods to approach the mind's problems. And he suffered perhaps his worst fate from the scientist who professed to be his ally and
student. In 1775, the sprawling and inconsistent *Observations* would
be popularized in a radical abridgement by the discoverer of oxygen,
Joseph Priestley. Priestly chose to drop the sections on physics and
theology, and left only Hartley's psychology intact. Hartley's grand
unifying system thus disappeared as did the author's intent to integrate mechanical and moral aspects of man. Unitarians in England,
influenced by Priestley, would adopt Hartley as a guiding influence
for their rational religion, but only after his mystical beliefs had been
forgotten.

And so, David Hartley would be remembered for the least original part of his project. He would be seen as simply an exponent of
Locke. He would be placed somewhere near the origins of British
associational psychology, a fertile tradition that commenced with
Hobbes and Locke, then later included James Mill, his son John Stuart Mill, Alexander Bain and doctors throughout Europe like Alfred
Binet and Sigmund Freud. That aspect of his work had been cherry-
picked from a much stranger assortment.

Dr. Hartley's clinical ideas were not so easy to purify. Disruptions
of the rational faculty, he concluded, were of two kinds. Children,
drunkards, those in their dotage or in a delirium all suffered from
bad vibrations emanating from immature or diseased nerves. Others,
through overexertion or violent passions, disrupted mental linkages
and began to judge events wrongly or act violently. Melancholia and
insanity were a mix of such bodily and mental troubles.

Most English doctors had not accepted Locke's claims for mental illness based on ideas and misassociations, but Hartley incorporated these theories into his account of nerves and brains. And he hoped his work would encourage others to follow him and to more closely examine thought disorders:

> An accurate history of the several kinds of madness from those physicians, who are much conversant with this distemper, is greatly wanted and it would probably receive considerable light from this theory. . . .

WILLIAM BATTIE WAS a diminutive man of good birth but small fortune. Born in 1703 to the vicar of a small parish, the boy lost his father when he was ten, leaving him in a precarious financial position for years to come. Nonetheless, Battie attended the prestigious Eton College, where he developed a reputation for being both brilliant and pugnacious. Spurred on by his need to win scholarships or sink, Battie's combativeness even spilled out into a memorable brawl with a rival who tossed the young boy—always said to be "of mean size"— headfirst into a wall. Battie's mother rose to her child's defense and smacked the offender, all of which left a powerful impression that would be revived with merriment years later after William Battie picked a fight that made him famous.

After Eton, Battie attended King's College Cambridge on scholarship and excelled in the classics, but his family's poverty did not allow him to pursue the study of law. Instead, he turned to medicine. He set up practice in Uxbridge, then decamped for London, where after a year he managed to be made a Fellow of the Royal College of Physicians. Erudite, quick to gaiety, pantomime, and crude humor, Dr. Battie made his way in the smoke-filled rooms of clubby London medicine.

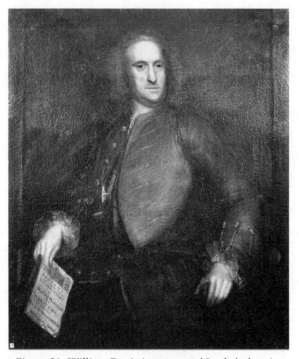

Figure 20. William Battie incorporated Locke's theories
of mind into the treatment of madness.

He would remain a well-connected representative of the medical
elite for the rest of his illustrious career. For example, from 1749 to
1754, Battie was chosen to be the prestigious Lumleian Lecturer, an
annual lecture established in 1582 to be given by a highly esteemed
member of the Royal College. Battie's seat near the center of power in
the Royal College also led to controversy, when that institution was
accused of anti-Semitism. An English doctor trained at Leiden, Isaac
Schomberg had been denied admission to the College after repeatedly meeting the normal requirements. His blacklisting prompted a
satirical poem entitled "The Battiad." An anonymous writer mocked
the puffed-up, well-fed doctors who sought to exclude Jews. And as
the title boldly declared, the main culprit was the censor of the College, the publicly solemn, privately lewd William Battie:

See him with aspect grave, and gentle thread,
By slow degrees, approach the sickly bed:
Then at his Club behold him alter'd soon,
The solemn Doctor turns to low Buffoon.

Accusations of anti-Semitism did not prevent Battie from rising in the ranks and serving as president of the College. Nor did the odd medical path he had chosen, for while his classical scholarship and interest in natural philosophy won him esteem at the College, Battie had tied his professional fortunes to the dubious treatment of madness. In 1742, he became one of the governors of Bethlehem Hospital; he helped set up the first apothecary for the asylum and was active in its general affairs. Around 1751, Battie purchased premises on Islington Road to set up his own private madhouse. The same year, he became physician for St. Luke's Hospital for Lunaticks, a new public institution for the impoverished mentally ill. Built in Moorfields next to the Bethlehem facility, this simple hospital rose up before ornate Bedlam like a stern reproach.

The contrast in styles was not accidental. In June of 1750, a group of London city merchants had come together in King's Arms Tavern in Exchange Alley to discuss the need for such a philanthropic endeavor. In addition to Bethlem, there were only two minor public hospitals that took care of the mad, one in Norwich and another solely for incurable women attached to Guy's Hospital. More was required. And so a year later, the hospital run by William Battie opened its doors. In a pamphlet, the founders of St. Luke's pointed to failures across the way. Bethlem had been unable to meet the needs of the impoverished mad; long waiting lists for admission meant many useful members of society were lost, increased public violence, and whole families thrust into poverty due to the great cost of caring for a brother or sister. Furthermore, it was not just more beds that were needed, but a wholly different kind of institution. St. Luke's would become a teaching facility and open its doors to "Gentleman of the Faculty to Study and Practice (of) one of the most important Branches of Physick, already too long confined (almost) to a single Person." This was a dig at the closed world of Bethlem, where one doctor, John Monro, long had ruled.

Seven years after St. Luke's opened its doors, William Battie reiterated these assertions in the first general medical book in English on madness. His 1758 *Treatise on Madness* proposed a new theory for insanity and rebuked Bethlem for their secretive methods. They did not share their procedures, experiences, and insights, did not teach other physicians, and did not welcome medical students. They operated as a lucrative guild. St. Luke's would differ: it would not strive to create a financial monopoly, but would open its doors for advancement and learning.

The *London Evening Post* dismissed these attacks on Bedlam as mean-spirited and nothing less than an attack on all royal hospitals. Others might have questioned whether Battie's criticism was merely self-serving. However, the book was not just competition for a bigger share of the market, but also cutting-edge medicine. Dr. Battie adapted David Hartley's project of marrying nervous physiology to a Lockean mind. To make a medicine of nerves and minds, the doctor dismissed a series of competing formulations. Theoreticians of nervous fluid were living in a dream; did the brain look like a big gland? "Let us quit enchanted ground," he wrote of these suggestions. Mechanists who imagined solid nervous ropes that sagged in madness were "extremely delusive."

As for those who had taken the anima of old, that life-giving soul, and redeployed it thanks to the unfortunate encouragement of Dr. Willis and Dr. Stahl, it was time to wake up. These were not just bad ideas but disastrous ones. Such unwarranted metaphors on the soul, consciousness, and intellectual agency were dangerous and may "become an instrument of death in the hands of a Madman," a seeming reference to the vicious measures advocated by Thomas Willis, who saw the doctor in combat with an out-of-control animal. The sentence bears rereading: the dangerous madmen Dr. Battie feared were deluded doctors.

Insanity was dependent on the way external stimuli created sensations that then got tangled up as they were processed. The essence of madness was the delusions that then emerged and structured the imagination, Dr. Battie declared, echoing the famed lines of Shakespeare in which the seething brains of lovers, poets, and lunatics were all driven by "shaping fantasies." Battie employed the latest developments in nervous physiology to flesh out these claims. As the Lumleian Lecturer, Battie likely learned of the groundbreaking experiments by Swiss scientist Albrecht von Haller, who in two seminal lectures in Göttingen, reported how externally stimulated muscle tissue contracted and was irritable, while nervous matter reacted with a sensibility that communicated impressions to the soul. Battie also probably knew of the work of Haller's Scottish rival, Robert Whytt, on sympathetic reflexes. Battie echoed these views and proposed that nerves were imbued with a unique capacity for sensibility. Pressure on nerves, not bad vibrations, led to distorted sensation, delusions, and madness. For example, a blow to the head might create the sensation of sound that excited the idea of a musical instrument and lead to the chimerical belief that violins were playing. False sensation excited associated ideas that solidified into insanity.

Unlike Haller, who proposed a clear division between brain disorders and soul afflictions, Battie proposed two species of madness that were both of this world. "Original" madness corrupted the nervous substance via heredity: it was incurable and generally could be managed by mercury for syphilis, opium for pain, and quinine for intermittent fevers. Madness might also be "Consequential," and occur when nervous substances were disturbed by external pressure. Culprits included head traumas as well as excesses of passion or reason, as best exemplified by violent rage or the incessant studies of "shattered philosophers." Delusions of this sort might be cured if the source of the trouble was identified and relieved.

That's where the new asylum came in. Active management in a therapeutic environment cured more often than medicines, Battie claimed. If faulty sensations and perceptions led to madness, controlled environments could be the cure. Temperance could be forced upon the indulgent, exercise on the slothful. Patients would be kept emotionally balanced somewhere between joy and rage, isolation and excitement. Clean air and an orderly atmosphere would exist for all.

Battie condemned Bedlam's practice of allowing tourists to gawk at patients: "(T)he impertinent curiosity of those, who think it pastime to converse with Madmen and to play upon their passing ought strictly to be forbidden." He voiced concern about visits from family members who might reinforce old associations and retard change. And while he concurred with the conventional wisdom regarding bleedings, emetics, cold baths, and other remedies, he warned that these treatments should be tailored to the specific cause of the insanity, not routinely administered.

When the British ambassador to Russia, Sir Charles Williams, became mad, he was given over to Dr. Battie. His treatment exemplified some of the precepts that Battie employed, and their great indebtedness to Locke. Doctors presented Ambassador Williams with a written compilation of his thoughts and actions, which detailed his mental errors. The patient was asked to respond in full, which he did, unfortunately for the doctors, with quite plausible counterarguments. Mental treatment would prove to be no easy game.

When William Battie's pamphlet on insanity reached the desks of mad doctors and the stewards of Bedlam, it caused a stir. Reviewed in March 1758 by the Scottish surgeon turned novelist Tobias Smollett, the book's shortcomings were rehearsed, including the doctor's failure to distinguish madness from things like melancholia, his unwarranted insistence that deluded imagination was central, his neglect of causes like the influence of the moon—"Everybody knows, that the raving fits of mad people keep lunar periods"—as well as his surprising omission of well-established cures like shaving the head to encourage perspiration. Dr. Smollett considered Battie's work, and the controversy it stirred up, so delicious that he copied whole passages of Battie into his 1762 novel *The Life and Adventures of Sir Launcelot Greaves.*

However, the novelist did the well-regarded Dr. Battie little harm, for he was a member of the Royal College, and a central figure in London medicine. His treatise was not predicated on vulgar opinion, but that of an English hero, John Locke, as well as the latest scientific physiology. It rejected clinical nostrums for tight logic on the nature of causality, a subject on which the author digressed for pages.

Four months after Battie's *Treatise* was published, the battle was joined. The superintendent of the famed asylum across the road, a man whose last name was synonymous with traditional mad doctoring, rose up to defend his institution and his predecessor at Bethlehem Hospital, who had been his own father. While Battie clawed his way to the top, his rival, Dr. John Monro, was to his station born. From a prestigious medical family, he took up his assumed role and jogged toward a professional life filled with victory. Groomed to take over for James Monro, the famed physician at Bethlem, he did so and similarly handed the same position over to his son, who would hand it to his own descendent. While private madhouses were businesses that often stayed within the family, Bethlem Hospital was the leading public institution in England dedicated to madness. Astonishingly, it would be run by a dynasty of Monros for over 125 years.

The Monros had landed in London when their Scottish forbearer Alexander was forced to leave Edinburgh because of his Catholicism and his Jacobite sympathies. The family became high Anglicans and spawned many men of the cloth. Alexander's son, James, however, went to Oxford and became a physician. In 1728, in a tight vote, he was chosen to become the doctor to Bethlem. He rose to prominence in London, and in magazines, newspapers, popular ballads, and light verse, he was known as Britain's Mad Doctor.

Not all the attention, however, was laudatory. Monro's harsh treatment methods were detailed in an embarrassing exposé written in 1739 by Alexander Cruden called *The London-Citizen Exceedingly Injured*. The respected compiler of a massive concordance to the Bible, Cruden sent an account of his imprisonment at a private madhouse to the nation's legislature in the hope that his story would convince them to regulate such establishments. Cruden had landed at Robert Wightman's madhouse, a place that had contracted the services of Dr. James Monro. There, Cruden was chained, handcuffed, straightjacketed, and ignored for long stretches. He portrayed Dr. Monro as aloof and disinterested: the doctor prescribed a medication a week before seeing the patient and briefly visited Cruden a week later without sitting down, like a "bird upon the wing." Others had complained of Monro's summary judgments, but Cruden's credibility plunged when he also announced that he sought to be appointed moral censor of the country and wished to be referred to as Alexander the Corrector.

James Monro's son John was born in 1715 and attended Oxford, where he secured the most prized fellowship, an extraordinary stipend that supported ten years of medical studies in England and abroad. This good fortune, it was rumored, had been engineered by his famous father. The medical student scurried off to Leiden, Edinburgh, France, Germany, and Italy, where this grandson of a Jacobite was said to dine with the Pope. This too may have been malicious gossip, but it reveals that for some, the family's political allegiances were in doubt.

After receiving his medical degree in 1747, John Monro assumed his place as a governor of Bethlem, then became joint physician of the asylum with his ailing father, and finally took over himself. In 1753, Dr. Monro joined the Royal College and immersed himself in music, literature, and art, a gentleman's pursuits. Like his father before him, John Monro never published a word on madness, nor did he present a report to the Royal Society. His views were traditional: bleedings, vomits, and fresh air would cure most forms of insanity, whatever the variety. Bethlem Hospital had been very good to him; he evinced no desire to alter anything.

William Battie's *Treatise* attacked these hidebound verities. Four months after this publication appeared, prompted into action by a furious board of governors, John Monro replied. He cagily refused to let Battie turn this into a quarrel between the modern scientific and Galenic conventions, for in 1750 assertions of tradition rarely were a winning argument. Instead, he sought to position himself as an empiricist, a man like Thomas Sydenham who sought to observe the facts and go no further. Proudly alluding to his extensive clinical experience, Monro rejected Battie's notion that madness was *always* marked by a deluded imagination. He picked this assertion apart, pointing to counterexamples such as men who run amok without fanciful hallucinations or paranoid plots in mind.

Monro challenged the notion that the imagination was faulty, rather than the madman's judgment. William Battie had avoided a confrontation with the Church by not directly linking insanity to the highest of man's rational functions: his judgment. Many theologians followed Aquinas and considered the imagination to be part of the sensitive, or animal, soul; thus, it could be sick without implications for the soul's immortality. A high Anglican, Dr. Monro took another route: he insisted that the mad "see right, but judge wrong" not due to any primary disturbance in their rational faculties, but secondarily due to some other bodily disorder.

A great deal was at stake in these small differences. By denying that his patients' judgment was itself diseased, William Battie like Locke preserved a modicum of reason for the mentally ill. That meant they could be talked to, taught, logically approached. For John Monro, since the capacity to judge was vitiated, madness represented a complete descent into unreason. It was not due to limited errors that might be corrected, but was a wholesale dehumanizing catastrophe. It made little sense to employ mental means with such a creature.

With regards to the nature of the mind, Monro pointed out that Battie, this "great man of learning," was quite baffled. He had confused sensation with perception, and imagination with judgment, while he pontificated about the rules of logic. And this know-nothing dared to suggest that his medical foes were crazed! Well, William Battie's arguments were at times so obscure that Dr. Monro felt sure they would be comprehensible only by "senior recluses" in Bedlam. Bewitched by fashionable notions of nerve physiology and Lockean associations, the St. Luke's doctor had succumbed to a madness often seen in asylums—that of the scholar whose speculation turned into delusion. "Theorists deserve the suspicion of insanity," Monro acidly wrote, citing an eminent colleague. The authority was, of course, William Battie.

Monro was not done. Madness remained unknowable, he continued, a Proteus of many shapes. Attempts to generalize about its causes were doomed. Treatments that so shocked William Battie—for instance, a regimen of forced vomits for a year—were not disturbing, because in fact, they worked. Patients improved from these regurgitations. And bleedings were surely required. Keep your theories, Monro declared, for I have seen what cures.

The public debate between these well-placed London physicians highlighted the tensions between modern approaches toward knowledge. The scientific medicine of Boerhaave and Haller relied on inductive and deductive logic to construct a guiding theory, while the empiricism of physicians like Thomas Sydenham eschewed such generalizations. Battie had embraced Locke's theory of thinking matter with a theory of nervous sensibility to understand illnesses of the mind. Other doctors believed such a theory was empty. In fact, William Battie would have been disappointed to find that one of his inspirations, Dr. Haller, did not approve of his efforts. "I have profited little from Battie on *Madness*," he wrote to a colleague in 1759; "it's totally pure theory, without the shadow of experience."

False conceptions of mental illness also meant that the doctors themselves could become deluded and dangerous. Extremes of either rationalism or empiricism, critics agreed, led to a kind of madness among the medical men. In speculating, mad doctors risked becoming no different from their own patients, like those mad scientists and insane geometers whose system-building left reality far behind. And by sticking too close to observable facts and experience, they might fall prey to the accusation that they simply regurgitated culturally shared prejudices and delusions from the past. John Monro's empiricism led to a kind of know-nothing conservativism that left no grounds to question what one's father or grandfather believed to be true.

The public quarrel between William Battie and John Monro highlighted these differences, but in other ways the two gentlemen weren't that dissimilar. In daily practice, Monro might have favored vomits more than Battie, but both approved of blistering and bleeds. Their great controversy was over the idea of mind, that newly proposed human essence that sat somewhere between the brain and the soul. Still, after their spirited quarrel, these London doctors collaborated on cases and jointly testified before the 1763 Madhouse Enquiry. In a lawsuit for wrongful imprisonment, Battie even came to Monro's rescue. His clever cross-examination of the plaintiff revealed that, in addition to his damning accusations, the injured party could speak to a special princess through cherry juice. The doctor from Bethlem was found not guilty, thanks to this demonstration of the patient's deluded imagination, a theory of madness he did not accept. Monro apparently contained his qualms long enough to be acquitted.

Despite his standing in the community of London's physicians, Battie's stew of philosophy, morals, and medicine initially remained uncomfortably foreign and unpalatable to his colleagues. In 1764, when he retired from St. Luke's, Battie left the field of battle to Monro, who clung to power at Bethlem until 1789. Only gradually did Battie's novel views find supporters. In 1755, Dr. George Baker, a student of Battie who would be knighted and serve as a physician to the king, argued that Battie's mix of mind and medicine was neither strange nor novel. "From the earliest antiquity, from the very cradle of philosophy and medicine, we learn that it was a regular thing for the princes and professors of philosophy . . . to practice medicine." The battle between passion and reason, Baker continued, could no longer be a concern just for the theologian or the moralist. When affections of the mind threw off the restraint of reason, rebellious behavior ensued, alongside mental disturbances. At these times, it was not Galen, but Socrates' medicine that was required.

Over the next two decades, others began to consider mental medicine. James Vere, a merchant and governor of Bethlem Hospital, conceived of mind disorders—"nervousness," he called it—emerging from the battle between the lower instincts and one's morals. As a few of these practitioners emerged, they were dubbed by one observer the "Antimaniac physicians."

While a minority, these doctors began to garner attention. In 1778, the owner of a madhouse in Kent, William Perfect announced great successes based on "the late learned and celebrated Dr. William Battie." In a book that went through seven editions, he insisted that deluded imaginations could be created by fervent reading and fanatical speeches, and that such zealots could be cured by an absolute restriction of inflammatory pamphlets. In this way, one could gradually right all the wrong associations.

Mental models were also announced by Thomas Withers, a founder of the York Lunatick Asylum, which opened in 1777, and William Pargeter. Other schemas emerged based on Locke, Hartley, and Battie, such as Andrew Harper's 1789 *A Treatise on the Real Cause and Cure of Insanity*, and James Adair's work on the natural history of the mind. Doctors no longer shied away from the belief that the mind's health, once a matter of theology and metaphysics, now rested on medical ground.

As these scattered voices emerged, John Monro steadily pushed back. After a tenure of forty years, Monro bequeathed his position to his son; Bethlem would mostly remain a bastion for traditional views of the brain and soul that did not make way for the mind and did not encompass mental medicine. Many doctors shared this view. Writing in the *Critical Review*, Tobias Smollett enjoyed the debate between Battie and Monro, those "rivals in fame," but ultimately he sided with the "manly resentment" and filial piety of John Monro. In the Royal College, a similar kind of piety meant doctors continued in their Galenic tradition. Hartley, Locke, and Battie would not be called on until a crisis emerged of the most staggering sort.

The Cure of a Lunatic King

A S NEW MODELS of mental medicine emerged, decades of mounting concerns over abuses in the for-profit madhouses of Great Britain erupted. As early as 1740, Daniel Defoe had written that these private establishments should be banned and replaced by licensed hospitals. Otherwise, there would be no end to the ugly game of husbands locking away wives to enjoy their mistresses, wives ridding themselves of their misters for gallants, and children whisking away their parents so as to enjoy their estates. However, it was not until 1774 that parliamentary investigations into such improper confinements resulted in the Madhouses Act, which required these businesses to become licensed and inspected by the Royal College of Physicians. A strict eye needed to be kept on "gaolers of the mind, for if they do not find a patient mad, their oppressive tyranny makes him so."

In a culture that embraced increased personal liberty, medical men were increasingly on the frontlines, asked to discern what kinds of extreme behavior and thought necessitated the limit or loss of one's freedom. Accusations of false confinement and wrongful imprisonment became commonplace in the press and in self-published pamphlets. Aggrieved ex-patients like Alexander Cruden looked to the courts for justice. And the doctors themselves sometimes found

these complaints to be sound. For example, both Drs. Battie and
Monro were called in by the court to examine a supposedly mad
woman named Mrs. MacKenzie, who had been repeatedly confined.
After examining her, they found no signs of illness.

Debates over asylums and mind medicine spread for another reason: despite their differing methods or perhaps because of them, Drs.
Monro and Battie conveyed a stunning optimism about their capacities to cure insanity. These beliefs caught the attention of a growing
group of philanthropists, the well-to-do who had benefited from
England's increased prosperity. Merchants and aristocrats had joined
the clergy to consider the care of the impoverished ill and the creation of hospitals. However, as a network of voluntary general hospitals sprang up across England during the middle decades of the 18th
century, they shared a similar restriction: no madmen or -women.
That, many believed, needed to change.

Charitable-minded elites began to consider separate hospitals
for the pauper mad. St. Luke's had established a workable model.
Through voluntary subscription, Battie's hospital raised more than
100,000 pounds, an astounding figure that allowed that hospital to
be built in a year, and expand from twenty-five patients to over four
times that by 1787. That same fund-raising approach was successfully
adopted in the provinces. Between 1764 and 1792, pauper asylums
opened in Newcastle-upon-Tyne, Liverpool, Manchester, and York;
they all combined curative care with custodial restraint, management with medicine. Appeals for private funds regularly reminded
citizens of both their humanitarian duty and the danger madmen
could pose for the community.

While a vibrant and profitable trade existed in private madhouses
for the middle class and well-to-do, these new charitable institutions
offered free care to the poor. At the center of each was a physician
whose expertise gave him authority over the lay governors of the
institution. Power struggles broke out between competing doctors,
who strove for these positions. When the dust settled, John Hall

in Newcastle, Alexander Hunter in York, and Thomas Arnold in Leicester, established themselves at the head of new institutions. All struggled to hold off naysayers and rivals, especially from established private madhouses, who perceived these institutions as a threat.

The most prominent of the new asylum directors was Thomas Arnold. Having inherited his father's madhouse in 1766, the high-minded Arnold took in up to ten impoverished patients whom the parish would not pay for, at a reduced rate, and kept two slots open for free care. He vigorously advocated for the creation of a Leicester Lunatic Asylum, which, after thirteen years of effort, opened in 1794 with Arnold at the helm. Arnold blamed some of the misconceptions of madness on the ignorance and greed of other madhouse proprietors. He believed that the understanding of insanity had benefited little from science because the mad were kept in establishments run by laymen, adept at bookkeeping and confinement but not natural philosophy or medicine. Arnold was determined to be different.

In addition to his practical initiatives, he embarked on a Herculean attempt to categorize and classify insanity. His teacher, the Scottish doctor William Cullen had created a gargantuan nosology of medical ills, with 4 classes and 150 genera. Cullen agreed that the mind's ills had been unjustly ignored and insisted that they should have a place in his system. While he ascribed "neurosis" to the nerves and body alone, in his nosology, Arnold would conceive of the mind as an active force that could drive illness and, conversely, could be harnessed to heal. As Thomas Arnold became a leading spokesman for mental medicine, he could not help but wonder aloud about "the boundaries between what may not improperly be called moral and medical Insanity."

Arnold's *Observations on the Nature, Kinds, Causes, and Prevention of Insanity* sought to clarify those confusing, common words: madness, insanity, and lunacy. Old distinctions would be tossed away, and new ones would be based on Locke and Hartley. Since ideas came from sensation and reflection, there must be a corresponding Ideational Insanity and a Notional Insanity. The first was characterized by hallucinations and illusions, while the second consisted of thirteen types of cognitive errors, including one with sixteen subtypes. Arnold pointed his finger at an array of mental causes: he worried about toxic vibrations and eighteen kinds of excessive passions. Arnold promised a 66 percent cure rate for that group whose minds were made ill by ideas.

In the second half of the 18th century, long after John Locke portrayed madness as a partial loss of one's faculties, the belief that madness was treatable in part by moral means gradually grew. The Vagrancy Act of 1744 had established that before a madman was sent to the poorhouse, there must be some effort to restore that sufferer to health. While many doctors still employed the standard purges, vomits, and bloodletting, along with medications like opium, a vocal vanguard emphasized mental cures based on a doctor-patient relationship. In this context, one could restore the balance of reason and passion through discipline, logic, stern lectures, threats, and intimidation.

Such efforts made sense only if patients had lost *some* but not all of their mental capacities. Thanks to this rationale, the brutal methods used to subdue the frenzied beast inside with terror and beatings could and should cease. John Ferriar of Manchester commented on the increased sensitivity to the management of the mind of the insane, the appeal to the sufferer's pride and honor, and the import of restraint from what he bluntly described as years in which confined lunatics were tortured and even murdered. From his faraway outpost in the Bahamas, Dr. Andrew Harper also decried confinement as mostly ignorant torment, sure to make matters worse. Attention to the ideas and impressions of the mind, conversely, offered hope. Moral management thus began to acquire a double meaning: it pointed to treatment of the "moral" or mental faculties of patients, while it demanded that caregivers refrain from inhumane violence and cruelty.

AS GEORGIAN ENGLAND became more secular, old supernatural explanations were ridiculed. In John Monro's 1766 casebook, he reported
a large number of sufferers who claimed to be at the mercy of the
Devil or filled with the Lord's spirit, explanations he waved away as
imaginary. Miss Compton of Argyle Street "fancied" herself to be
wicked, while Mrs. Blinkhorn "imagines" she hears voices, and a
young lad "fancied the Devil had been talking to him." Monro gave
this no credence at all. Even religious leaders no longer believed in
the inspired members of their flock. One Nonconformist preacher,
called in to see someone who had become touched by God, packed
the young fellow off to Dr. Monro, telling the mother to use his
name as a reference, since he had sent many others to Bedlam. To
the horror of John Wesley, who heard this tale, Monro asked the boy
to stick out his tongue and without further delay declared him mad.

Interest in mind illnesses were also stoked by celebrated cases,
such as that of the writer Christopher Smart. Born to a family filled
with Dissenters, this hard-drinking, fast-living Cambridge poet cut
a dashing profile in London, thanks to his supercharged ways. He
picked public scrapes, started a fashionable literary magazine, and
was a much-commented-upon figure who spent lavishly and lived
eccentrically. His friend the poet Thomas Gray recalled that, while
at the theater, Smart would make a spectacle of himself as he howled
with laughter before punch lines were delivered and sought to mimic
and play all the parts on stage himself.

At the age of thirty-four, this literary maverick fell into a full-
blown frenzy. Smart was brought to a doctor who offered little and
a priest who recommended prayer. So Smart prayed fervently, incessantly, excessively, whether he was in the midst of a conversation, in
a store, or in the middle of London's streets. He had taken St. Paul's
advice to the Thessalonians literally: pray without ceasing. Admitted

to St Luke's, the patient who decades earlier might have been deemed holy was labeled incurable by William Battie. Transferred to a private madhouse in Bethnal Green, Smart was confined, though not in harsh conditions. His room adjoined a small garden, and he was allowed to have a cat as well as access to a library. During this time, he wrote stirring poetry, such as his 1756 "Hymn to the Supreme Being on Recovery from a Dangerous Fit of Illness":

> *When reason left me in the time of need,*
> *   And sense was lost in terror and in trance,*
> *My sick'ning soul was with my blood inflam'd.*
> *   And the celestial image sunk, defac'd and maim'd.*

As his "nerves convuls'd," he wrote, his "mind lay open to the powers of night."

One of the most popular poets of his day, William Cowper was known to have fallen mad. In 1763, suffering from depression, he made a number of suicide attempts. Desperate for help, he consulted a Dr. Heberden, who advised country air. Cowper ended up in Dr. Nathaniel Cotton's Collegium Insanorum in St. Albans, a place noted for its enlightened care. After his recovery and release, Cowper fell under the thrall of the Reverend John Newton, author of the hymn "Amazing Grace," a former slave-runner-turned-minister of a sect called the Church Militant. In 1773, Cowper again became delusional, and Newton countered Cowper's scary belief that Providence wanted him sacrificed like Isaac by forcing the writer to submit to a series of sadistic trials. When finally separated from the brutish Newton, Cowper recovered. Cowper described these struggles in "Lines Written Under the Influence of Insanity," in which his dark depression made him feel "in a fleshy tomb . . . /Buried above ground."

None of these celebrated cases compared to one that shook the foundations of Great Britain when, in the winter of 1788, King George III became insane. All of England was stunned to hear that their Soveriegn, not long ago considered divinely endowed, was sweating and singing and raving in his bedroom chambers. Stories of his bizarre behavior were avidly reported in the daily press. In the *London Chronicle*, the *London Gazette*, and the *Morning Chronicle*, readers were transfixed by the mental collapse of their monarch. Gossip of a deranged king filtered through Europe. The crisis that ensued, at once medical and political, put the country's fate in the shaky hands of its doctors.

The king's malady had developed slowly. In the last months of 1788, the fifty-year-old George began to experience insomnia, excessive talking, and confusion, while also complaining of stomach pain. However, in some circles, it was said that by then the king had not been well for a few months. After all, he was noted to be acting

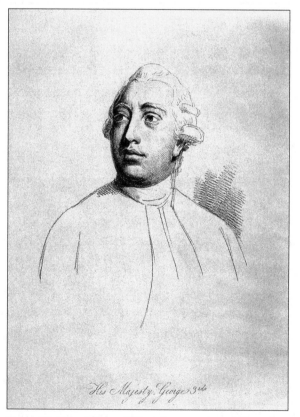

Figure 21. King George III's madness captivated his nation.

oddly earlier, when for example, he had tried to run a race with a horse and had accused an innocent fellow of eloping with the king's first love. He was also spotted merrily playing an imaginary fiddle.

By the time Sir George Baker, president of the Royal College of Physicians, was called in, the king was in the clenched grip of fury. During this consultation, the king pulled off the doctor's wig. This former student of William Battie, who had delivered a thoughtful address at Cambridge on diseases of the mind but in truth had little experience treating such disorders, was quickly overwhelmed. Others were called in, including Dr. Richard Warren, a society physician to aristocrats, including the Prince of Wales, the king's impatient heir. The king refused to see Warren, who nonetheless sped off to inform the prince that the king's life was in danger. To the Duchess of Devonshire, Warren penned these three explosive words: *Rex noster insanit*—The king is insane.

The terrified queen grew to detest Dr. Warren, whom she believed was swayed by political motives. If the king was insane and incurable, a Regency would be required, which would give the Prince of Wales his father's throne. The queen frantically searched for alternative advice. Lady Harcourt consulted one of Battie's old students, William Fordyce. The king's loyal prime minister, William Pitt, added his own physician, a seventy-five-year-old general practitioner who forty years earlier had spent seven years running a private madhouse. The royal physicians grew to be seven in number, alongside two surgeons and two apothecaries. However in this battle, madness, it seemed, still was winning.

While doctors milled about and were abundant, the traditional caretakers of the soul were conspicuously absent. No priests, exorcists, or conjurers were called in. While such services still were employed in the general populace, the time had passed for those in elite circles to suggest that the king's convulsions and fiery talk had anything to do with his soul. Instead, this group of doctors huddled and desperately debated what had gone wrong. Dr. Warren first proclaimed the disorder to be either ossification or water pressure on the brain, or perhaps morbid humors. William Pitt's doctor agreed. In the end, all the doctors save for one, agreed to round up the usual suspects. One of the humors must be out of whack, they concluded, and they predicted that the sovereign would never recover.

The consequences of such grim prognostications were awful for the king and the nation. Increasingly frantic, the queen, on the recommendation of Lady Harcourt, called in Dr. Francis Willis. Born in 1718, Willis was a distant, not terribly distinguished descendent of the famed neuroanatomist. Slated for the church, he was sent to Oxford and took holy orders before he turned to medicine. At the age of forty-one, after practicing for years without a license, he finally received his doctor of physic degree. As a physician in Lincoln, he developed a reputation for curing the mad. In 1776, he moved to Greatford, where he opened a private madhouse that catered to the well-to-do.

Visitors remarked on the way patients in Greatford worked as gardeners, thatchers, and threshers, attired in the same smart black and white outfits. The Duchess of Devonshire noted the kindness of the doctor's care, which included the courtesy of keeping a pack of hounds, so patients might enjoy a hunt. In the battles over madness, Dr. Willis had clearly positioned himself alongside William Battie; he built a madhouse around optimistic notions that the management of mental and moral life should be combined with traditional medical interventions. He practiced these methods and, like most of his peers, wrote almost nothing. He seemed destined for obscurity.

The queen's call to this undistinguished doctor must have come as a great surprise. And when the seventy-year-old arrived at Kew Palace in December of 1788, the royal physicians no doubt shared this astonishment. Willis was not even a member of the Royal College of Physicians. Still, the new arrival encouraged the queen and her staff. "Dr. Willis is a man of ten thousand; open, honest, dauntless, lighthearted, innocent, and high-minded," wrote the second keeper of the robes, Fanny Burney, in her diary. He was said to blend intelligence with "placid self-possession." Some were reassured that the Reverend Dr. Willis united medical and ecclesiastical capabilities in his person. Even more welcome was this: despite the patient's violent deterioration, Dr. Willis proclaimed that the king would be cured.

To the dismay of Warren and the other Royal physicians, this upstart moved to the front of the pack and, after a series of struggles, was given carte blanche at Kew Palace, where since November 27 the king had been sequestered. Dr. Willis would need every bit of this authority to execute his audacious plan. The doctor brought his son, Dr. John Willis, three assistants, a new invention from France called a straight waistcoat, and the conviction that he must exert total control over the man who controlled Great Britain. In addition to the emetics, blisterings, chemicals, and other measures aimed at the king's body, Willis initiated a rigorous form of mental therapy.

What ensued over the next ten weeks was a fierce, at times bizarre, struggle between a provincial mad doctor, a gaggle of envious, enraged society physicians, a scheming prince too eager for the crown, a prime minister determined to protect the king's rule, and a monarch whose every word was once a divinely authorized command and now could only be heard as gibberish. Accounts of the ensuing events would be skewed by where the reporter stood in this carousel of jealousy, greed, and fear. One member of the court recalled that Willis warned the queen that to effect his cure, he would need to establish empire over this patient as if he were the "meanest" of individuals. Another horrified colleague claimed Dr. Willis casually confided that his method was not dissimilar to breaking an animal, the same brutal analogy that led his forbearer Dr. Thomas Willis to "therapeutic" acts of stunning viciousness. In actuality, however, Willis's methods were more mixed than that. The monarch would not be subjected to torture. However, Willis insisted that the insane be treated under his own absolute authority, so as to restore their capacity for self-restraint. He would employ his commanding presence to force a realignment in King George's mind.

In fact, after the initial shock of ordering the monarch about, the other doctors had not been so passive or gentle. When called in, Dr. Warren had been "the first to be severe" with George. And the Opposition doctors, as they came to be called, at times accused Willis of being too lenient. When Willis sought to reward behaviors and allow the king to see the queen or his little girl, Princess Amelia, or take a walk, Dr. Warren and his allies would pounce upon this imprudence. Reports circulated that read: "Willis let the King see the Queen. He is much worse." They did not seem to comprehend that Willis had a rationale based on theories that they did not share about the workings of the mind.

The once-majestic royal was now led about by a doctor emboldened by his belief that he could straighten out crooked thoughts and return reason to the insane. Dr. Willis's series of rewards and punishments, freedoms and coercions, replicated in microcosm the balance that he hoped the king would soon possess. The Opposition doctors were scandalized when Willis tried to win his patient's trust and allowed him to wield a razor to shave himself. However, at other times, Willis was quick to have the king punished and laced up in the waistcoat. Commanded to restrain himself, an angry and at times unhinged George grew to deeply resent the bullying tactics of this lowly doctor, though he did note moments of kind concern.

Meanwhile, calls for a Regency were growing louder, propelled by the other medical personnel who kept up a stream of bleak pronouncements regarding the king. The madness of King George inaugurated a debate in which each physician's position on insanity could be seen as motivated by political affiliation alone. The squabbling medical men were soon sorted by the public into Tories and Whigs. Warren accused Willis of distorting the medical record and disgracing his profession for political purposes. The accusation was quickly tossed back at him.

The House of Commons called the doctors to testify. The discussions and cross-examinations were tense, but not without an absurd kind of comedy. The king was not getting better, Dr. Warren solemnly swore. Warren had consulted with the aged Dr. Monro and followed that Bethlem doctor's position: vitiated reason meant any bit of madness was a symptom of total insanity. Therefore, the king's increasing stretches of repose and rationality under Willis's care meant nothing. King George was gone. Cross-examinations by the king's allies in the House were withering: Did Dr. Warren mean to say that one mad word meant a man was fully insane? Did he truly mean that the insane rave and moan and then, in an instant, recover all at once?

Dr. Willis then assured the House committee that their monarch was much improved. He could read a few pages, where before he read none. He had longer periods where he uttered astute and highly reasonable observations. Insanity was a partial failure of reason, as laid out in William Battie's treatise. To return the king's mind to balance, Dr. Willis would continue to increase the power of reason against the "gusts of passion." Following Dr. Battie, this new doctor believed that the king's crazed errors could be corrected by a rational capacity that, while compromised, had never been completely lost.

The House of Commons was thus presented with utterly contradictory opinions. A member sympathetic to the king asked the generalist Dr. Warren if it was not so that specialists of this branch of medicine were more knowledgeable than doctors like himself. Not if they were less intelligent, Warren snapped. Others pressed the society doctors to comment on Dr. Willis's twenty-eight years of experience with madness and his purported cure rate of nine out of ten patients within six months. The opposition doctors were exceedingly dubious, especially after Dr. Willis admitted he had no records to document these success stories.

While the inquiry focused on the king's prognosis, it also touched upon the causes of this catastrophe. In addition to theories of brain damage and humoral disregulation thanks to wet leggings, a critical concern was whether this delirium was due to fever and hence not really insanity. Drs. Willis and Warren here agreed: that was wishful thinking. The Whig politician and writer Richard Sheridan grew frustrated and asked the doctors to distinguish classes of madness that recovered from those that did not. Surely, cheap talk about recovery might not apply to the king. William Pitt squashed any such discussion.

In the end, Willis suggested the king fell ill due to too much work, severe exercise, too great abstemiousness, and too little rest. In Battie's terms, this was consequential madness and thus curable. George's sensory experiences should be highly controlled; he should be in an environment of limited emotion. The other doctors agreed on this last measure and accused Willis of being too lenient. Warren described his horror when he entered the king's chamber and found that he had been given a book to read, and not just any work, but of all things *King Lear*, the heartbreaking tale of a mad monarch. Willis admitted that he had been outfoxed by his erudite patient. While George's initial request for that play was rebuffed, the well-read king asked for a volume by a lesser-known author who, unbeknownst to Willis, had also tried his hand at Lear.

The harshest cross-examination of Willis came from the writer and parliamentary statesman Edmund Burke, who was horrified to hear that the monarch was allowed to shave himself. What was the doctor to do if his patient went berserk with the straight edge? An observer reported Dr. Willis's reply:

"Place the candles between us, Mr. Burke," replied the Doctor, in an equally authoritative tone—"and I'll give you an answer. There, Sir! By the EYE! I should have looked at his thus, Sir—thus!"

Dr. Willis was known for the paralyzing power of his stare. An opponent, the Duchess of Devonshire described him as a "fierce looking man with a commanding eye by which he manages his Madness." He believed this gave him a form of emotional control that surpassed the straitjacket. If sensation was disordered, this intense glare from the authoritative physician forced itself through hallucinations and delusions. The doctor would glare his way into the patient's awareness. External scrutiny would become internalized and this would become the "principal means used for recovery."

This notion of a piercing eye was not Dr. Willis's invention. Others had come to the conclusion that the doctor must somehow make his presence felt in the disordered sensorium of the mad. The gaping eye had been employed by William Pargeter, who claimed that ferocious eyeballing of the disturbed made chains unnecessary. Called to see a maniac who was ripping apart his cell, Pargeter "suddenly unlocked the door—rushed into the room and caught his *eye* in an instant. The business was then done—he became peaceable in a moment—trembled with fear, and was as governable as it was possible for a furious madman to be."

That was not the only means of mental therapy. As the king began to slowly recover, Willis took great effort to follow the advice of Locke and Battie. Dr. Willis confronted the king over lingering fancies and delusions. No, sir, nothing improper had transpired with Elizabeth, Countess of Pembroke. Absolutely no plans were afoot to remove the king back to Hanover. Wrong ideas and false associations from the acute phase of his illness were to be broken down at all costs, or else they might settle into fixed delusions. Willis and his team employed stern lectures, frank challenges, and the use of countervailing proof when possible. Elizabeth herself was dragged before the king to confirm that he had done nothing improper to her.

Demands for a Regency remained, but as February came, Dr. Willis and the king's allies seemed to be winning. As George's mental state improved, a last-ditch effort to install a Regency was averted, and on March 14, 1789, the king returned to Windsor, a cured man. The nation had followed the tense and dramatic battle between the doctors, a national restaging of the quarrel between Monro and Battie with much higher stakes. And Dr. Battie's ally, Dr. Francis Willis, had won and become a national hero. Willis did not lose the opportunity to sing his own praises: he minted a coin with his own profile, which on the back read: "Britons Rejoice Your King's Restored, 1789."

King George III would remain well for twelve years, years that cemented the impression that Dr. Willis and his optimistic colleagues who studied this branch of mental medicine had made a great advance.

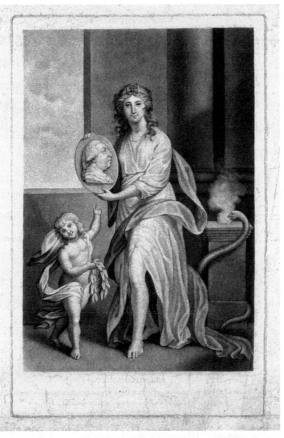

Figure 22. The goddess of health, Hygieia, holding a relief of King George III, commemorating his recovery, 1789.

Traditional physicians had publicly demonstrated their powerlessness over madness. Though the controversy continued, the highly publicized recovery of King George decisively tipped the balance in favor of a new guard who believed in minds and their fragilities.

Across Great Britain and the Continent, news spread of this curative mental method for madness. The famed Dr. Willis and his sons would be paid enormous sums for their care; they received a fortune of 20,000 pounds to travel to Portugal and treat the mad queen. A startlingly new vista had opened up: lunatics could be cured by methods Battie, Willis, and others prescribed. General doctors with their standard array of Galenic cures were not only no longer appropriate for the treatment of these illnesses; their treatments were reframed as cruel and useless torture. Specialists in mind medicine were required, and, increasingly, more and more men sought to earn their living filling this demand.

Old-guard mad doctors—those who positioned themselves against Locke, Battie, and Willis—struggled. After John Monro died, his son Thomas took over Bethlem, where he and allies like John Haslam, the asylum apothecary, did their best to resist these new trends. Decades after the king's treatment and his subsequent relapses, Haslam still attacked Dr. Willis as a fraud whose cure rates were lies. Willis's grandson rose up to defend his illustrious forebearer and claimed the doctor meant he had cured nine out of ten cases of *delirium*, which was much more feasible, since these states were known to pass. And in 1810 when the king had a relapse, the new doctor called in to assist, Dr. Matthew Baillie, desperately asked his wife to pull his copies of both Battie and Monro to try and get his own bearings.

After the recovery of King George, others could not help but seriously consider the methods of Dr. Willis. Once, the rational soul combated the animal passions, but mental medicine conceived of madness as a breakdown that could be reformed by ideational and behavioral means. The Philadelphia doctor Benjamin Rush wrote to inquire about Willis's methods. From Paris, Dr. Philippe Pinel studied this new form of medicine.

King George III would again find himself at the center of another debate between madness and medicine when, in 1800, James Hadfield tried unsuccessfully to assassinate him. Hadfield's lawyer proved his client was delusional, subject to religious mania. The fervor of his ideas about God were proof, not of his devotion, but that his mind was ill. The assailant was acquitted on these grounds. With no legal provision to lock Hadfield up, the Act for Safe Keeping of Insane Persons was passed, and the would-be religious murderer—now considered a madman—was sent to Bethlem.

⸱⸱⸱

A YEAR AFTER the king's recovery, another case of mental illness had dramatic consequences. A melancholic Quaker widow from Leeds named Hannah Mills was hospitalized in the York Asylum. Then suddenly, her family was informed that the woman was dead. She had been allowed no visitors, and her tight-knit community was outraged and suspicious.

Only thirteen years earlier, this asylum in York had opened with great fanfare. This charity would care for the insane poor "with all the tenderness that is compatible with a steady and effectual government." York's physician, Alexander Hunter, conceived of himself as an advocate for the new, moral medicine. He told subscribers of a case from 1778, a seafarer who sustained a terrible loss that operated so violently upon his mind that he was instantly deprived of his sanity. Dr. Hunter studiously avoided traditional bleedings and emetics, got his attendants to feed and clothe the man like a baby, and patiently waited five years for the sailor to return to health. However, the death of Hannah Mills called into question just how tenderly patients were treated in the York Asylum.

Suspicion was heightened because of Hannah Mills's religion.

For many, the Quakers were the original religious madmen, enthusiastic Nonconformists who once horrified the young John Locke.
However, during the ensuing century, these once-fearsome radicals
had shifted into a more quietist stance. While Quakers intermarried,
maintained strict rules of behavior, and often kept to themselves,
they also became businessmen and professionals, as well as activists
engaged in prison reform, educational initiatives, abolitionism, and
poor relief.

The death of Hannah Mills gave the Quakers in York pause.
If their beliefs were considered lunacy by the broader community,
then what kind of cure could they expect in a madhouse? In the
17th century, Nathaniel Lee worried that he had been declared mad
by the vote of an insane majority. Similarly, a minority with a different belief system might be considered by their very identity to
be mentally abnormal. Quaker elders began to hatch plans for their
own place of healing, not an asylum, but a retreat. The York Retreat
would not open for another six years, but when it finally did, it
embodied a bold step forward.

The founder of the retreat, the tea merchant William Tuke, did
not seek to establish a religious place of healing. He appointed a doctor and a surgeon as his superintendents and never denied that the
illnesses involved were natural. However, the Quakers stood against
corporal punishment and chains, so this institution like its rival,
the York Asylum, aspired to use no physical restraints, an ideal that
nonetheless they found impossible to attain. Like many other asylums, the York Retreat used straight waistcoats and even employed
bloodletting. In these practices and on paper, the York Retreat did
not seem to differ much from the York Asylum.

What distinguished the retreat was its eagerness to place moral
and behavioral forms of treatment at the center of their institution.
If mental ills came from disruptive experiences, then it made sense
that contrary experiences might allow for amelioration. The York
Retreat institutionalized a system of environmental and psychologi-

cal interventions that became their credo. While moral management for the nearby York Asylum mostly meant, do no harm and let nature heal, the Quakers institutionalized aggressive mind cures. At times, they found it hard to rely solely on this—for instance, they despaired about the patient who could not be shaken from his belief that he was a pillar of fire. Nonetheless, they believed ill Quakers—for a long time, all their patients were church members—had lost governance of themselves and could regain it through methods of persuasion alone.

While the founders of the York Retreat took some encouragement from Locke's notion that insanity was mental and partial, the Society of Friends were closer to the theories of Scottish thinkers like Francis Hutcheson. Quakers were always encouraged to embrace the Inner Light, a belief that seamlessly merged with Scottish theories of an inborn morality. Since Quakers were unable to attain Oxbridge educations, one of the earlier doctors at the retreat, Dr. George Jepson, was influenced by medical models of sympathy that he had learned in Edinburgh.

At the York Retreat, the wild eye of Dr. Willis was replaced by an army of eyes, all imploring one to act correctly and regain one's balance. Such surveillance, *pace* Locke, could penetrate the mind and modify behavior, a belief that also inspired Jeremy Bentham's 1787 utopian penitentiary, the Panopticon in which prisoners behaved due to the gaze of the jailor. At the York Retreat, a strict system of rewards and punishments also enforced conformity with community ideals. Individual pride and honor would be stimulated to motivate the deviant and disturbed. In matters of masturbation, the reading of dangerous literature, the drinking of spirits or taking of opium, Quaker caretakers and patients kept each other in line.

Unlike religious sanctuaries or medical asylums, the York Retreat and its brand of "moral treatment" consolidated a century of thinking on the mind, its ills, and remedies. While a physician was in charge, this experimental commune relied on social cohesion and the power of emotional ties in groups to assert a strict moral code. That would bring order to the odd, the weird, the lost, and the broken. There was no inquiry into the nature of one's delusions and wrong associations, no attempt to fathom that individual reality. Thanks to their uniform religious convictions, the staff at the York Retreat approached behavior with a clear set of rules. Thus, their moral treatment differed from the individual reeducation advocated by John Locke or the mental medicine touted by William Battie.

For most British mad doctors, the York Retreat was not a fascinating experiment; it was a threat. If some had made the case for adding mental causes to the brain and body, this Quaker institution had gone much further, making traditional medical practices seem secondary. Even Dr. Francis Willis, the grandson of the king's healer, denounced those whose absurdly exaggerated models of madness called for all moral engagement and no medicine.

In 1813, Samuel Tuke, the grandson of the York Retreat's founder, wrote a pamphlet that advertised the origins, method, and success of their establishment. Fatefully, the leaders of the York Asylum took umbrage at the mention of Hannah Mills's death. They too considered themselves moral and humanitarian. Their loud protestations brought public scrutiny to their institution. Godfrey Higgins, a magistrate, bought his way onto York Asylum's governorship and quietly began to poke around. What he discovered was horrific. He tallied 144 unexplained deaths that had been covered up, and discovered four secret cells filled with human excrement. As his inspections became public knowledge, a suspicious fire broke out in the asylum that killed four more patients.

The York Asylum, built on the high hopes raised by mental management at St. Luke's, was shut down as a shameful failure, while the York Retreat stood as a paragon of humanitarian care. Samuel Tuke became a highly sought-after consultant, whose models for mental hospitals spread from Philadelphia and Aberdeen to Glasgow and New York. Asylums began to rebrand themselves as "Retreats." Tourists who once flocked to Bethlem now changed their itinerary. By the 1820s, over four hundred visitors a year made a pilgrimage to the York Retreat to see how vigorous moral treatment could right a mind gone wrong.

PART III

FROM FRENCH *ESPRIT* TO ALIENATION

Here is the book.
But where is the reader?
The reader is the book itself.

—DENIS DIDEROT,
on the mind

The French Sensationalists

B RITISH DEBATES OVER the nature of the soul and mind filtered into France during the first decades of the 18th century.
There, advocates of modernism self-consciously billed themselves as
lumières, lights unto the darkened superstitious land; they were also
variously *savants, philosophes*, and the *éclarés*, leaders of the Enlightenment. They often looked to England for inspiration, and so became
engaged in the heated arguments that surfaced with the work of John
Locke.

Followers of British intellectual fashion faced a barrier in Europe:
few on the Continent read English. If Latin once functioned as the
language of all learned people throughout the Western world, the
moderns now wrote mostly in the vernacular, with French first
among these national languages. Only it could pretend to a universality among elite European readers. And so, if French authorities
could keep their own language from being sullied with these texts
from Locke, Hume, Mandeville, and Shaftesbury, they would effectively eliminate the spread of seditious notions regarding the soul.

And in fact, these seminal English texts faced vigorous censorship
in France. Ideas that challenged absolute monarchy and Catholicism
were not permitted. Thus, the earliest acknowledgments of Locke
and controversies over the soul were strictly condemning ones. In

the 1737 *Treatise on the Soul of Animals wth Reflections both Physical and Moral,* the author took great pains to denounce an unnamed author who suggested that matter could think. Another essay lectured some vague group of thinkers who dared to apply mechanical operations to the soul. In 1744, the reviewer of *Philosophical Inquiries* by St. Hyacinthe took the time to condemn the wild notion that matter could reason, remarking that this would mean all matter, including rocks, should be able to cogitate. Readers might have been excused for asking these cryptic authors, but who was it that ever said matter *could* think?

If censorship still made such names unmentionable in France, in cities and towns circling its borders, there lived a battalion of radicalized, former French subjects, many of whom detested the government and its Church. These Huguenots had been exiled from their homes after the Revocation of the Edict of Nantes. They settled in Switzerland, Holland, and England and became central to a vibrant, though illicit, French book trade. Protestant literati, they took a special pleasure in translating works that questioned Catholic dogma, including English works on the nature of the soul. They were happily aided by Protestant entrepreneurs, who seized the opportunity to market works in France that were illegal in their former homeland.

In Holland, the Huguenot refugee Jean le Clerc founded his journal *Bibliothèque universelle et historique.* His *confrère,* Jacques Bernard, started the *Nouvelles de la république des lettres.* These early publications contained abstracts, excerpts, and reviews of English books and pamphlets by Locke, Newton, and Shaftesbury. Le Clerc even printed a French extract of Locke's *Essay* before the book ever appeared in England. Meanwhile, Pierre Coste, another Huguenot who settled in Holland, decided to teach himself English by translating Locke into French. His bumbling translation of the *Essay* snaked into France through an underground network and brought these subversive writings to an eager public that ranged from provincial bourgeoisie to the enlightened royals of Europe.

Anonymous essays, satires, polemics, and treatises emerged from freethinkers and libertines who challenged, parodied, and at times viciously lampooned cherished beliefs of the *ancien régime*. A raft of underground publications included *libelles* and *chroniques scandaleuses*, biting portraits of eye-opening indulgence and perversity in the court of Louis XV. Political gossip and mockery mixed with scatological and pornographic assaults on the Church. Licentious lesbian nuns shared the stage with horny priests and virgins debased by aristocratic pimps. While proper views dominated public discourse, these shocking works flowed through subterranean channels into private salons, as well as taverns, cafés, and bookshops.

By 1720, Descartes's dualism—once a scandal itself—had become French orthodoxy. His compromise between mechanistic science and eternal souls was parroted in official circles and taught in schools. However, in clandestine publications, mockery of his immaterial Cogito abounded. This ethereal idea was parodied by characters who were, in their deepest essence, lusty, grinding bodies in motion. Such was the message of the illicit best-seller, *Thérèse the Philosopher,* published in 1748. In this novel, Father Dirrag first delivered a Cartesian lecture on the purity of the soul, before furiously screwing the innocent Eradice, all the while telling her that that thing she felt between her legs was the holy cord of St. Francis's robe. While in the act, Thérèse exclaims, "What mechanics!" As she builds toward orgasm, she blurts out, "I sense that my mind is completely detached from matter!" This sacrilegious work portrayed the Cartesian soul as a low ruse. All was matter and motion, hedonism and bodily need. And the book found its way into many hands; the celebrated Parisian salon wit, the Marquise du Deffand, friend of Voltaire and lover of Horace Walpole, recommended it to Jean-Baptiste le Rond d'Alembert, though she asked him to keep this endorsement to himself.

Anonymous pamphlets more directly attacked the division between body and soul. *The Spirit of Spinoza* supported the radical materialism of the Dutch thinker. *The Material Soul* seconded

Thomas Willis's notion that the *anima* was fire in the blood, and thought was the result of the brain and animal spirits. The 1743 work *New Liberties of Thought* turned to medicine to support the notion that the mind of man was mechanical. And Jacques Pernetti's *Philosophical Letters upon Physiognomies*, published in 1746, argued that the soul must depend on the physiological functions of the body.

After Jean le Clerc had introduced John Locke's *Essay* to French readers in 1688, and Coste had published his full translation in 1699, the English thinker became the most important source of opposition to Cartesian verities. A growing Anglophilia pushed Locke forward, and acolytes pressed his case. Coste wrote essays that highlighted controversies over thinking matter. In 1736, the Marquis d'Argens— thought to be the secret author of the novel *Thérèse the Philosopher*— helped promote the cause with a best-seller, *Jewish Letters,* followed by a glowing account of Locke's life and thought.

Locke's most influential, early French admirer was Voltaire. After a quarrel led to his imprisonment, Voltaire, then France's foremost poet, escaped to England. When he returned home years later, he illicitly published *Philosophical Letters*. In this influential 1734 collection, Voltaire painted a glowing portrait of free scientific, intellectual, and political life in England. Liberty of expression, freedom of the press, religious toleration, and that great scientific trio of Bacon, Newton and Locke—my Holy Trinity, Voltaire would joke—all stood in stark contrast to the deadened state of affairs in his homeland.

Voltaire's account riveted readers and infuriated the authorities, who had the book burnt. With characteristic wit and élan, Voltaire demolished long-standing verities and cast a dark shadow on life in Catholic, absolutist France. Liberal toleration had resulted in innovation and modern advances. The author especially lauded Locke, the thinker who had "given a pretty good proof" that the soul and thought were not the same thing. The Englishman had vanquished Descartes with a devastating attack on innate ideas, and the proposal that thought had been superadded to matter by the Divine Maker.

Voltaire's essay on Locke was so popular that it was reprinted alone as "Letter on the Soul"; it also stirred a number of young thinkers from their slumber. Denis Diderot was transformed by the book and commenced a lifelong attempt to find the proper place for soul, mind, and body. Jean-Jacques Rousseau credited Voltaire's book with launching him on his pilgrimage. And Émilie du Châtelet was even more deeply moved by Voltaire, for the two became lovers and collaborators at her country chateau in Cirey, where he took refuge after the firestorm created by his book.

Once a Cartesian, the brilliant Châtelet immersed herself in Locke, Newton, and the new wave of English and Scottish thought. She took up the translation of Mandeville's *The Fable of the Bees*, attracted to his radical critique of ethics, since present conventions denied women the right to be equal, thinking beings. While reading Dom Augustin Calmet's vast exegesis of the Bible, Emilie also took it upon herself to pen a radical analysis of Christian morals. For over 700 pages, in blistering prose, she highlighted contradictions, impossible claims, and absurdities in the Holy Book. There was not enough water on Earth for the Flood, snakes do not eat dirt, and the Sermon on the Mount was filled with "fairly ridiculous things." Jesus's injunction to a leper to keep his cure a secret, provoked this rejoinder: "It is pleasing to come to convert the world and to hide one's miracles." This outwardly devout woman dared not publish her shocking attack on religion, but it was passed around her circle, while Châtelet moved on to what would be her great life's work, a translation and in parts a correction of Isaac Newton's *Principia*.

UNABLE TO STAUNCH the tide of illicit publications, French authorities loosened their grip. In 1750, a new *directeur de la librarie* and chief censor, Chrétian-Guillaume de Lamoignon de Malesherbes was appointed. With that, a fox was handed the keys to the henhouse.

Malesherbes was a modern, who made it clear that anything short
of overt calls for atheism or regicide would be countenanced. Over
the next twenty-five years, he found ways to circumvent or ignore
prohibitions, and was not above tipping off endangered authors when
his own office was after them. While the full seal of approval was
withheld from heterodox works, publishers now understood that
they would not be prosecuted if they received some tacit nod from
Malesherbes' office. Unapproved but tolerated works quickly shot up
from a few dozen to over three hundred by the 1760s. One censor
candidly admitted that any self-respecting Frenchman must read the
clandestine literature. How else, he asked, was one to know what
was modern?

A wave of epochal publications now rushed into France. These
works reinterpreted French law, politics, and theology. However, the
arguments over the mind and soul faced an additional problem for
French *savants*. Pierre Coste, the novice translator, had discovered
that his project was stymied again and again by John Locke's words
for inner life. As the Englishman created neologisms and took the
liberty to redefine old words, his translator fell into great confusion.

The Académie française had been founded to establish and
enforce linguistic purity; since 1694, their dictionaries officially listed
and defined French words and their usages. Confronted with Locke's
weird terms, Coste could get no help from officialdom. What was he
supposed to do with "consciousness," or worse, "self-consciousness,"
things Locke claimed should become central to the definition of
personhood?

In a footnote, Coste dutifully informed his French readers that
the word he chose for consciousness—*la conscience*—really was not
synonymous with the English term, which—in addition to moral
self-observing functions—included wider matters like human sentiment and conviction. The French *conscience* from the Latin *con-
scientia*, had been clearly defined by the Académie française as the
internal light by which man recognizes good from evil. In French

as in English, conscience implied such ethical awareness. Locke's claim that identity depended on consciousness was thus muddied and incorrectly circumscribed.

The treacherous problems of translation did not end there. Locke employed terms like "perception," "uneasiness," and "reasonableness" that simply had no equivalents in a French dictionary. The translator concluded he had no choice but to break away and coin new words for these English terms. However, in perhaps the most important choice, Coste did not dare to offer a new word for "mind," the central term for Locke's thinking thing. The Latin *mentis* did not exist as a noun in French, so what was one to do? Coste could rely on *mentalité* for a way of thought; however, for that thinking thing, he had nothing to turn to. Voltaire's claim that Locke had written a natural history of the "soul" was one the English author would reject: his history was of the mind. Nonetheless, like Voltaire, Coste translated "mind" with *âme*—soul—thereby obscuring the central distinction that Locke intended, the break he hoped to make between a natural thinking entity and the spirit of God in man.

To make matters worse, Coste translated "mind" not just as *âme*, but also as *esprit*. *Esprit* came from Greek and signified breath. And every day across King Louis's realm, children and adults recited the Lord's Prayer, where *le Saint Esprit* referred to the Holy Spirit of the Trinity. *Esprit* also could be used to refer to the incorporeal substance of God in man. In 1751, the famed biblical scholar Dom Augustin Calmet, wrote a book on spirits, such as ghosts, revenants, and vampires. He had little reason to worry that the *esprit* in his title would be confused with anything other than those otherworldly beings that zip about in the night. Adding another layer to the rich connotations of this word, Descartes and his followers christened man's immaterial, thinking being the *esprit humain*—the human spirit.

To make any sense of Coste's usage of *esprit*, readers of the Academy dictionary would have to work their way past the first seven definitions of the word, all of which referred to celestial beings, good and bad angels, and animal spirits. Only then would they encounter the Academicians noting that sometimes the word referred to the faculties of the rational soul.

And so as rational scrutiny of psychic life gathered momentum in France, there would be this paradox. The central terms Locke proposed for consciousness and the mind, pivotal concepts he employed to naturalize aspects of the rational soul, would grow dark as they were given over to French words that also implied their antithesis. Consciousness might also be conscience, and mind was linguistically indistinguishable from soul and spirit. While considering the most common word for mind, *esprit*, Voltaire threw up his hands. Everyone's *esprit* differed, he confessed—the term was fatally vague.

Watched by the authorities, some radicals may have taken comfort in such double-talk, for it preserved enough room for deniability if one was accused of heresy. For others, the language of the mind had become a mirror, dark in its recesses, reflecting more than enlightening.

IN THE FRENCH Court and in royally sanctioned publications, English debates about the nature of the mind first could be heard as faint whispers. However, far from the censor's stamp, a new social forum had emerged, filled with constant chatter over such controversial subjects. In France, literary and philosophical salons had begun to emerge, which in a semipublic manner, brought together not just nobles, but also philosophers and writers as well as visitors from abroad. If the goal was once hedonistic pleasure in food, wine, flirtation, and assignations, it had transformed into a movable feast of discussion and debate, much of which concerned modern views. Through these salons, news spread about forbidden writings that challenged the status quo.

The salons were curated almost exclusively by women, a number of whom were writers themselves. One of the first literary salons in Paris was the creation of Madame de Tencin, a freethinker who had taken her orders as a nun only to then be officially secularized by the Pope in 1712. In Paris, she embraced a freethinker's life, had affairs and became pregnant with a child that she abandoned, who nonetheless grew up to be one of the most influential Enlightenment thinkers, Jean-Baptiste le Rond d'Alembert. Tencin became a novelist and regularly hosted gatherings of French literary figures as well as a procession of English visitors. And she mentored Madame Geoffrin, whose wildly popular salon on the Rue du Faubourg Saint-Honoré became one of the most sought-after invitations in Paris.

Similarly, other freethinking women created literary salons and fostered protégés who went off and founded their own circles. The playwright and novelist Françoise de Graffigny created a well-known salon in the 1740s and matched her cousin's daughter, Anne-Catherine de Ligniville, with one of its habitués, Claude-Adrien Helvétius. Madame Helvétius in turn set up her own glittering salon of *philosophes*. Madame Geoffrin's great rival, the Marquise du Deffand, entertained a more aristocratic crowd, and so her protégé, Julie de Lespinasse, spun off to form her own distinct group.

These salons created a network that encouraged and supported readers and writers. They facilitated the spread of cutting-edge thoughts and incendiary notions, and provided an audience for those who might consider writing such a work. Thus, the great debates that ensued between Enlightenment French writers were arguments that, not infrequently, were staged after dessert.

One avid salongoer was Charles-Louis de Secondat, Baron de La Brède et de Montesquieu. Trained as a lawyer in Bordeaux, Montesquieu served in the local Parlement and was active in the Bordeaux Academy of Sciences before he became a celebrity for his 1721 novel, *Persian Letters*. After traveling extensively, including a two-year stay in England, Montesquieu returned to France and began what would be a protracted labor—he claimed the writing almost killed him—on his 1748 masterpiece, *The Spirit of the Laws*.

Motivated, some say, to counter the mechanistic materialism of Hobbes and Spinoza, Montesquieu set out to establish a natural foundation for self-guided individual action and governmental rule. According to the baron, different kinds of governments—republican, monarchial, and despotic—possessed different principles and different animating spirits. Climate, religion, local histories, habits, and other such factors play a role in what general spirit pervades a particular place and its people. Thus, this epochal work boldly insisted on the relativity of laws from different cultures, and undermined the universality of Christian ethics.

At the same time, Montesquieu's work did not fully establish what exactly he meant by that increasingly tricky word in his title, *esprit*. In the text, he used the word promiscuously to refer to the spirit of commerce, aristocracy, the republic, justice, equality, inequality, and the nation. Montesquieu also spoke of the soul as a God-given universal, as well as a thing formed by its environs. In manuscript form, this work was read by the baron's friend, the wealthy denizen of Parisian salons, Claude-Adrien Helvétius, who was both inspired and concerned. Much later, he told David Hume that he advised the baron against publication for fear of the harm it would cause him. And in fact, the book was placed on the Index of Forbidden Books and its author would face intense hostility.

A decade later, another anonymous work began to circulate in France, which could be read as a follow-up to *The Spirit of the Laws*. Simply called *De l'esprit*—literally, *On the Spirit*—it was initially approved by a careless censor. Swiftly, however, the book's *privilège du Roi* was revoked by Malesherbes, who suspended all publication and demanded changes, including the elimination of passages that showed that classical authors and some Church Fathers considered the soul to be corporeal. Condemned by Pope Clement XIII and the

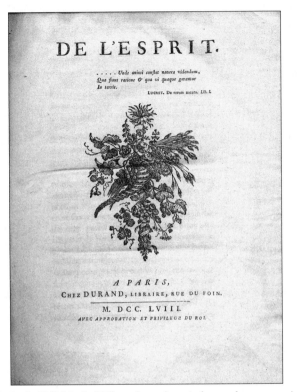

Figure 23. C. A. Helvétius's 1758 work on the mind caused an uproar in France.

Parlement in Paris, the book was burned on February 6, 1759. The salons buzzed, and those who devoured banned books found their appetites whetted. Between 1758 and 1759, fourteen revised pirated editions reached eager readers intrigued by the scandal. A mysterious author had tried to define *esprit*. As to whether the human spirit was material or spiritual, he shockingly dodged, saying "who knows?"

However, the cloaked author then proceeded to promote a theory of society that was dependent on individual psychology, and material notions of human inner life obviously indebted to John Locke. Thought was based on sensation, memory, and the assemblage of ideas in new combinations. Human understanding did not depend on inborn ideas or faculties. Reason, reflection, and judgment were complex transformations of what was seen, heard, tasted, smelled and felt. Behavior was driven by hedonism and corporeal sensibilities, the desire for good feelings and the avoidance of bad ones. Ethics were a rationalization for such a pleasure principle. Societies created ethical rules that justified what was desired and condemned what was not. Virtue was merely a fig leaf for these deep demands.

This assault on moral life was stunning, if not totally novel. For some time, *philosophes* had been contemplating reports filtering back to Europe about distant societies of Native Americans, Chinese, Africans, and others, whose conventions and rules seemed to work well despite their lack of Christian ethics. Pierre Bayle's once-scandalous hypothesis about an ethical community of atheists transformed into questions about these foreign heathens. Voltaire wrote of an American Indian who calmly explained why their tribe dined on enemy soldiers that had been killed in battle. The horror Voltaire initially felt dissipated as this woman rationally explained that if not for this custom, wild animals would tear these bodies to shreds. Authors began to use the trope of the far-off land, where impressions *naturally* led to different moral rules, as an implicit attack on the absolutist claims of the *ancien régime*.

Thus, the arguments in *On the Spirit* blended well with those of Montesquieu, and for good reason. This outrageous model of inner life was the brainchild of Montesquieu's friend, Claude-Adrien Helvétius. Condemned as dangerous, sacrilegious, and subversive, *On the Spirit* generated a storm of protest throughout Europe while being recognized by the likes of David Hume as a work of genius. Inevitably, a clamor built against the author. While his wife lobbied the censor and Voltaire fought to save the renegade writer, a 1760 Parisian theatrical satire, *The Philosophers*, ignited the public's wrath against Helvétius. Voltaire advised his friend of the growing danger, the writer got the message, and he fled to England. However, his book remained on French soil and became a steady underground best-seller.

While being titillated, French readers of *On the Spirit* were also befuddled. "Soul" and "spirit" were terms with which one prayed, spoke of one's spiritual essence and one's relation to God. With these newer secular definitions, it seemed the same words could be employed for all-too-human purposes. Was conscience—the inner experience by which a good Christian considered good and evil— now also some broad description of a human's awareness of herself? The slippage between these definitions tossed readers back and forth between Heaven and Earth. From the Lord's Prayer to Helvétius, French readers vertiginously spun.

A telling confusion awaited Helvétius when the author sought to translate his book into English. Voltaire wrote to his befuddled friend, whose English was poor, to warn him that *esprit*, a word so equivocal in French that it might signify the soul or the mind, had no such ambiguity in English. Voltaire advised, that any English translation of his title must refer to human "understanding." And in fact, in 1759, the translator simply rendered the title as *Essays on the Mind*. In his *Pocket Philosophical Dictionary*, Voltaire further addressed this confusion with his French readership and asked: "And what is it that, for want of a better term, you've called 'intelligence,' *esprit*, from the Latin *spiritus* ('breath')? You haven't a clue, have you?"

And yet a great deal was at stake in having a clue. While professors and theologians continued to use Cartesian notions of the soul and spirit in schools, claims regarding thinking matter, a seemingly nonspiritual spirit, and a natural, even potentially material, soul began to infiltrate French life.

John Locke continued to be the central authority associated with the mind in France. As French thinkers sought to popularize and simplify his thought, Luc de Clapiers, the Marquis of Vauvenargues, a friend of the ubiquitous Voltaire, anonymously published *Introduction to the Knowledge of the Human Mind* in 1746. That same year, another unsigned work made the rounds. *Essay on the Origin of Human Knowledge, Where We Reduce to a Single Principle All that Concerns the Human Understanding* advertised its wares well. The author promised to bring clarity to the brilliant but sloppy Locke. The result led to accusations that the author was a plagiarist, and in England, this new book would be published with a subtitle, *Being a Supplement to Mr. Locke's Essay on the Human Understanding.* However, while this author considered himself a follower of Locke, he proposed a drastic and consequential alteration to the Englishman's theory.

Étienne Bonnot, the Abbé de Condillac, was an abbé in name only, for he was a freethinker. Condillac revered John Locke, but when he referred to the mind as *l'âme*, his choice was not slippery or passive, but based on a theological justification. While Locke posited that men received ideas from both passive sensation and their capacity for active reflection, Condillac proposed that while Adam and Eve may have possessed both of these modes of knowledge, after being banished from Eden, human beings lost their reflective capacity. Since the Fall, humans possessed only the limited capacity to know the world through the passive processes of their senses. They could not consider and reflect and judge. And if he was accused of eliminating the active mental element that allowed for moral choice and free will, Condillac could simply blame that on Adam and Eve.

Thus, humans strode out into the world, naked and with minds that were emptied, blank slates. Everyday experience swarmed them with impressions, many of which were instantly lost. However, through the connection of these ideas and the use of signs and language, faculties of the mind were gradually constructed, such as attention, perception, and consciousness, then memory, imagination, and reflection. Hence, Condillac, that determined "Lockist"— Voltaire contrasted him with "Asininists"—differed from his teacher in this way. He did not believe that there was an autonomous capacity for reflection. Humans no longer enjoyed such power.

With that one change, the French sensationalists were born. A group of thinkers emerged who considered all human knowledge and interior life to be exclusively due to external impressions. In

1754, Condillac made this case more vividly, with an extended thought experiment that would come to symbolize his beliefs. Imagine a statue, he began, endowed with the love of pleasure and the hatred of pain. Next, give that otherwise inert thing the capacity to smell. Then add sight, touch and, one by one, the other sensations. What kind of mind would result? The answer was our minds: "The statue is therefore nothing but all that she has acquired," the abbé concluded. "Why is this not the same with man?"

These conclusions struck many as too mechanical and at odds with free will. Condillac's statue, like Descartes's theory of the animal machine, clearly referred to the water-powered automatons that stunned audiences throughout Europe. However, evidence of other kinds also influenced Condillac and his followers. For example, in London, a surgeon, Dr. Cheselden, had pulled off an astonishing feat: he restored sight to a man who had been blind since birth. This recovery offered an extraordinary opportunity to test one of Locke's theories. And in fact, the patient displayed no sense of extension and space. These were, Cheselden seemed to prove, purely learned.

Condillac knew of the English blind man, as did his coterie of allies, brilliant writers like a young Jean-Jacques Rousseau and Denis Diderot, who regularly huddled with him at the Hôtel du Panier Fleuri. Diderot embraced these ideas; after all, he had inspired Condillac with his own attempt to dissect the sensory components of the psyche in a series of philosophical essays on the blind, the deaf, and the dumb. But Condillac's imaginary statue unnerved Rousseau and made him concerned that such a line of thought could only end in apostasy.

Of course, the abbé did not seek to depart from Christian ethics. In an addendum to his *Treatise on the Sensations*, he insisted that human will was free. Man repented, deliberated, and chose between desires. He had the capacity to be moral. Nonetheless, there was something contrary, even uncanny and unacknowledged, in Condillac's insistence that this sensing statue possessed the capacity for intentionality. "Once our statue realizes this power," he wrote, "it realizes it is free."

Condillac's statue captured others' imaginations. From Geneva, Charles Bonnet had run the same thought experiment, and expressed shock that another's conception of the mind was so close to his own. Man, he wrote, was an organic statue until he opened his eyes and ears and mouth. Bonnet had anonymously published *Essay on Psychology* in 1755. In this, perhaps the first modern work of French "psychology," Bonnet adopted Lockean presumptions but explicitly considered the thinking faculty to be immaterial soul. In his 1760 work, *Analytic Essay on the Faculties of the Soul*, however, Bonnet sought to reduce the operations of the soul to its parts, search for relations between these pieces, then map out the effects of each. Soul analysis, he insisted, must resemble the anatomical interrogations of a physician. If that sounded like an atheistic taking-apart of the soul like it was a clock, Bonnet was ready. He had dissected the soul's operations, not its immaterial essence. Still, as the author excitedly discussed the amazing mechanical duck built by Vaucanson, one could only wonder how far an ingenious inventor might go.

Despite himself, Bonnet's attempt to pursue how the soul and the body influenced each other also led to a creeping mechanization of inner life. Newtonian conceptions as employed by, among others, Leiden's doctors like Boerhaave, had the potential to extend into traditional soul functions, as was evident in Guillaume-Lambert Godart's 1755 book on the physics of the human soul, or Claude-Nicolas Le Cat's 1767 book on sensations. Le Cat, a physician from Rouen, said that the soul's actions on the body were mysterious, but pushed on to argue that reason was so deeply predicated on the body as to be at times its equivalent. If this was not across the line, it was very close.

Bonnet's "psychology" was born into this confused world. The term was not his invention but one that dated back to the late 16th century when it denoted the study of the soul. In England, Thomas Willis had used it decades earlier, and, more important, it had been heralded by the German philosopher Christian Wolff, whose influential work filtered into France during the 1730s. Because of his praise of Chinese morals, Wolff was run out of Prussia by the bloodthirsty Friedrich Wilhelm I, only to be urged to return home and head the Berlin Academy after the king's rebellious son took power. By then, Wolff had published two books, *Empirical Psychology* and *Rational Psychology*. Bowdlerized texts of these works made their way into France after the philosopher's death. Wolff's inquiries began with the reality of consciousness, which he equated with the immaterial soul. Much as with prior authors from the 16th and 17th centuries, for him, psychology remained the study of soul-consciousness.

Thanks to Helvétius, Condillac, Diderot, Bonnet, and others, an approach to the mind emerged in France. Sensationalist models of inner life often hedged on the materiality of the mind, but went further than Locke by eliminating innate capacities for reflection. These theories predicated knowledge on the fallible process of sensation, and hence shook beliefs in any invariable truths that could emerge from human understanding. If varied experiences made for different ideas, morals, and minds, who was to say which was wrong? Between Chinese morals and those of the Jesuits, who knew? Surely, Voltaire's Indian cannibal would be a crazed monster if she were dropped into the world of Versailles. However, French aristocrats would seem insane if transplanted to a tepee in the New World.

Such questions on human nature would grow in importance as some reformers and radicals began to reconsider France's political and ethical life. If laws were not innate, soul-based, or divinely inspired, if they were not God-given revelations, but rather rickety, man-made impressions, then surely they could be wrong. For Voltaire and other reformers, sensationalism thus supported a wide-ranging attack on religious fanaticism, magical claims, bigotry against other religions, and morals predicated on the hereafter. If knowledge was always contingent, then there could be no incontestable basis for these things.

Radical sensationalism contained other powerful, destabilizing, implications. If all knowledge came from all-too-human capacities like seeing and hearing, was it possible that "reality" itself was a grand illusion? In the hands of the British philosopher George Berkeley, it seemed so. Influenced by Locke, Berkeley, the Lord Bishop of Cloyne, allowed that blue was the color our senses assigned to the sky, nothing more. The sole absolute truth was in ideas, and thus his brand of idealism put his followers back inside Plato's cave. Was the verity of our experiences really just a long, strange trip into hallucination? Voltaire scorned such sophistry and worried it would let the credulous believe any old thing. Strolling with James Boswell, Samuel Johnson shared Voltaire's disgust. When discussing Berkeley's belief in the unreality of the world, he struck his foot with "mighty force" against a stone, and triumphantly declared, "I refute him *thus*."

Matter was not the only thing that could melt away in the realm of ideas and senses; radical sensationalism meant minds had no active power; hence, all the previously assumed faculties of the mind, such as memory, reason, and imagination, were erased. The mind might weave complex entities, but it possessed no intrinsic capacity for judgment, rational choice, or ethical deliberation. And if this was so, it also meant that humans routinely and rather grossly deceived themselves. Their narratives of deliberation and choice were fictions.

Helvétius recognized that his own model eliminated free will. How could there be liberty "if as Mr. Locke has proved, we are the disciples of friends, parents, books and, in fine, all the objects that surrounded us? All our thoughts and wills must then be the immediate effects . . . of the impressions we have received." Armed with his beliefs in the mind's capacity for reflection, John Locke himself was in no such corner. However, French sensationalists having rid themselves of any overarching intelligence, faced charges of fatalism. Helvétius weakly declared that philosophers could treat the effects of liberty, not its causes. Voltaire also tried to wiggle out of this bind: "Liberty is nothing but the ability to do what I want," he offered.

However, he did not refute the belief that what one *wanted* might be fully determined.

Questions regarding human freedom were not academic. Liberty as a human right was becoming a growing political concern for the *lumières*. How could one advocate for individual political freedoms if men and women possessed no such capacity? Religious tolerance, individual rights, voting rights, and a liberal state were all predicated on a belief that women and men could act on their intentions. It made no sense to seek to liberate a statue or a whirring contraption.

⌒

THE POLYMATH DENIS Diderot spent much of his adult life wrestling with the conundrums posed by fatalism and free will, materialism and living beings, and the mind and its place in Nature. The son of a cutler who made surgical instruments, Denis trained in the Jesuit school in his native Langres, then settled in Paris, where he received a masters of arts degree from the University of Paris in 1732. Ultimately, however, the boy could not abide his family's expectations to become either a clergyman or a lawyer. Disowned by his father, Diderot began to eek out a living as a tutor, translator, and pen for hire. He churned out sermons, translated Shaftesbury, and then was hired to translate that symbol of Enlightenment, the dictionary.

Publishers had decided that a French edition of Robert James's *A Medicinal Dictionary* would be profitable. The British inventor of the Fever Powder, along with his childhood chum Samuel Johnson, had churned out three thick volumes of information that covered much of medicine. To do so, they had made use of the common, if slimy, strategy of plagiarizing works from foreign languages. Since most of their readers had no access to foreign works, there was little risk of being found out, that is, until this French edition was proposed. Diderot and Dr. James's other French translators realized that they were translating stolen French sources back into French.

During this time, Diderot was also translating himself. Once a committed Cartesian, he read Voltaire's seminal essays on the English and promptly embraced Locke and the Newtonian form of Deism that his French compatriot did so much to promote. In 1746, Diderot anonymously put out *Philosophical Thoughts,* essays that argued, among other things, that Christians were led by inspired madmen called "prophets" and obsessed with a delusion about reincarnation. Such beliefs, the author believed, provided no bulwark against atheism. Only a unitary God who designed a law-bound world could do that.

Banned and burned, the book, though unsigned, made the author's reputation in the salons of Paris, where the young Diderot's omnivorous intellect thrived. He made the rounds at different venues and bedazzled audiences. His circle of admirers grew. Encouraged by a low-life publisher, the still-impoverished Denis whipped off the novel *The Indiscreet Jewels,* his 1748 stab at the thriving genre of philosophical pornography. In this work, one character proposed that the soul started in a newborn's feet and worked its way up toward the head, but that in certain voluptuous women, it got stuck in their "jewels" and lingered there evermore. A year later, the young pornographer took a strictly philosophical approach to the question of human sensation with a work on blindness. Considering this deficit, he concluded, might highlight what vision provided for our inner lives. A blind man, for example, would have no shame in his own nakedness. Thus, he concluded, moral absolutes might be provisional, accidents of our senses. Meanwhile, Diderot had discovered Spinoza and adopted the radical materialist's view that spirit and matter were one and the same. In such a determined universe, free will was a cosmic jest.

This dazzling thinker soon found his own freedom at risk. The police had been watching him for over a year. Joseph d'Hémery, an officer who specialized in monitoring the book trade, found it possible to tolerate and even admire a number of *philosophes*. Diderot, he concluded, was "a very clever boy but extremely dangerous." In July of 1749, Denis was imprisoned in the *donjon* at the Château de Vincennes. His crimes were ones of thought and expression: his erotic novel and his philosophy of the blind made him a risk to morals. More particularly, the well-informed policeman, who filled his files with the writer's' profane jokes and lewd songs, likely culled from spies at different salons, noted that Diderot "prides himself on his impiety, very dangerous, speaks of the holy mysteries with scorn."

After a short time in the *donjon* and a longer period confined to the château, Diderot was released. While he would continue to pursue his concerns about the mind and Nature in works that combined his deep knowledge of the sciences and medicine with his adroit literary style, he would not risk incarceration. Instead, his sarcastic and biting critiques would be passed around in clandestine literary circles and only published after his death.

By the time of his release from Vincennes, Diderot had more than his own skin to preserve. Before being imprisoned, Diderot had been engaged in a massive project that had been approved by the censors: he hoped this work would become a public monument to the progressive, rational worldview he espoused. Initially, he had been chosen by a publisher to produce a French version of Ephraim Chambers's English *Cyclopaedia*. A highly successful reference work, Chambers had, like Robert James, simply helped himself to a great deal of writings from Europe. After his experience with the James book, Diderot made the case that a translation of Chambers into French would just be in good part a retranslation of French sources. It would elicit scorn and rage from the authors whose work had been pilfered. He convinced the publisher to sponsor a new work to compete with the *Cyclopaedia*.

Diderot was a superlative choice for this massive undertaking.

His command of science, philosophy, and literature was vast, and he sat at the center of a network of writers who could be recruited for help. In addition to Jean-Jacques Rousseau and Condillac, he was so close to Helvétius that many whispered he had been involved in the writing of *On the Spirit*. He was also a regular at the influential salon of Paul-Henri Thiry, the Baron d'Holbach. After arriving in Paris in 1749, the baron regularly opened his sumptuous mansion to a glittering array of libertine playwrights, poets, doctors, journalists, and freethinkers. He himself had fallen under the sway of mechanistic philosophy as a student in Dr. Boerhaave's Leiden. In 1770 when he anonymously published his *System of Nature*, this atheist opened his argument by swiftly dismissing the soul and insisting that all was due to matter and motion, the fundaments of Nature. Men had been deluded to think their inner impules emerged from some immaterial source, rather than simple, internal motion. Such a prejudice only led to delusion and unhappiness. This work was immediately condemned and burned; equally quickly, it leapt to the top of the list of desired illicit books.

With approval from the royal censor, the *Encyclopedia, or Dictionary of the Sciences, Arts, and Trades, by a Society of Men of Letters* recruited articles to encompass all that was known, and more slyly to introduce and advocate for the new philosophy of reason championed by the *lumières*. Along with his coeditor, the mathematician Jean-Baptiste le Rond d'Alembert, Diderot began the daunting task of ordering and categorizing all of human knowledge.

To do so meant wading into dangerous waters. As the police reports show, a great deal was tolerated with regard to new scientific discoveries and social perspectives, but attacks on the soul and the mysteries of Christianity, while paraded about in illegal writings and elite salons, were still publicly unacceptable. And yet, any work that proposed to organize and unite all of knowledge needed to face the divide that moderns had encountered since the collapse of the scholastic system. How would they link soul and Nature, revelation and reason, religion and science? And how would they do this without the censors shutting them down?

This delicate task called for Diderot's terrific linguistic capacities and rhetorical sophistication. However, when an overarching introductory statement came due, the mastermind of the *Encyclopédie* was shut up inside Vincennes. His junior partner, d'Alembert, who had been recruited for his precocious scientific acumen, not his philosophical talents, set to work on their blueprint for modernity.

Abandoned by Madame de Tencin, the renegade nun who found her métier as a wealthy *salonnière*, Jean-Baptiste le Rond d'Alembert grew up to be a prodigy who won fame at the age of twenty-six through innovative work on Newtonian dynamics. Now seven years later, he had been asked to find a way to unify all knowledge. Surprisingly, the result was a stunning success, a far-reaching manifesto that drew applause from the likes of Voltaire and Frederick the Great. The *Preliminary Discourse* would also be an effective piece of advertisement that inspired a small army of volunteers who now offered their services to this massive project. And while it elicited concern from Jesuits, d'Alembert was sly enough to give the censors no obvious cause to halt the operation. Perhaps this is what the persecuted Montesquieu meant when he congratulated d'Alembert for a work that was nervous yet precise and contained more thoughts than words. By craftily zigzagging, the author of the *Preliminary Discourse* managed to avoid a premature showdown between the old and the new.

On June 28, 1751, the *Preliminary Discourse* appeared with the first volume of the *Encyclopedia*. D'Alembert billed his preface as nothing less than a "philosophical history of the *esprit*." But what did he mean by *esprit*? In his short history, he lauded Locke as the thinker who held up a mirror to man and created an "experimental physics of the soul (*âme*)." Physics of the soul? For those who expected the author to elaborate, there was little more. D'Alembert would not land in the *donjon*, for he expressedly employed supernatural notions of the soul and the spirit, though he himself grew confused about when to use *esprit* or *âme* and, in later editions, went back to change one word for the other.

Nonetheless, this history of all that was known could not avoid the obvious: it would be predicated on the editors' beliefs in the capacities and limits of human understanding, the very question that pushed Locke to posit the mind and the one that became heated with the rise of the French sensationalists and their fight with Cartesians. Would the immaterial soul be at the base of all knowledge?

The editors did what they needed to do: they dodged. All knowledge could be thought of as related, one, part of the same tree with different branches. The idea of a Tree of Knowledge was not original: Chambers had used it, and he himself had borrowed this analogy from Sir Francis Bacon, whom d'Alembert invoked. However, the roots of Bacon's tree in 1605 were not in question. Human knowledge, he had confidently asserted, was based on the traditional faculties of the rational soul. The soul's capacity for memory gave rise to history, its imagination created aesthetics, and its reason produced philosophy. By following Bacon, d'Alembert and Diderot now seemed to predicate human knowledge on faculties that—as followers of Condillac—they believed were neither innate, nor God-given, nor real.

Nonetheless, d'Alembert's tree mirrored Bacon's, rather than introducing a mind based on new principles. The study of Nature was given over to science, but when it came to the science of man, the editors cautiously divided things up in the orthodox manner: studies of the body were for medicine, and studies of the soul were for metaphysics. *Pneumatology,* or soul science, was dutifully listed as the way to comprehend rational and sensitive souls.

While Francis Bacon's schema was a step away from those who considered knowledge to derive from a tree in the Garden of Eden, a century and a half later, the authors of the French *Encyclopedia,* by reproducing Bacon's assumptions, risked building their entire edifice on what many savants now considered to be thin air. While call-

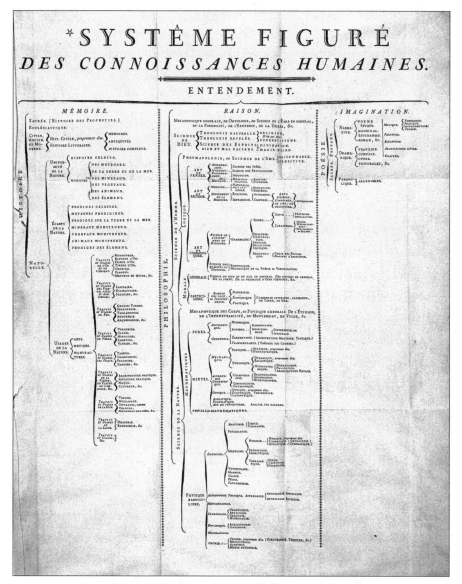

Figure 24. In their *Encyclopedia*, Diderot and d'Alembert divided all knowledge according to the faculties of memory, reason, and imagination.

ing for the advance of reason and science, they continued to employ supernatural categories that made it seem as if the last century of debates about the mind added up to nothing.

Such contradictions were the price of publishing in absolutist

France. However, in a series of asides, d'Alembert winked at his readers. In a discussion of religious authority and its history of stifling honest inquiry, he turned to Sir Francis Bacon and granted that while this great thinker broke free from many shackles forged by the scholastics, he was, alas, still enchained. It was left to the reader to guess what those shackles might be.

And later, d'Alembert took back some of the ground he had ceded to tradition. His march through human history showed that progress was based on faculties of knowledge that were built up through sensations. He claimed that the first human sensations led man to recognize the existence of God, the immortality of the soul, and other church truths. Having gotten that out of the way, he argued that, since the Renaissance, humans had accumulated more and more experience that resulted in the perfection of their mental capacities, which undercut any notion of innate, God-given faculties! D'Alembert even suggested that ethics were founded prior to Christianity. Thus, it was not the soul and revelation that taught men how to behave, but the growing, sensing, and perceiving mind.

"The universe, if we may be permitted to say so," he allowed, "would only be one fact and one great truth for whomever knew how to embrace it from a single point of view." However, while resurrecting the possibility of a modern Great Chain of Being, he kept to Cartesian dualism: the unbridgeable divide between matter and consciousness. Rocks, bees, mankind, and God could all be linked someday, but for now Nature and the soul would remain distinct.

In the end, despite some discordant notes, when the censor closed the *Encyclopedia* after d'Alembert's introduction, he could rest content. Only those who made their way into the reams of verbiage contained in the forthcoming volumes discovered more disturbing things. The *Encyclopedia* grew to some 74,000 entries and articles, in which named and anonymous authors proposed points of view that ranged from the conventional to the radical. Scholastic, Cartesian, Lockean and more obscure views jostled alongside each other. In the end, d'Alembert's *Preliminary Discourse* served, intentionally or not, as a Trojan Horse: inside its conventional framework lurked a vast range of opinions, including some spear-throwers dedicated to toppling the status quo.

The most important of these hidden radicals was none other than Denis Diderot. In the first volume, he signed a 27-page entry on the soul, the supposed foundation of all knowledge. Throughout this extensive essay, the author made it clear that the most impressive challenge to reigning doctrines came from Baruch Spinoza and his belief that the universe was all one substance. In Diderot's sweeping account, he included appraisals of materialists from Lucretius to Hobbes, but again and again, the central authority that he considered over the first fifteen pages was the scandalous Spinoza. After much careful deliberation, Diderot distanced himself from that thinker, but his extensive, respectful exposition spoke for itself. With enemies like this, the Jesuits might have muttered, Spinoza needed no friends.

Denis Diderot's omnibus essay also demonstrated how much would need to be rethought if in fact man did not have a soul. If that knot was untied, new accounts would be badly needed for matter and universe, thought and mind, the difference between the living and the dead, as well as the animal and human. New explanations would be needed for Nature and the possibility of free will, ethics, the afterlife and mortality, the relationship between body and consciousness.

Within the *Encyclopedia,* numerous thinkers weighed in on these problems. While overtly bowing to the immortal soul, many hurried on to consider what the world would look like if everything was known through sensory experience. One unsigned essay on logic, one of the rational soul's central functions, stated that understanding of this "operation of the soul" was perfected first by Locke, then Condillac, which meant it took place because of sensations. Buried in this and other seemingly traditional accounts, there were enough little flickers against *ancien régime* to start a fire.

The *Encyclopedia* was an instant success. Over 130 contributors authored thousands of articles. Readers no longer needed to turn to illegal literature to read long essays on archheretics like Hobbes and Spinoza. While most accounts sought to diminish these materialists, some, such as the author of the entry on liberty, did not. Condillac wrote no articles, but was referred to in many. Conscience, the source of moral and religious life, was given a common definition, but then was considered through the lens of John Locke and the sensationalists.

For a while, the powers being challenged did not seem to notice. Then in 1759, an abbé from Prades plagiarized whole paragraphs from d'Alembert's preface for his own thesis. Horrified that the new philosophy had found its way into the thought of one of their own students, the Church protested. The censor's approval for the entire project was rescinded. Eventually, d'Alembert abandoned the project, leaving Diderot alone to toil on this *summa* of modern knowledge. He would soldier on for thirteen years and produce twenty-eight volumes. Despite their heterogeneous nature, these books would become central to the dawning of an Age of Reason, one predicated less on belief and revelation, and more on an entity that, though still called the spirit or the soul in French, had taken on distinct characteristics of being a sensing and perceiving mind.

11

Vitalism, the Missing Link

D URING THE EARLY decades of the 18th century, French anatomists took up Descartes's quest to find the seat of the soul, and by 1750, enough seats had been found for a dinner party. In his essay on the soul for the *Encyclopedia*, Diderot showed off his learning by surveying these findings. After Descartes's now discredited claims for the pineal gland, a Dr. Vieussens had pinned the *pneuma* down in the oval center of the nervous system, while Dr. Petit pointed to two eminences at the anterior of the ventricles. Others fingered the cerebellum, and Le Cat, the surgeon from Rouen, raised the flag of victory when he discovered the soul in the tissues that covered the brain, the pia mater and dura mater. Diderot himself sided with King Louis XV's trusted surgeon, Dr. de La Peyronie, who by a careful process of elimination seemed to prove that the soul resided in that tough tissue between the two cerebral hemispheres, the corpus callosum.

However, French doctors could not avoid the problems that emerged from a neat divison between soul and matter. Dr. Stahl's *anima,* instead of maintaining those two categories, gave the soul back its power to determine bodily illness and health. Meanwhile, a growing body of evidence seemed to undercut the medical mecha-

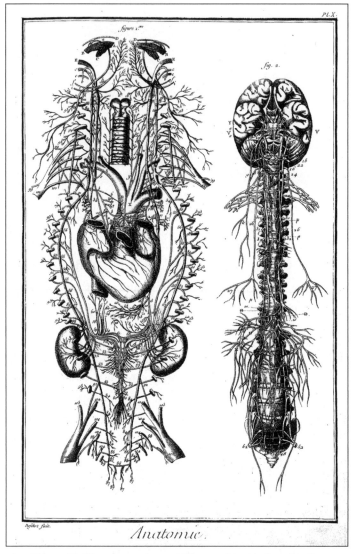

Figure 25. The nervous system illustrated in the *Encyclopedia*.

nists' view of the body. After the Dutch Antonie van Leeuwenhoek stared through his microscope at microrganisms wiggling about, after Jan Swammerdam demonstrated that muscles still responded to nervous stimuli even after they were severed from the spinal cord, and after experiments showed that cut-up polyps still contracted, it became increasingly troublesome to claim the body was a passive machine. Rather, it seemed to have some inner force that as early as 1672 the English doctor Francis Glisson had called irritability. Even in Catholic France, some began to think that it was not enough to defend Descartes's division. A new theory was required that remade the bodily machine and, with it, the soul.

RAISED IN SAINT-MALO, a port city in Brittany, Dr. Julien Offray de La Mettrie was a rebel and a publicity hound, just the kind of man to shout out what others only dared to whisper in private. In doing so, he created a *succès de scandale* and catapulted the debates over the nature of the body and the soul into the glare of French public awareness. His notorious work assaulted the delicate boundaries that separated science and religion, and forced more French doctors to enter the soul debates, if only at first to violently denounce this colleague.

Born in 1709, Julian considered a life in the clergy, imbibed a Cartesian curriculum at the Collège d'Harcourt, then decided to try medicine. After some years in Paris, he went to Leiden and took in Boerhaave's approach to human physiology and illness. Won over to mechanical theory, La Mettrie dedicated himself to translating the Leiden master. In his translations of Boerhaave, La Mettrie incorporated the commentary of the famous Swiss doctor Albrecht von Haller, then added a few shocking thoughts of his own, namely that the faculties of the rational soul could be seen in mechanical terms.

Returning to France, the young doctor won a post as a military surgeon. During the War of the Austrian Succession, he contracted an illness and during a febrile delirium had an epiphany. As overheated hallucinations danced before his eyes, he concluded that all thought and understanding must be predicated on the body. This, by itself, was not news. Both Galenic and Cartesian doctors believed that fever and other bodily factors could disrupt the immaterial soul and make for madness. La Mettrie, however, was eager to push this further.

In 1745, *The Natural History of the Soul* appeared in print. The book was attributed to an Englishman, "Mr. Charp," and was purported to be translated by an unnamed member of the French Academy of Sciences. Amid this subterfuge, the book was dedicated to a real person, Pierre-Louis Moreau de Maupertuis, a famed natural philosopher also from Saint-Malo, who literally traveled to the ends of the Earth to prove Descartes wrong. Maupertuis had made an expedition to Lapland to take measurements and confirm Isaac Newton's contrary theory that the earth was flattened at the North and South poles. What the public did not yet know was that in private, this Frenchman also rejected Cartesian dualism and suggested that all animals possessed degrees of intelligence. With its title, *The Natural History of the Soul* seemed to promise a voyage like Maupertuis's, one to the farthest reaches of the inner world, in the service of dismantling Descartes's immaterial soul.

However, the title was misleading. This was no natural history, but rather an abstruse, at times confused, discussion of the soul's forms and its relations to matter. The author employed scholastic notions only to then demonstrate that they had been demolished by Locke. Mr. Charp dismissed innate ideas and considered the possibility that the mind's contents were only due to sensations; however, he would go only so far. The author mocked simpletons who would follow Spinoza and consider man to be but a machine. He would soon regret this display of contempt.

Two years later, when *The Natural History* was reprinted, a new personage appeared near the title page. Mr. Charp's work was now preceded by a critical letter written by an obscure doctor named Julian Offray de La Mettrie, addressed to Voltaire's lover, Émilie du Châtelet. Scholars suggest the two may never have met, but the familiar tone and the belles-lettristic tradition of dedicating works to one's mistress, said otherwise. In this faux letter, the doctor expressed shock over the many absurdities hazarded by Mr. Charp! He assured this lady that he himself had examined the same exact questions and had come to precisely opposite conclusions.

All this audacious catch-me-if-you-can trickery must have made for much private amusement, but if La Mettrie was ever convinced that his theatrics fooled anybody, he was wrong. *The Natural History of the Soul* was condemned and burned, and its true author was identified and forced to flee to Leiden. Enraged by this turn, the author picked up his pen again. The result would almost uniformly bring forth condemnation and horror. Before going public with his new outrage, La Mettrie scurried back to his earlier book on the soul. He deleted that short sentence in which he mocked those who considered humans to be machines, then he published *Man-Machine.*

The French doctor would become equated with the wild provocation in this title. Disgust and hatred rained down upon him. In Holland, *Man-Machine's* publisher hurried to save his own skin: in an advertisement placed at the front of the book, he disavowed the doctor's views, and in case there was any doubt, wrote a treatise called *Man More than a Machine.* Banned in France and even Leiden, La Mettrie's book was burned in The Hague. German reaction was particularly negative, once it was known that the author of *Man-Machine* had taken refuge in the court of the Prussian king Frederick the Great. Of all the troublemakers that this monarch gathered around him, to many, this one seemed to be the most unforgivable.

Lost in the uproar was the inherent ambiguity of La Mettrie's infamous title. By affixing man and machine, was he hoping to materialize the soul or animate matter? For many, the answer seemed clear: his title referred back to Descartes's "animal-machine," and therefore this renegade sought to extend mechanical thinking into the soul. However, for those who read beyond the title page, the author's position was not so clear. La Mettrie used the term "Man-Machine" just as John Locke had juxtaposed opposites with "thinking matter." At times, it seemed that he sought to fuse incompatible terms into something that modified and altered what it meant to be both a machine and a man. Was this mechanistic materialism, or a new kind of animism, or perhaps a jester's paradox?

La Mettrie seemed to support all of these points of views. In one passage, humans whirred like a set of levers and pulleys; in another they burned with inner force. *Man-Machine* forced forward the question that John Locke left to God: how *did* thought and active powers of reflection emerge from matter? Instead of repeating that the Maker simply made it so, La Mettrie looked to medicine. He chided those who were not physicians from daring to even discuss such a topic. Philosophers were handicapped by their ignorance of the body, while doctors alone could grasp the mixed nature of mind, matter and soul.

For La Mettrie, medicine taught that the body held the power of self-movement. Man was a weird, organic, alive kind of machine. Thus, older conceptions of mechanics needed to be revised into more dynamic models to explain human beings. Man was a "machine that winds its own springs." While La Mettrie still used *âme* to signify mental events, for him, this was an active principle, the mule pulling the cart. Hence, men and women were enlightened machines, the outcome of self-moving soul matter, replete with thought and feeling. When he died in 1751, La Mettrie left behind near-unanimous disgust that drowned out such subtlety.

However, inquiries continued into the meeting of man and machine. The precise medical source for La Mettrie's self-starting mechanism could be found in *Man-Machine*'s warm dedication. This kiss from the reviled outlaw landed on the cheek of the pious Albrecht von Haller. Dr. Haller recoiled and quickly denounced La Mettrie as possessed, if not by Lucifer, then at least by Lucretius. Adding insult to injury, Haller did not deign to refute La Mettrie in his scientific writing, but only in his theological essays. For he continued to maintain a hard line between biology and theology that fell precisely in front of the human soul. La Mettrie was a heretic and an idiot, a Spinozist and mechanist who didn't understand the limited implications of mechanics. This atheist forgot that machines can't build themselves and can't make for conscious experience.

Despite these protests, Haller could not fully disown La Mettrie. For whether he liked it or not, Haller had mapped out a way to merge science and the rational faculties of the soul. Unwittingly, his research seemed to create the posssiblity of a natural bridge between thought and matter.

MONTPELLIER SITS IN the southern outback of France, a broad swath of terrain far from Paris in the Languedoc province. Facing the Mediterranean, the city also looks east to Italy. Founded in the 13th century, Montpellier's medical school benefited from these nearby influences, taking Renaissance advances from Italian anatomists and developing a strong botanical tradition, thanks to Arabic innovations. Granted the right to dissect one criminal a year by the local Duke of Anjou, Montpellier built its own anatomy amphitheater in 1556 and created its Jardin des Plantes in 1597. Doctors in Paris could not boast of such facilities for another half-century.

A bastion of Huguenot sentiment, Montpellier became a boomtown in the late 18th century; mortality rates dropped, the population grew, as did its wealth. As this provincial administrative center increased in stature, so too did its medical school. While the Faculty of Paris strictly enforced its orthodoxy, Montpellier medicine became known for its openness to alternatives such as Paracelsian chemistry. And with patients, these innovators seemed to rival the more established Paris physicians. While Montpellier graduates were not formally allowed to practice in Paris without recertification, their best and brightest often found favor in royal courts, including the king's. Thus, in one fell swoop, they would be granted the right to practice throughout the country.

In the 18th century, Montpellier became the center for an alter-

native medical ideology that linked the mind and the body. Montpellier physicians snaked their way between Stahl's animism and
Boerhaave's mechanism, so as to account for human beings and their
inner lives in one unified model. In the process, Montpellier's leaders
were forced to reevaluate commitments that for decades had been
considered foundational for natural science. Most strikingly, they
dared resurrect a hated notion from Aristotelian science.

The elimination of teleological reasoning had been a huge
advance for modern students of Nature. Comets did not streak the
sky to achieve a final cause. Bacon, then Boyle and his colleagues,
sought to rid science of such claims. However, in Montpellier this
was challenged, at least for biology. The first leader of the Montpellier school scolded "the Moderns" for dismissing purpose in Nature,
and thereby cleared the way for Stahl and his soul-directed explanations. While some in the Montpellier school veered toward such
animism, others stuck to a more moderate path. The Montpellier
doctors recognized that there must be an active force in living matter, something that did not just react, but contained the power to *act*.
The body, the Montpellier theoreticians would argue, was a composite of living parts that, in sum, created something qualitatively new.
This challenge to reigning theories would be called vitalism.

Montpellier's turn toward vitalism began during the 1730s with
the arrival of François Boissier de Sauvages. Sauvages discovered that
the medical faculty was devoted to Cartesian medicine, much like
the rest of France. He was not impressed. Years earlier, as a medical student at Montpellier, he had written a thesis on the passions
and their affect on illness, than traveled to Paris where he became
immersed in the taxonomic study of plants at the Jardin du Roi. As a
young medical practitioner, he often found himself lost in a tangle of
symptoms. He yearned for a coherent nosology and began a lifelong
attempt to classify disease.

In 1731, Sauvages returned to Montpellier and quickly became
a highly influential professor, who advocated a new path in physi-

ology. As Sauvages attacked Descartes, he was surrounded by acolytes devoted to Stahl's theories, a spiritually based teleology without
constraints. Dr. Stahl believed one's God-given soul orchestrated all
bodily functions and acted to preserve health. Sauvages eventually
posited a more restrained theory, a mix of Stahl, Newtonian medicine, and the thought of the German Christian Wolff. The moderns,
according to the Montpellier doctor, had followed mechanistic materialism into fantasyland. By ridding Nature of teleology, they ran
into a dead end, because in fact, the body jumped with the power of
purpose, force, and intention.

Sauvages still attributed these forces to the soul. It was the soul
that knew, desired, and moved. These basic functions could be
divided: reason and reflection were conscious and strictly human,
while sensation, memory, and imagination were unconscious and
common to all animals. This last point was critical, for it answered
challenges from physiology. Did the soul really monitor each beat of
the heart, and each rise of the diaphragm? Where was this soul when
men slept? Dr. Sauvages answered that the inferior soul uncon-
sciously managed these tasks. However, a researcher then demonstrated that the heart could pump after death; that is, the cardiac
chambers pumped for a while *after* the human soul had departed.
Shaken by this discovery, Sauvages wrote to the Rouen surgeon Le
Cat to express his disbelief. Somehow, he insisted, these movements
must stem from the soul.

Some of Dr. Sauvages' students were open to other solutions. A
third way between mechanism and animism emerged among them.
While the 17th-century Cambridge doctor Francis Glisson was
credited with the notion that living matter may possess a distinct
"irritability," it was Haller who popularized this notion. His studies
showed that flesh possessed "irritability" and "sensibility." The first
was characterized by the retraction of muscle fibers from a stimulus.
The second represented the way nervous tissues transmitted this contact to the soul.

In 1752, Haller presented these ideas in two influential papers at the Royal Society of Sciences in Göttingen. Soon thereafter, he fell into debate with the man who had come closest to these conclusions, Scottish professor of medicine Robert Whytt. Whytt also advocated for a sentient principle in animal life: by studying vital and involuntary motions, he concluded that irritability was always attached to sensibility. However, Haller defended the notion that irritation was a quality of inferior biological beings, such as eels and mollusks, while sensibility was exclusively human.

As these debates swirled, Sauvages sent a distressed letter to Haller. Those who do not "believe in the power of the soul over the body," he worried, would employ these ideas and end up as "materialists, fatalists, Spinozists." His concerns were not ill founded. Even Sauvages began to move in a more secular direction. In his first nosology of illness, written in 1732, Sauvages had called for a class called "Spiritual Maladies," which he distinguished from madness, but by 1763, his nosologies omitted the soul entirely.

Sauvages and Haller were both devout men, but their eye-opening physiological studies of force and activity in the body upset the Cartesian balance between Nature and God, the body and the soul. Sensibility seemed to be a physiological function that made it possible to conceptualize higher intellectual functions and active capacities like will that had long been reserved for God. Theories of sensibility made one consider a totally new kind of machine, a dynamic, self-winding, partly autonomous one that possessed capacities like consciousness and reflection.

The dedication of *Man-Machine* to Albrecht von Haller was thus appropriate, for that pious physiologist had unwittingly cut a path for renegades to consider a fully humanized, thinking animal. And there was more that heretics could thank Haller for: the Swiss-born physiologist had postulated that different qualities were felt in different regions of the brain. Therefore, he had concluded that the seat of the soul—though *not* the soul itself—must have extension.

Characteristically, Julien de La Mettrie refused to dance around with the issue. Haller, he bluntly declared, had proven that the soul was a *thing*.

⸺

AMBITIOUS AND YOUNG, Théophile Bordeu plotted his escape from the provinces for years. Born February 22, 1722, near Pau in the Pyrenees, Bordeu was the son of a local doctor who had recently converted from Protestantism. The boy attended a Jesuit school, then studied medicine in Montpellier, and soon thereafter, like a number of ambitious Montpellier graduates, he began to dream of freeing himself from the petty professional rivalries he encountered in Pau, by making a big move.

First, Bordeu's ambitions sent him back to Montpellier for further studies. However, life there was distinctly unattractive, for religious strife had broken out. This Huguenot stronghold was periodically roiled by insurrection. In 1744, a year before Bordeu returned, a twenty-five-year-old charismatic Protestant pastor named Mathieu Majal had begun to attract massive crowds, estimated at 4,000 to 5,000. The king sent in troops, who arrested some 10,000 Protestants; the pastor was executed, as was his doctor. Bordeu's letters home are filled with the news of this crackdown, after which proof of being Catholic was required for even the most minor bureaucratic matters, including getting one's grades at school.

In medical school, Bordeu studied with Sauvages and was impressed by the debates between mechanists and supporters of Stahl's *anima*. In 1742, he completed a thesis on the topic of sensation, in which he rejected Boerhaave's views, thus alienating a number of the older Montpellier faculty. He suggested that the human body was not a machine but, as once imagined by Menenius Agrippa, more of a republic, composed of many living parts whose activity was regulated by sensibility imbued in the brain and nerves.

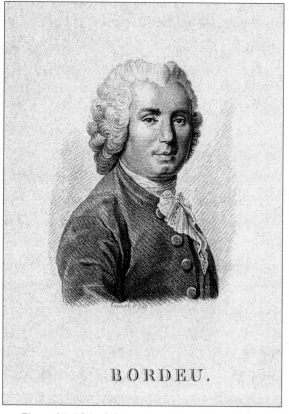

Figure 26. Théophile Bordeu, Montpellier vitalist.

With these ideas buzzing in his head, Bordeu began to dream of a change. He would go to Paris and, if given the chance, show all the Parisian charlatans and fashionable, money-hungry poseurs how to truly practice medicine. In the fall of 1746, Bordeu arrived, thanks to the support of his well-off cousin, Louis de Lacaze. For six years, the unlicensed Bordeu laid his hopes for fame and fortune at the feet of Lacaze, a successful Montpellier graduate and the only doctor in the capital he knew.

Dr. Lacaze was happy to take on his relative in exchange for an odd form of payment. Théophile was forced to ghostwrite a medical treatise for his mentor. At first, Bordeu was deeply grateful and considered the book "our project." However, over time Bordeu became embittered, then enraged, by this odd apprenticeship. By 1754, the younger man complained of this crazy doctor, who imagined he would create a new kind of medicine and exploited him for that purpose. Lacaze chastised this impudent ingrate. However, by then Théophile had made enough contacts of his own in Paris to survive. He broke free of his forced labor and cozied up to Denis Diderot and some of the most famed freethinkers in Paris. Bordeu cast off this "mad liar," who he believed had tried to enslave him.

Bordeu was not the only one acting as Lacaze's scribe. He had a similar arrangement with another young Montpellier medical graduate, Gabriel-François Venel. Venel later became famous for the bubbly water—"seltzer"—he discovered in Selz, Germany. However, he too made good use of his time as an apprentice and found his way into the salon of Baron d'Holbach. A friend of the encyclopedists, Venel became the editors' trusted contributor on *materia medica*, dietetics, and chemistry and contributed a staggering number of pieces, more than 700, to that enterprise.

Bordeu's collaboration with Lacaze appeared in print in 1755 and immediately was hailed as epochal. Granted approval by the royal censor, *The Idea of Physical and Moral Man: To Serve as an Introduction to a Treatise on Medicine* bore an epigraph from Lucretius and no author's name. The title announced a reframing of the battle between body and soul, mechanics and theology. Without siding with either camp, this new work proposed a full medicine of man, one that included the physical and the moral in its purview.

The guiding assumptions of the book, not surprisingly, came from Montpellier. First, there was the title, which offered new terms for a human science, one that dropped the old, freighted dichotomy of body and soul for a new, less charged one. In 1691, the Académie française defined "moral" as that which concerns the conduct of life. "Moral" generally alluded to, but did not directly refer to, conscience and the soul. Maneuvering into that grey zone, Lacaze and Bordeu proposed medicalizing the arena of good and bad habits and behaviors.

By proposing a unified medicine of the moral and the physical, Montpellier doctors could attempt a synthesis, a unification of bodily animal functions with mental life. Over the next decades, a number of French writers avoided the language of body and soul and pursued instead the physical and the moral. Lacaze and Bordeu argued that dividing mankind into a bodily machine and a soul destroyed the complex whole. Reductive mechanics typically broke a circle of causes and effects at some arbitrary point. To pull a force out of this complex chain and call it *the* cause, was to risk simplifying and worse, it led inevitably to confusing causes with effects. Autopsies studied dead bodies, not dynamic living beings. Baconian experimentation and empiricism alone made it difficult to recognize the big picture. Man was an elaborate ensemble of sentient, interacting parts, linked by sympathetic and antagonistic actions. Medical research should focus on the laws that governed the whole, what the Montpellier school had dubbed the "Animal Economy." This intricate assemblage linked the physical and moral aspects of humans in sickness and in health.

According to Lacaze and Bordeu, sensations affected the inner organs thanks to the nerves, which sent oscillating currents into the brain. The brain then acted to regulate the entire bodily system. This nascent psychophysiology seamlessly merged with French sensationalists, but in addition to outer influences, these doctors proposed that a "sentiment of our existence" sat at the center of experience. This state of consciousness originated in childhood, became organized around memories of pain and pleasure, developed into personal habits and organized one's choices and voluntary actions. When the mind was in a state of reflection, it produced electric currents that led to nerve sensation and then willful action. Thus one's mental state could deeply affect the animal economy, as demonstrated by the effects of terror on respiration, heart rate, and the skin.

Lacaze and Bordeu did not hesitate to draw out the political implications of their theory of moral life. Individuals' sensibilities determined their character. Overly sensitive persons too often served their own passions, much like primitive savages. Civilization helped develop restraints that held hedonism in check, even for these individuals, thereby changing their natural disposition. Reflection, the aspect of the mind that Locke foregrounded and Condillac dismissed, was the saving grace of cultured Europeans. Reflective capacities dominated the reactions of the civilized, who could resist their own emotions. However, these restrained beings were also prone to suffer from too much civilization; they could be excessively inhibited and develop nervous disorders. Mental disease did not result from Lockean misassociations, but rather from the overflow of sensibility or conversely, its excessive restraint.

While Lacaze's grandiosity annoyed Bordeu, the older man was not wrong to believe that French medicine was ripe for such a synthesis. For decades, the mechanists and animists had staked out contrary positions that made each other's vulnerabilities apparent. This holistic approach, pieced together from Sauvages and the Montpellier school, held out the possibility of incorporating mechanistic notions into a broader, complex system without resorting to supernaturalism.

The novelty of Bordeu and Lacaze's model became apparent when compared with the work of another supposed maverick, Antoine Le Camus. His 1753 *Medicine of the Spirit* also called for an integration of physical and moral medicine. Dr. Camus sought to unite medicine and metaphysics, and like La Mettrie, he insisted that this synthesis come from doctors not *philosophes*. Physicians needed to establish the operations of cerebral anatomy, discern the physical causes of human differences in *esprit*, and create therapies for *l'esprit*.

Given that the doctor employed Locke for his model of cognition, it might seem that this was also a call for naturalists to freely pursue mental therapeutics. It was not. In the end, Camus's book was a dizzying mix of brain fibers and souls, Locke and innate ideas, Galenic nonnaturals, biblical revelation, and new physiology, a staggering, uncoordinated attempt to found moral medicine. Always ready with his verbal dagger, Voltaire made quick work of this troubled effort. "Ah! Monsieur Camus," he quipped, "you haven't put much spirit into the Medicine of Spirit!" Adding to the embarrassment, in his second edition, published after La Mettrie had created a storm, Dr. Camus declared himself a faithful dualist.

By the time Lacaze's work was published, his coauthor had risen to some prominence. In *Anatomical Research on the Position of the Glands and Their Actions*, Théophile Bordeu argued that glandular activity was due not to mechanical forces like blood velocity, but rather a sensitivity inside living matter. Stahl, Sauvages, and Robert Whytt also subscribed to this view; however, they believed God's force was inside the body, a position that Bordeu mocked. He sketched out a fully materialist theory of sensibility based on the animal economy.

John Locke refused to elaborate on the link between body and mind. However, like Whytt and Hartley, Bordeu and Lacaze now dared to consider this question. They navigated away from Stahl, Sauvages, and mystical notions of the soul, and sought to naturalize the mind with the aid of an inherent force, a sensibility that resided in human physiology and could conceivably account for active mental processes like reflection, ethical choice, and free will.

Montpellier's materialistic vitalism began to take off in Paris. Bordeu's views began to be repeated in salons and journals, and he and his colleagues became allied with Diderot, d'Alembert, and Montesquieu. Editors of the *Encyclopedia* turned to Montpellier graduates, who began to offer this alternative perspective on a range of subjects.

Take, for example, Haller's notions of irritability and sensibility. Readers of the *Encyclopedia* discovered that the Montpellier school had eliminated the first term. Under "Irritability," three lines simply instructed one to turn to "Sensibility." Bordeu's student, Dr. Fouquet, contributed a lengthy exposition on sensibility and sentiment, as synonyms for the *agent conservateur* of life, that singular aspect of Nature that allows for animate action. A quick history moved from traditional views of the sensitive soul to Dr. Thomas Willis's nervous flame to the work of Bordeu and Lacaze.

In the *Encyclopedia*, a great expositor of the Montpellier school was Bordeu's acolyte Jean-Joseph Menuret de Chambaud. This doctor would contribute over eighty entries, including one on "Animal Economy" that alerted the reader to Lacaze's work, and insisted that the line between matter and mind needed to be breached. While medical philosophers were often accused of atheism, he wrote, to be a good moralist, it was necessary to be an excellent physician. The holistic theory of an animal economy allowed for this, by bringing to light the importance of self-regulation, a branch of medicine so often neglected. Such a perspective allowed one to consider managing "sensations from the passions, in a manner so positive and so clear, that it results in a medical treatise on moral life and happiness."

As theories of sensibility took center stage in Montpellier, these doctors evinced great interest in the passions. Menuret de Chambaud penned the entry on "Mania." The periodic fury, the singing, shouting, and quarrelsome behavior, even the prophetic enthusiasm, was ascribed to disruptions of one's sensibility. These occurred due to passions, forced studies, profound meditations, anger, sadness, fear, burning sadness, and lost love. While the actual derangement of the brain remained unknown, these complex disruptions left their mark and could be found on autopsy. As for treatment, Menuret de Chambaud highlighted the Montpellier school's skepticism about the standard medical reign of terror like induced dysentery, and instead looked to Nature to slowly regulate and heal.

Menuret de Chambaud noted mania's periodicity, which fit well with Bordeu's theories of physiological dysregulation. In "Crisis," his essay in the *Encyclopedia,* Bordeu argued that unlike a broken machine, the human body periodically fell into dysfunction and then could adjust and repair itself. This essay drew much attention and was excerpted in the *Journal des sçavans* and the *Journal économique*. Its call for gentle treatments and natural cures made Bordeu highly desired

among some highly placed aristocrats, most importantly Madame du
Barry, Louis XV's favorite mistress. Thanks to her, the provincial
doctor from Pau entered the king's Court.

Diderot and many of his fellow encyclopedists lived in danger,
while Bordeu now became a dignitary. He joined the Medical Faculty of Paris, and after 1770 was in line to become the king's physician. Bordeu's theories became so popular that he could hear them
echoed in his own mistresses' whispers. For instance, the Marquise
de la Vaupalière wrote: "Oh my dear Théophile, what pain your
absence makes for me both morally and physically." Indeed.

In 1768, Madame du Barry moved to Versailles and her physician
accompanied her. That year, he also sought to consolidate Montpellier's ascendancy by publishing a history of medicine that led inexora-
bly to their innovations. Through a materialistic vitalism, medicine
was poised to move beyond bodily ills to tackle not just individual
but also social problems. Medicine offered insights into the understanding of man's passions, habits, and temperaments, which were the
fundament of a nation. While French doctors like Louis XIII's personal physician, Marin Cureau de La Chambre, had written on the
maladies of the soul, the great breakthrough came with John Locke,
who, Bordeu reminded his readers, was both a doctor and a visitor
to Montpellier. Now doctors and philosophers must join together
and profit from Locke's advances by founding a truly philosophical
medicine.

Philosophers studied man, his passions, his society, and the revolutions of states. However, since there was no distinct soul and body,
only a mix of moral and physical elements in mankind, these thinkers were badly in need of medicine to ground their theories. Which
approach to medicine should be adopted by this new breed, which
Bordeu called *les médecins philosophes*?

Montpellier had adopted a naturalistic model, in which all movement was based on sensibility and sentiment. This was a synthesis, equally hostile to medical animism and mechanism. Heartbeats,

the blood pulse, and liver secretions were not externally driven but rather caused by inner sensibility. The mind also emerged from animal economies and their inner sensibilities.

For Bordeu, Fouquet, and Menuret, the living body was like a swarm of bees that hung from a tree, each with a life of its own, but in sum something quite different: a functioning hive. When in harmony, that hive was the model of health, while its disruption resulted in illness. Single, mechanical explanations missed the interactive nature of such living systems, what Lacaze called the "circle of action." The mind emerged from the sensitive interplay of the body. God did not need to superadd thought to matter, for out of those buzzing bits, reason and reflection were readily born.

〜

BY 1770, THE Montpellier school of Lacaze, Bordeu, Menuret, Venel, and others helped promote the exploration of "the physical and the moral" aspects of everything from gender difference to delirium to laughter. These arguments, which linked physiology and the self, compelled these doctors to be philosophers, and their conclusions pressed philosophers to consider medicine.

Vitalism of this sort steered clear of dualism and reductionism; it rescued consciousness from being either supernatural or a delusion. In the Montpellier model, consciousness was simply *ur*-sensibility, the most refined manifestation of that biologic building block. Locke's great dodge, his inability to justify the link between thinking and matter without recourse to God, now had a plausible natural grounding. Sensibility provided the missing link. It solved Mersenne's riddle by placing an active, natural force within the body's machinery. In this way, one could imagine that something like volition, reflection, and morality might exist within Condillac's statue.

Even though this link was hypothetical, it was treated as a breakthrough. Theories of sensibility suddenly opened the door for an embodied mind. Perhaps man did not reduce down to a ticking contraption, but rather the very idea of the body must be expanded to possibly include complex, dynamic functions, including wanting, thinking, and choosing.

In the salons of Paris, the *philosophes* took notice of these profound claims but no one more so than Denis Diderot. Diderot would later claim that the most interesting debates of his time involved medicine, and his fascination led him to radically alter his philosophical views. Early on, Diderot's reading of Voltaire's essays had made him embrace Deism. As he began work on the *Encyclopedia*, Diderot had become convinced by Spinoza that we exist in a monistic universe where mankind could exert no free will. However, over the next decade, Diderot's study of his close friend Bordeu and the other Montpellier encyclopedists persuaded him of their position. While early medical entries in the *Encyclopedia* came from a broad range of doctors, after 1765, Diderot relied heavily on contributors from Montpellier. He began to reject Spinoza's view that human action and choice were all illusions.

Diderot's hilarious novel *Jacques the Fatalist* mercilessly ridiculed such positions. Jacques' head, the author informed his reader, had been stuffed full of the opinions of Spinoza. Therefore, every decision that this hapless hero considered was also one he knew to be thoroughly out of his own control. It was to be, or it was not to be, he assured himself as he ran directly into one calamity after another. However, despite his philosophical education, this poor being could not rid himself of the silly illusion that he possessed the power to alter events:

> He said thank you to anyone who extended a helping hand, so that the helping hand might be extended again in the future. . . . He was often inconsistent, just like you or me, and inclined to forget his principles, except in some circumstances where his philosophy clearly had the upper hand. It was such

times that he'd say: "Such and such had to happen, for it was written on high that it would."

At the story's end, Jacques settled down to raise his children as disciples of Zeno and Spinoza. And he consoled himself. If fate dictated that his wife would cheat on him, she would, and if not, she would not.

Diderot was not eager to test his own fate. Closely watched by the police, he circulated this comical meditation in private. Nor did he publish his next attempt to grapple with philosophy in fiction. Written in 1769, *D'Alembert's Dream* featured a character named Dr. Bordeu, who offered up answers regarding the essence of life and the nature of the mind. For this fictional Bordeu, the mind was a web of nerves that at its center held a spider, which was active consciousness. The analogy perfectly captured the viewpoint of the Montpellier group.

However, before Diderot could fully accept such views, he needed to unwind some of his older positions. Rumored to have aided Helvétius during the writing of *On the Spirit*, an older Diderot returned to that work to privately unwrite parts of it. In dense annotatations of his copy of that book, he now demanded to know how education and experience alone could account for all human differences. How could Helvétius ignore inner forces like health, sickness, and the differences of physical and moral makeup? And when Helvétius at times seemed to allow that the qualities of thought were not consistent with those of material objects, Diderot countered that matter was active and could easily account for mental action. There was no need to divide mind and body; thought was based on sensation, which was itself seamlessly rooted in physical sensibility. As to the ultimate nature of sensibility, the *philosophe* conceded that its workings were mysterious and he invited "all physicians and chemists" to focus on this magical property of organized matter, one that anyone could witness if they watched an egg transform from gooey matter into a furry chick.

This most medically oriented of the *philosophes* spent his last years trying to delve into this riddle himself. At his death, Diderot left behind an uncompleted manuscript, *Elements of Physiology*, in which he leaned on Haller, Bordeu, and others to argue for a biology based on sensibility. He embraced the Montpellier stance on the emergence of a complex biologic organization, and conceived of the mind as an active, sensing machine, capable of reflection and conscious choice and action. Aware of the paradox inherent in a model of the mind in which the subject was also an object to itself, Diderot expressed it in the form of a riddle: "Here is the book. But where is the reader? The reader is the book itself."

Nervous sensibility organized in the brain allowed for the emergence of memory, thought, self, and consciousness. Nature and mind were inextricable; in the aggregate, physical and moral life were one. That did not mean one couldn't distinguish parts of mental life that were mechanized and outside individual control, and others that were freely willed. To do so required a new kind of study that allowed for both possibilities. As with other 18th-century thinkers, philosophy had led Diderot to medicine, and medicine had led him back to philosophy.

By the time of Diderot's death, it became increasingly common for French writers to claim that philosophy and medicine should be entwined, especially when it concerned matters of morals, behavior, and intellect. If Descartes and Montesquieu enlightened philosophy through medicine, one physician wrote, Montpellier shined the light of reason on medicine through its use of philosophy. However, the results were not always enlightening. Consider the medicophilosophical work of one of Bordeu's acolytes, Pierre Roussel.

Another doctor from the southern Languedoc region, Roussel finished his general education in Toulouse, then turned to medicine, in the belief that it offered vast philosophical opportunities. He studied in Montpellier, trekked to Paris, then became close to Bordeu, whose practice he covered when the older physician was out of town.

In 1772, devastated by the death of his benefactor and perhaps worried about his own survival, Roussel threw himself into writing a provocative book that would make his name.

"I have always been convinced," Roussel wrote, "that it is only within medicine that one finds the foundations for good moral philosophy, and that if anything can lead medicine to the state of perfection, it will be the care that medical thinkers take never to lose sight of the internal force that governs animated beings." By distinguishing sensibilities—crude and refined, sensitive and dull, rational and irrational—one could help medicine reach beyond the sickbed to heal whole cultures. Armed with this assumption, Roussel set out to comprehend the lives of women.

While doctors in the Cartesian tradition considered bodily differences of the two genders, the souls of all God's children were left to the Scriptures. Of course, Christian theology did not treat the daughters of Eve equally—far from it. But in their holy essence, everyone's soul was the same. Now, the Montpellier vitalists—by proposing that the mind was embodied—opened the door for theories that differentiated male and female sensibilities, ethics, habits, proclivities, and minds. Roussel's 1775 work, *The Physcial and Moral System of the Woman,* was a landmark in the often dubious effort of establishing a medical anthropology of females.

For this lifelong bachelor who shuddered at the notion of marriage, the choice of subject matter required explanation. His eulogist, J. L. Alibert, concluded that the doctor had been spurred to study women after heartbreak. Whatever the motivation, Roussel's conclusions ran against the egalitarian models put forward by French sensationalists, who following Locke and Helvétius, saw men and women as blank slates whose differences could be accounted for by cultural influence and education alone. Dr. Roussel did not agree. He concluded that after puberty, men's sensibilities became firm and resistant, while women's turned vulnerable and overwrought. The former stood ready for rational enlightenment; the latter did not.

And so, in what would prove to be a recurring risk, prejudices as old as Adam and Eve were naturalized and given some scientific legitimacy by this medicine that included inner life.

Roussel's anthropological ambitions had been encouraged by Bordeu and another advocate of a philosophical medicine, Paul Joseph Barthez. Born in Montpellier, Barthez studied philosophy and rhetoric in Narbonne and Toulouse, then returned to his birthplace to study medicine. A year after he graduated in 1753, he followed Bordeu to Paris with his Montpellier credentials in hand. Fortune smiled upon him when he was received by an established Parisian doctor, Dr. Camille Falconet. Originally from Avignon, Falconet was a medical consultant to the king and, according to Friedrich Melchior Grimm, a father figure to many Parisian *literati*.

Armed with Falconet's introductions to literary salons, Barthez dazzled these audiences. As one awed observer noted, this doctor seemed to know math, medicine, and all languages, living and dead. He had read everything in all genres and, even among the wise encyclopedists of Paris, was classified as an "Astonishing Genius." D'Alembert befriended Barthez and became his patient. The young doctor contributed essays to the *Encyclopedia* on subjects as diverse as countertenors, the supposedly supernatural phenomenon of fascination, and animal force. In 1759, thanks to his wide-ranging intellect, Barthez was appointed medical coeditor of the *Journal des sçavans*.

In 1760, while his star was still rising, Barthez surprised many when he chose to leave Paris to accept a chair at the medical school of Montpellier. For the next two decades, he taught medicine and rose in the ranks until he became chancellor of the university. In 1772, he announced a great discovery; he had found a general vital principle in all life. A single, global sensitivity, he claimed, worked on the animal economy the same way that gravity worked on matter.

Barthez anticipated that many would scoff and insist this was merely a renaming of sensibility. And they did. From Paris, Dr. Bordeu sneered at his colleague's claims and insisted this so-called

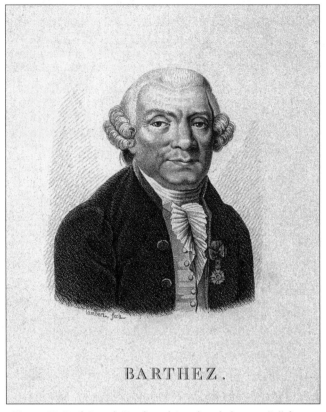

BARTHEZ.

Figure 27. Paul-Joseph Barthez claimed to deduce an "x" factor
that made matter active.

vital principle was just a dressed-up version of his own theory. Furthermore, Bordeu had conducted extensive experiments to validate
claims of sensibility in specific glands and organs, while Barthez
breezily claimed that he had inferred this unitary life principle.
When Barthez sent word of his discovery to Albrecht von Haller, he
received no garlands in reply. The best the Swiss physiologist could
muster was the assurance that the Frenchman's proposal would not
ruin their friendship.

A proud man, Barthez didn't give up. Instead, six years later he
produced *New Elements of the Human Science,* which heralded the
birth of a new field. Human attributes would be known, not through

metaphysics or Cartesian pirouettes, but as part of man's animal economy. If the physical and moral were intertwined, a new science based on this premise was required. It would pay off by creating new paths to health, happiness, morality, wisdom, and the good life.

For Barthez, the key remained his unifying vital principle. This vital principle was—as the doctor later explained—like an x in an algebraic equation; while its true identity remained mysterious, its presence was required for the equation to make sense. It did not matter if one called it a Vital Principle, the Soul, Nature or something else, the author rather scandalously observed. These were just words that marked the missing ingredient, the one that unified atoms with a conscious mind and made the bodily machine into a human being.

Barthez's restraint in defining the vital principle pointed back to the thought of Pierre Gassendi, whom the Montpellier doctor cited approvingly. However, this doctor did not fill his cloud of unknowing with God. Instead, this friend of d'Alembert insisted that the vital x principle be closely studied in its effects, not lost in abstractions. Metaphysics of that sort were only meant to delude and confuse. However, even as he explicitly positioned himself against soul forces, Barthez's vital principle approached the very same notion. For he did not believe this force necessarily resided in matter; it might be an independent substance or a mode of organic matter, who knew?

Like Whytt in Scotland, Barthez focused on the interactions of organs and nerves as they worked sympathetically together. The body harmonized its functions, in what Barthez called a "synergy." Disease was a form of global disharmony. Nervous disease, such as vapors, mania, hysteria, and melancholia were due to a breakdown of the interactions that regulated the animal economy. Illnesses of this sort should be expected to reveal nothing on autopsy, for they emerged from a dynamic disruption of the vital principle.

Barthez was careful to insist that the immortal soul still belonged to theologians, but there was no doubting that his human science greatly diminished that domain. The source of life, the human capacity for conscious thought, and free choice were all stripped from the soul. Furthermore, Barthez dared to claim that his science would lead to moral and happier lives. While he equivocated in a manner common to works that passed through French censorship, Barthez pushed forward with his pursuit of a science of human existence that would mostly supplant religious teaching. Judgment, reason, imagination, and reflection were modalities of organized matter. Human science would focus on individuals and their sensibility, nervous integrity, temperament, anatomy, gender, race, and developmental stage.

Upon its publication, *New Elements of the Human Science* was greeted by a slew of attacks. Despite approval from the French royal censor, the Vatican accused the author of heresy. Numerous deliberations ensued before Barthez was finally vindicated in Rome. In 1781, this increasingly famous Montpellier physician was summoned to Paris by Louis XVI, not to be punished, but to serve as one of his royal physicians.

This triumphant return would lead to riches, then ruination. In 1783, the doctor was accused of killing his dear friend d'Alembert. He successfully fended off these condemnations, and grew wealthy as a doctor snug in the king's court. However, just before the Revolution, Barthez penned a poorly timed *apologia* for royalty. It cost him his fortune, though not his life. Barthez retreated back to his native Languedoc and holed up in the fortified medieval village of Carcassonne. From there, he worked on a vastly expanded and bolder second edition of *New Elements of the Human Science*.

Even as Barthez became marginalized, his long tenure as a professor in Montpellier ensured that his ideas would not be quickly forgotten. Eighteenth-century medicine, once stuck between mechanists and animists, now had an alternative path forward, thanks to philosophical-minded doctors from Montpellier and their medical-minded philosopher friends. They tried to bring behavior and mental life into the realm of medicine and science. All this was made possible by their postulate of an active, vital force in animal matter. For some, this was the missing link between Nature and man, matter and consciousness. It was the missing piece that John Locke did not possess, the one that explained how brute matter could think.

CHAPTER

12

Honest Jean-Jacques and the
Morals of Sensibility

THIS NEW VANGUARD of eighteenth-century *médecins-philosophes* did not neglect their Hippocratic duties: Montpellier doctors considered illnesses of the animal economy based on irritability and sensibility, a paradigm that made them especially attuned to nervous conditions. Graduates of Montpellier became popular for holistic therapies that excited hope and offered a respite from the standard bleedings and vomits. Often, they sought environmental alterations that might reset the pathological sensibility behind illness.

In 1753, the Parisian doctor Antoine Le Camus had previewed some of the same ideas when he focused on climate, diet, and the power of moral and physical education to modify human temperaments and disease. As a lone maverick, Le Camus could not rival the entrenched Medical Faculty of Paris, but the Montpellier school gradually posed exactly such a threat. Self-styled as members of the medical opposition, they bucked the dictums of Paris. Montpellier's theories of nervous ailments were promoted in the *Encyclopedia*, where alongside conventional humoral descriptions of hypochondriasis or hysteria, the reader might also happen upon a quite different take on, for example, "satyriasis." The author Paul Jacques Malouin described a vicious disposition that led to excessive tension and sensibility in the male sexual addict. Similarly, the entry on "Mania," composed by Menuret in 1765, proposed that the illness must combine a brain disposition with an excessive sensibility. Beings of exquisite mental capacity—geniuses, poets, philosophers, and mathematicians—were all susceptible to mania. And all present medical interventions were frauds. For Menuret, the only helpful treatment was moral and focused on the moderation of the emotions.

Barthez concerned himself with the individualized treatment of nervous and mental disorders. The vaporous, hysterical, or melancholic patient must have his or her sensibility restored through moral habits, kind society, peaceful baths, and a soothing diet. In this way, treatment would strengthen the realm of the mind, much as rest cured the enervated. Based on a logic that emerged from the idea of sensibility, Montpellier vitalists advocated for mind-body cures that were attuned to the interplay of inner and outer forces. They could not have predicted how their model would help underwrite a new vision of morality, sanity, and human interiority, thanks to the efforts of a hypochondriacal Swiss orphan.

ONE OF THE most celebrated physicians of his time, Samuel-Auguste-André-David Tissot used theories of sensibility to medicalize a number of behaviors formerly simply considered immoral. Of Italian stock, but French-speaking and Swiss by birth, Tissot was tutored by his uncle, a Protestant minister, then schooled in the Genevan academy founded by Calvin. In 1745, as an extension of his service to the Great Physician, Jesus Christ, he trekked to Montpellier to study medicine. The seventeen-year-old lived with Boissier de Sauvages, whom he revered. However, during his years of training, he grew disappointed by his professors, who seemed ignorant and mercenary. He read what he could, then when the sun went down, this Swiss villager began to head for the city's bright lights. Tissot fell in with frolicking drinkers and gamblers, and immersed himself in theater, cards, and billiards. Later, shamed and much chastened, Tissot would characterize this as the saddest period of his life.

Tissot's wild times led to a burdensome family debt and an extra year to finish his medical training. When he graduated in 1749, the embarrassed young doctor returned home, carrying these disturbing experiences with him, along with the most modern advances in medicine. A dedicated follower of Haller, he won the privilege of translating that scientist's seminal lectures on sensibility into French. Tissot was rewarded for this task when Haller, who increasingly towered over continental medicine, praised the translation as one touched by genius. However, unlike Haller, Tissot had already looked beyond nerves and muscles, and manifested an interest in the way diseases of sensibility could disrupt reason in his thesis on mania and melancholia.

After his training, Tissot began professional life as a Swiss country doctor, but that would not last long. Smallpox outbreaks pushed him to advocate for vaccination, an innovative practice not widely accepted in Europe. This, he believed, was science in the service of mankind, the Enlightenment in action. Soon, his consultations became highly sought after. In 1751, he moved his practice to Lausanne, where he became official doctor to the poor. Again, his penchant to break with tradition became clear when an epidemic of bilious fever broke out: he recommended a fruit diet rather than bleedings and purgings. Bern authorities posted Dr. Tissot's remedy in its villages.

Meanwhile, Tissot's ambition led him to become a voracious reader and an eager correspondent with Johann Georg Zimmermann. Their relationship would last over forty years and become, by Tissot's admission, one of the *douceurs* of his life. Zimmermann was Tissot's double, a Swiss doctor with outsized philosophical ambitions, stuck in a provincial town. Born in the German-speaking part of the Bern canton, he had studied philosophy before choosing to go to Göttingen to study medicine with Haller. Zimmermann became Dr. Haller's assistant and in the process rose to fame himself when, in 1751, he established the irritability of cardiac tissue. A few years after this taste of fame, however, Zimmermann found himself back in Brougg, his hometown. In 1754, he and Tissot met and became fast friends.

In animated letters, the two discussed Boerhaave, Bordeu, patients and remedies, political gossip, and most of all books. Each man considered himself a citizen of the Republic of Letters. They gobbled up the latest from Voltaire, Diderot, Helvétius, and countless others. Zimmermann wondered if his true calling was to be a poet. He and Tissot shared incredulity over supernatural beliefs, debated morals, and proposed theories for the reform of society. When their philosophizing became too heady, Tissot reminded his friend that they were but small town doctors. Offended, Zimmermann urged his colleague to make his mark on the ages. Gradually, Tissot began to more fully inhabit the identity that was already available to men like him and his friend, as a *médecin-philosophe*. In a short autobiography written for Zimmermann, Tissot placed himself in a lineage that began with John Locke and Julien de La Mettrie, who in Tissot's view was the only one "who dared to speak the truth."

In 1761, moved by his encounters with poor sanitary habits, ignorance, and lack of access to medical care that afflicted the poor in isolated villages, Tissot broke with his guild's dictums and published one of the first serious medical self-help books. In the spirit of the *lumières*, Tissot penned *Advice to the People* not in Latin, but in French in the hope that literate laymen would read the book and provide for the illiterate especially in the remote, mountain villages of Switzerland. Skeptical of chemical prescriptions that his colleagues doled out, Tissot advised readers to manage diet and hygiene. Strikingly, despite his prior interests in nervous and mental troubles, Tissot ignored these topics in this book. Later, he made it clear that stoic mountain folk had a hundred problems and nervous disorders were not one.

To Tissot's shock, *Advice* became a best-seller, snatched up by rich and poor alike throughout Europe. Eager for pragmatic information about their own health, readers ran through sixteen French editions, and intense demand led to over a dozen translations. While *Advice* was not devoid of some old humoral strategies, its touting of diet with preventative measures, and its resistance to overtreatment with prescriptions, marked its difference.

Thanks to this work, Dr. Tissot moved to the center of the European medical stage just as he had also developed ideas about the nervous system and the mind. As early as 1754, he had told Zimmermann that he longed to use his friend's ideas of irritability in clinical practice. And medicine of the *esprit* was the most interesting aspect of their field. Tissot even pressed a skeptical Albrecht von Haller to consider William Battie's mind cures.

In 1758, Tissot announced plans for a new work on nervous diseases that resulted from pernicious behaviors. If sensibility was central to illness, then different habits, which provoked nervous reactions, could foster illness. That year, he affixed a brief tract on such matters to an unrelated one on bilious fever. Unlike his self-help book, this new pamphlet was written in Latin and discreetly directed to medical colleagues. It focused on a shameful sin that the doctor now reframed as an illness. When an unauthorized French translation hit the bookstores two years later, it caused panic.

The biblical sin of Onan, or masturbation, was traditionally a matter for the clergy. However, that had begun to change. In 1716, medical interest in this subject had been stoked by an anonymous English publication, *Onania*, which warned that masturbation was a moral plague that carried terrible physical dangers. An equal mix of medicine and theology, this book circulated widely. Taking up the same subject, four decades later, Tissot assailed the chaotic logic of this text and conducted a cooler medical appraisal on sexual self-stimulation. New physiological models of sensibility, he suggested, allowed for a purely scientific understanding of those pale, stricken young men and women. Their nervous systems had been ruined, not by their immoral defiance of biblical law, but the disruption of a fragile balance. Unbeknownst to them, these onanists were marching down the path to insensate states like blindness, madness, and sudden death.

Given Haller's framework, Dr. Tissot's turn to varieties of overstimulation, including those involved in sex, seemed obvious, though that subject meant risking the Church's ire. However if this act was no sin, there was still little comfort for onanists to be found in Tissot. *Onanism* calmly announced that this nervous disorder was a drawn out act of suicide. Constant irritation of the genitals, the intense mental focus on amorous situations, and the terrible loss of seminal liquor accompanied by that convulsion of orgasm, all combined to destroy the balance of the nerves and the mind. In terrifying case reports, Dr. Tissot portrayed such beings who had succumbed to bodily temptation and ended in ruin.

Dr. Tissot did have some trouble explaining why, by the same rationale, any kind of sex was not pernicious. Haller himself considered an orgasm to be a kind of epilepsy that weakened the nervous system. However, unlike Haller, Tissot crossed over from the nerves to the mind to make his argument. In a line of thought that would hold among experts on sexuality for a century, he argued that masturbation was worse than intercourse in so far as it taxed the individual's imagination. In this way, nervous irritation was compounded by mental strain. Masturbation disrupted the animal economy and made for melancholia and epilepsy. While Boerhaave had grimly concluded there was no cure for this illness, Tissot was less pessimistic: he dismissed emetics, purgatives, and bleedings and placed his therapeutic emphasis on environmental cures, including that most effective remedy, the freezing-cold bath.

In medicalizing what were considered moral failures, Tissot joined a host of secularizing contemporaries, such as his British counterpart George Cheyne. However, the big man from Bath, old-line Galenists, and the medical mechanists had no model to account for human intention and therefore could not truly explain how moral choices made for illness. For them, free will and moral choice resided in the pure and unsullied soul. However, the Montpellier model allowed Tissot to cross over from nervous stimulation to psychic causes and effects. And while the Swiss doctor quickly denied being a metaphysician, he insisted that the physical and moral, the body and its highest mental functions, were so intricately enmeshed as to be one. Sensations affected nervous fibers that then registered in the brain; the mind resolved these inputs and took action. "The mind agitates the machine," he wrote.

Tissot turned to other afflictions of excess mental stimulation. He had followed the emergence in Great Britain of new ideas about mental medicine and had even pushed his friend Zimmermann, who was then working in a mad hospital, to take off where William Battie stopped and develop a new medicine for madness. Tissot himself first focused on life styles that any good Protestant might condemn—the wealthy and sedentary, the indolent and the hyperrefined. In 1766, Tissot also put out a tract that warned the *gens de lettres*, those *philosophes* who made progress and the Enlightenment possible, that their mental overexertion would stretch their imaginations to the breaking point. Upon reading this, Zimmermann wondered if he would have to abandon medicine to save himself?

Four years later, Tissot continued his assault on excessive stimulation and pleasure in *An Essay on the Diseases of People of Fashion*. There he detailed the cost of greed, envy, and jealousy among the *gens du monde*. The high life stimulated excessive ambition, vanity, and destructive passions that led to nervous diseases, including sudden death. Among the elite, such passionate agitation was dangerous, never more so than when vanity was humbled. Tissot ticked off prominent leaders who departed the world in a flash, thanks to a sudden assault on their pride.

During this time, Tissot's expertise was severely tested when his dear friend Zimmermann collapsed into a morbid depression. In 1767, melancholia descended upon him and deepened. Desperate, Zimmermann begged Tissot for help. The two doctors agreed that his sickness came from unremitting concentration on sad ideas. Suicidal, Zimmermann turned to religion, but nothing relieved his emptiness and pain. Tissot sent letters of hope and advice. Afraid to open one of these envelopes, feeling what lay inside might hold his life in the balance, Zimmermann finally tore open one envelope to find Tissot's prescription. There was no talk of bleeding, emetics, or purgatives, no herbal remedies. Relief would come by reorienting his mind through an immersion in Horace, Petrarch, Montaigne, and Voltaire. Zimmermann was crestfallen, then enraged. He curtly informed Tissot that such weak medicine would never be enough to counter the imbalance of his passions.

Zimmermann's depression dominated the later years of his life. Though hypersensitive to criticism and at times barely functional, Haller's former student was appointed Hanover physician to George III. His psychological writings on solitude and national pride were translated into numerous languages, but Zimmermann himself tottered on the edge of sanity. In his later years, he remained prone to intense sadness and paranoid fears regarding a secret order of Illuminati started by a Bavarian professor, Adam Weishaupt. However, Zimmermann's prestige as a doctor did not diminish; he even attended Frederick the Great on his deathbed. Tissot's continual attempts to help his dear friend reinforced a stark truth. When Zimmermann was acutely suicidal, he and Tissot had to admit the impotence of their therapeutic methods.

By 1770, Samuel Tissot was one of Europe's greatest doctors. Before he died, he would put forward one of the first descriptions of migraine headaches and some of the most accurate considerations of seizures. He would be lauded by scientific societies and world leaders like King George, Maria Theresa, and even Napoleon Bonaparte. The aristocracy of Europe eagerly sought him out, so that his clinical notes from 1775 to 1780 record him caring for the Prince of Beauvau, the Princess of Poix, the Duchess of Chaulnes, and sundry other royals. When Pierre Beaumarchais wrote an introduction to *The Barber of Seville* in 1775, he could safely assume that an inside joke about the Swiss doctor would amuse his audience. Tissot's views had become famous. What most did not know was that this doctor of temperance was involved in a behind-the-scenes effort to save a thinker so despised that even Frederick II of Prussia wanted nothing to do with him.

TISSOT'S INTEREST IN the health of philosophers was not based on conjecture alone, for a number had sought him out. A stormy Voltaire worried Dr. Tissot when he morosely signed off as "Le Malade Voltaire." The doctor heaved a sigh of relief after a colleague let him know this disgruntled genius *always* claimed to be mortally ill, thanks to "always irritated bile and his always irritated nerves." In fact, the Marquise du Deffand had noted this same tendency many years earlier. After another one of his farewell letters, she told Voltaire that his reports of being dead were the best proof of the immortality of the soul, since no one living being ever displayed more spirit than he did in the grave.

Tissot's encounter with Voltaire was passing; Voltaire dismissed the physician as less devoted to his patients than to his books. However, another *philosophe* so touched Tissot that he called their meeting one of the pivotal moments of his life. That patient was Jean-Jacques Rousseau. Born in 1712 to a Genevan watchmaker and the daughter of a Calvinist preacher who died soon after giving him life, little Jean-Jacques learned to share his father's pleasure for reading in a strictly puritanical environment where amusements like theater were illegal. He was abandoned by his father at ten and miserably apprenticed. At the age of sixteen, sick of the scolding and abuse, Rousseau abruptly left Geneva and commenced a life of wandering.

In nearby Annecy, the adolescent was taken in by the Baroness de Warens, or "Maman," as he called the woman who adopted him, became his surrogate parent, and for a brief time, his lover. Warens recently had converted to Catholicism and received a pension for her troubles. She decided that this boy from Calvin's hometown should switch sides too. The penniless Rousseau's conversion was more a matter of the stomach than the heart. Like the ragged whores and con men who joined him in Turin to undergo this reeducation, the helpless orphan desperately needed financial support. His Calvinism was one of the few things he had to sell. He did so. When he returned to Madame de Warens and settled in at Annecy, he became a passionate reader, discovered a deep love for music, studied math, physics, and chemistry, and stumbled upon Voltaire's letters on the English, which inspired him to become a writer.

During this time of great growth, Rousseau also began to be plagued by melancholy, headaches, and bodily pains. In 1737, dejected and fatigued, Rousseau was encouraged by Maman to make the arduous voyage to Montpellier to get medical help. He was cured on the carriage ride to that medical Mecca when he met a divorced woman. Pretending to be an Englishman, Rousseau had the most gratifying sex of his life and, miraculously, it rid him of his pains. By the time he was evaluated in Montpellier, Dr. Antoine Fizes congratulated the young man; he had "the malady of happy people." He was a hypochondriac. Rousseau remained in town a bit and amused himself by drinking with medical students before heading home.

In 1739, Rousseau's life took a sudden turn when his relationship with Madame de Warens ended. After vagabonding about, the broke, thirty-year-old autodidact landed in Paris, where this one-time valet, clerk, apprentice, and tutor tried to scratch out a living alongside the poor and desperate. He met a barely literate laundrywoman, Thérèse Levasseur, with whom he quickly sired and just as quickly abandoned five children, a choice that would long thereafter haunt him and give ample ammunition to his enemies.

Rousseau also made his way into salon life and befriended a group of radical thinkers that included the Baron d'Holbach, the editor of *Literary Correspondence*, Friedrich Melchior Grimm, and the post-Lockean sensationalists, Helvétius and Condillac. However, perhaps his closest attachment was to that confident prodigy Denis Diderot. Despite being a year younger than Rousseau, this writer acted as a mentor to his sporadically educated friend. Rousseau eagerly absorbed all he heard, so much so that later an embittered Diderot would complain that his one-time student was a viper that sucked up his teacher's ideas, then spat them out as his own.

Rousseau, Diderot, and Condillac met regularly for dinner at a tavern called Panier Fleuri. Later, d'Alembert joined their brainy group. Like his *confrères*, Rousseau took interest in the latest developments of a wide array of subjects, including natural science, especially chemistry, which offered deep insights into life, and medical views that debunked de Warens's herbalist potions. As the *Encyclopedia* took shape, this insecure composer and writer sat at the hub of the action.

A hungry, intense, and loyal friend, Rousseau took long hikes outside of Paris to visit his beloved Diderot after he had been imprisoned at Vincennes. On one long walk to the château, Rousseau claimed to have had an epiphany. In the *Mercure de France,* the Academy of Dijon had offered a prize for the best essay on the question of whether the restoration of the arts and sciences tended to purify morals. Rousseau decided the answer was . . . no! A lightning bolt of inspiration had struck him as he walked to Vincennes, which led him to explore this contrarian stance, or so Rousseau recalled. Diderot told a different story. As one who delighted in turning over ideas to consider them from many angles, so much so that his central positions often remained debatable, the philosopher told friends that he had dissuaded Rousseau from taking the boring and obvious affirmative position. If so, Diderot certainly lived to regret this piece of sophistry, for his sincere disciple set himself against the moral value of enlightenment and never let up.

Rousseau's essay contra the *philosophes* flattered the provincial grandees in Lyon, who awarded him the 1750 prize. His conclusions could not be called original—French moralists long decried the vanity of fancy knowledge, and religious apologists routinely cast reason as the enemy of faith. Rousseau's path to this conclusion, however, was different. He proposed that modern views of morality were vicious. Hobbes, he claimed, believed that men ate each other without squeamishness, while the twisted Mandeville dared to call vice the basis for virtue. Perhaps worst of all, the demonic Spinoza destroyed all morality by making everything material, even God. Rousseau proposed that men, in their original presocial state, were good. The savages of North America lived peacefully in nature, without trousers. Uncorrupted by society, human beings were simple, noble, and kind. As for any science of morals, that was impossible, oxymoronic. Science did nothing but destroy morals.

Rousseau's diatribe was not taken seriously by his coterie. Life in the salons was filled with ironic gamesmanship and playful intellectual display; many assumed Jean-Jacques was exaggerating for effect. No one could predict that this little essay would launch a lifetime quest in which Rousseau explored the way rationalism led to the destruction of childhood innocence, the corruption of natural feeling, moral failure, and grave pathologies. Eventually one by one, d'Holbach, Diderot, Grimm, and others would come to realize that their friend was deadly serious in his opposition to their core beliefs. An icy Voltaire vowed to destroy this traitor.

During these years, an increasingly isolated Rousseau continued to be troubled by concerns regarding his health. In the 1750s, he developed a chronic urge to urinate that led him to numerous doctors and, ultimately, resulted in a daily routine of catheterizing himself, a form of self-torture he considered necessary. He returned to Geneva and restored himself to his original faith, then found refuge with a new matron, Madame d'Épinay, who put him up outside Paris at the edge of a forest in Montmorency, where he contemplated a critique of political institutions and morality.

Jean-Jacques Rousseau had proclaimed that no science of morals was possible. However, like other *lumières*, Rousseau was well versed in physiology and medicine. He knew of the findings of Haller on irritability and sensibility, and the innovative work on the animal economy by the Montpellier school. Their belief in a pre-

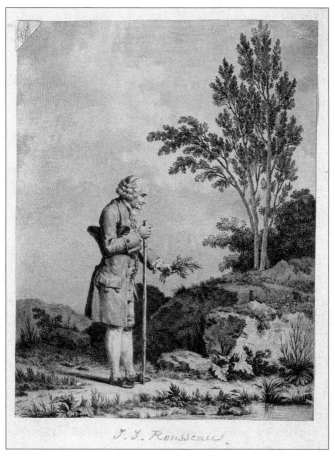

Figure 28. Jean-Jacques Rousseau turned to theories of natural sensibility to reframe ethics.

existing sensitivity in the living body corresponded perfectly with his own notions. In 1756, Rousseau conceived of a book that would knit together the moral implications of sensibility. It would be entitled *The Morals of Sensibility; or, The Wiseman's Materialism*. Rousseau dreamed that this work would be of the utmost practical utility. Natural morality rooted in the body and mind would banish falsity, unreason, and vice.

The 17th-century French writers on "la Morale" had developed a beloved ironic tradition; La Rochefoucauld and others pilloried heroes of restraint as possessing an extra dollop of self-love. Love was the greatest victory for vanity, and generosity was masked self-satisfaction. All this surely was a challenge to the puffed-up Versailles court and the satin-robed Catholic hierarchy, but some had gone beyond satire to claim that such moral failings actually led to illness. Vanity caused madness, envy led to jaundice, ambition stoked fever, and love "alone had produced more ills than all the rest together."

Jean de La Bruyère's lifelong project, *The Characters; or, The Manners of the Present Age*, presented a typology of human character based on the ways reason and passion consolidated into a personal style. Rousseau believed different styles were created by impressions from the outside that were modified continually by our senses and organs, so that without perceiving it, we are affected "in our thoughts, our feelings, and even our actions." He dreamed of writing the rules of human conduct in a way that exploded long-held lies and truly supported virtue: "From what errors would reason be preserved, and what vices would be choked even before birth, if one knew how to compel the animal economy to support that moral order which they so often disturb?"

By referring to the animal economy, Rousseau signaled his indebtedness to the Montpellier school in his *The Morals of Sensibility*. For his moral science, he needed a model of natural man that included passions and reason. In this, Cartesians offered no help, but Bordeu and Barthez did. In 1759, after Rousseau collected examples and created an outline, he suddenly abandoned the project. Nonetheless, its assumptions would continue to guide him.

Rousseau moved to Geneva with deeply misplaced hopes for a better relationship with Voltaire. By 1760 the elder statesman of the *lumières* had become "madly irritated" with him. Voltaire concluded that this attention-seeking idiot was a turncoat who was subverting the *philosophes'* project from within. Voltaire's stinging sarcasm finally led a jittery Rousseau to declare: "I do not like you, Sir," and then, as if he had not been clear, "I hate you." More of this was to come.

ADMIRED BY THE French royal censor Malesherbes, and protected by the Duc de Luxembourg, in 1762 Rousseau published a shocking work of moral reform. *Émile; or, On Education* was a philosophical fiction, a book that reimagined childhood and therefore proposed a new method of upbringing. The core beliefs were the same ones that inspired *The Morals of Sensibility; or, The Wiseman's Materialism*. Having absorbed Montesquieu's ethical relativism and the sensationalism of Helvétius and Condillac, and knowing enough about the physiology of inner sensibility, Rousseau offered up a vision of a child not as a fallen soul filled with original sin, nor as a statue stirring and coming to life, but rather as a noble little savage, a natural being whose innate sensations combined with external influences to create, over time, a distinct and fully formed personality.

Rousseau placed great emphasis on childhood development, but mocked *au courant* Lockean pedagogy, in which little tots were fed complex logic whether they could understand syllogisms or not. Endowed with inner sensibilities, children were no idea machines, but beings who were deeply affected by their environments. Before ever possessing a moral life, a child's natural sensibility was often distorted by the adult world, which turned him away from the harmony his sensitivities would otherwise naturally seek.

Everything from Émile's nurse and her milk to the patterns of behavior he witnessed and the assumptions of his culture would make their mark on him. They would create Émile's habits, his morals, his character, and his self. Blameless, born free, this child had entered the world with a range of inner reactions that offered widespread potential; however, soon he found himself—like the political subject of his time—everywhere enchained. He took in the ways of the world, which were enslaving, disorienting, and alienating. Nature had endowed him with the gift of sensibility, but civilization managed to transform that into anxiety and sickness.

Chief among the culprits in the deformation of children were doctors:

> Medicine is all the fashion in these days, and very naturally. It
> is an amusement of the idle and the unemployed . . . such need
> doctors to give them the only pleasure they can enjoy, the plea-
> sure of not being dead.

Doctors corroded happiness and created joyless worriers. Medicine instilled cowardice, anxiety, credulity, and the fear of death, rather than bravery and acceptance. "Live according to nature; be patient, get rid of doctors; you will not escape death, but you will only die once while the doctors make you die daily through your diseased imagination. . . ."

Natural men did not suffer from such pathologies, in which their inner sentiments turned against the self. Rousseau's goal was to raise such liberated men, though he did not think the same could be hoped for with women. In line with the misogynistic Pierre Roussel, Rousseau proposed a much more conventional upbringing for Émile's female counterpart, Sophie. To the disgust of those freethinkers who followed Helvétius's egalitarian view of gender, Rousseau's Sophie was encouraged to take up the masks of her decadent culture. She should not be expected to strive for the same natural goodness and authenticity, but should learn to wear the lies of civilization well.

In much of his argument, Rousseau echoed the Scottish critique of Locke: reason was our capping achievement, but it could be employed only after the successful development of sensitivities and feelings. Dr. Boerhaave, Rousseau pointed out, believed that many children's diseases originated from convulsions due to their excessively sensitive nervous systems. One must be gentle with Émile. Teach him to consider intense rage and anxiety as kinds of sickness. "I picture little Émile at the height of a dispute between two neighbors going up to the fiercest one and saying in a tone of pity: 'You are ill, I am very sorry for you.'"

Similarly, Émile's teachers would painstakingly endure the child should he become furious. During an outburst of temper, Émile would not be subdued by force or fear. Evil could never correct evil; rage could not heal rage. When Émile hollered, his caretakers would be quiet and calm. Do not raise your voice, Rousseau counseled; take away objects the boy might break. Should he smash up the windows, allow him to sleep in the cold for a few days, but do not scold him, for the intensity of your passion will only incite more of his own. After a few days, silently repair the windows. Should the wild child shatter the glass again, inform him that the windows are your possession and that you must keep them safe. With that, place Émile in a windowless room. While he may howl, finally he will repent. And when he does, quickly release him. Should he offer up an apology and some compensation, clasp him to your breast and forgive him.

This method of treatment was not geared toward the forces of reason, but rather the developing sensibility of the child. They would model the values of modesty, moderation, and benevolence.

This strategy for treating out-of-control children could be also applied elsewhere. Those in charge of prisons should consider these ways, and doctors could use this gentle approach with the furious and the mad.

Émile represented Rousseau's promise of a sage materialism, thanks to the use of sensibility as a link between body and mind. Should a boy follow his natural sentiments and be treated thusly, he would become brave, courageous, reasonable, and deeply moral. If you wanted proof, Rousseau advised, search out little Émile. He existed in the lucky lands where there were no doctors, philosophers, or priests.

The 1762 publication of *Émile* received tacit permission from Malesherbes' office. Why not? Rousseau was a celebrity, whose novel a year earlier, *Julie, or the New Héloise* was a sensation. However, the censors badly misjudged public reaction. Volcanic protest rose up against Émile and transformed the remaining years of Rousseau's life. From here on, he would be pilloried, reviled, hunted, exiled, and constantly discussed. Before this book he was famous. Now he was also infamous.

At the heart of much of *Émile* was a question that Rousseau did not have to directly answer, thanks to the ambiguities of the French language. What was one educating when one taught a young child? Was it their mind or their soul? Rousseau used the term *âme* liberally and skirted any debates over the soul and its immateriality. Yet, it was hard to miss the fact that his model for most of Émile's inner life derived from physiological notions of the child's sensibility and post-Lockean sensationalism. Character and morals developed from this mix of inner feelings and external impressions. Rousseau might allow that all this took place in the "soul," but it was no soul that the Pope would recognize.

A long section of *Émile* entitled "Profession of Faith by a Savo-yard Vicar" had directly taken up the spiritual education of the child. Here, Rousseau genuinely advocated for the soul's immortal life,

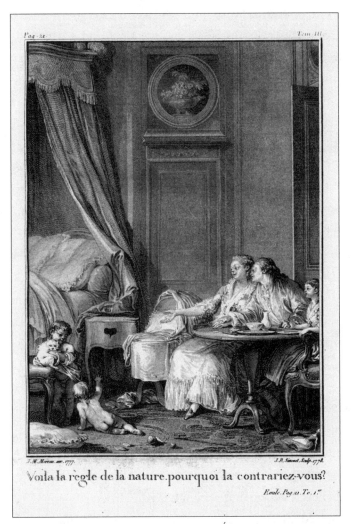

Figure 29. An illustration from Rousseau's *Émile*. The caption reads:
"Here is the law of nature, why do you contradict it?"

something he believed was a needed consolation for the harsh trials of existence. However, in his discussion Jean-Jacques managed
to scandalize priests and *philosophes* alike. He bluntly dismissed all
conventional religious teaching. Children's innate spirituality was
corrupted by churches; the three monotheisms were all bitter, small-
minded sects. "Natural religion" could suffice for the developing of
a conscience. If this seemed like radical materialist talk, Rousseau

rebuffed that notion. Philosophical atheists were, in his view, no different from their enemies. They too were fanatics.

Published in May, *Émile* was denounced by the Sorbonne in June.
The Parlement of Paris condemned the book to an auto-da-fé and
called for the author's arrest. Rousseau scampered out of France to
Switzerland, but there too he was a marked man. Geneva condemned
his book and Bern soon followed. The author had become a fugitive.

In 1762, the same year that Rousseau challenged the Church,
he published his reconsideration of political authority, *Of the Social
Contract; or, Principles of Political Right,* a work with clear connection
to little Émile and the corruptons of society that afflicted him. The
book memorably began: "Man is born free, and everywhere is in
chains." Divine right was a sham, he declared. Each individual was
morally and legally equal; the authority of the sovereign came only
from their combined "general will."

Thinkers puzzled over Rousseau's general will, but for the theoreticians of sensibility and sympathy, it made great sense. Much as
Adam Smith considered sentiments to merge and guide complex
human economic interactions through an "invisible hand," Rousseau
saw them flowing together, uniting and creating something larger.
In the same way that the fibers and sensitivities resulted in a general
living whole, animal economies in sympathy with others could melt
into one communal being with a will.

Jean-Jacques Rousseau had now stuck his thumb in the eye of
clerics, monarchists, rationalists and liberal savants. If he was desperate for attention, he now got plenty of it. The Republic of Letters transformed into a village of scolds and gossips. Writers buzzed
with news about the hunted man, his purported whereabouts, his
fate, his character and the opinions of this personally shy, publicly
fearless writer. Tarred as no different than the Jesuits, many *lumières*
grew to detest Rousseau. Voltaire decried that crazy "little monster."
Diderot wondered where his former friend's excesses would land
him. Counts, barons, marquises, princes, duchesses, and royals from

France, Luxembourg, Holland, Scotland, and Prussia, read Rousseau and joined in the debate. Some called for his head, while others passionately swore they would do anything to protect him.

⌒

AMONG THE PARTICIPANTS in these heated discussions over Rousseau's fate were a small group of enlightened Swiss physicians. Some angrily demanded that Rousseau be forced out of their country, but Dr. Samuel Tissot was not one of them. He hoped to save Rousseau from others, and even more so, from himself.

In July of 1762, soon after the order of *arrêt* in Paris made Rousseau return to Switzerland, Tissot met him. For the doctor, the experience was transformative. In Rousseau, he had found an ideal, the "first of men," humble and honest. "How I love those people who have the courage to listen to the interior cry of Nature in favor of the rights of men," the physician wrote.

With the writer now facing exile, Tissot took up his pen to plead for support from colleagues like Hirzel and Zimmermann, as well as Albrecht von Haller. Haller, now a baron in Bern, the man who helped spawn theories of sensibility, was quite firm in his conviction. From orders given by the Lord God himself, every Christian prince must mark their indignation against this blasphemer. To the baron, exile seemed a quite modest punishment. Tissot replied that Jean-Jacques was not irreligious, for he allowed for God, the spirituality of soul, and its immortal life.

Unbeknown to Tissot, Haller was simultaneously being lobbied by another Genevan thinker. Two years earlier, Charles Bonnet had published his seminal book on psychology, an analysis of the functions of the soul, in which he maintained strict distinction between the soul's functions, which were analyzable, and its essence, which was mysterious and immortal. Bonnet believed his psychology conducted its soul analysis while maintaining the verities of the Bible.

Hearing of Rousseau's 1762 publications attacking Church and State, Bonnet was at first tentative and asked Haller for his opinion. Soon thereafter, Bonnet made up his own mind: he advised Comte Charles de Geer that Rousseau sought to undermine the belief in the eternal life of the soul. *Émile* and the *Social Contract* attacked the fundaments of religion and government. Another letter to Haller soon followed to warn that this enemy of the aristocracy was now heading to Bern, no doubt to seduce others with extreme notions of liberty. Prussia's King Frederick, Bonnet sneered, protector of that devil La Mettrie, would probably take him in. And so one of the founders of psychology, thanks to his commitment to soul-body dualism, became one of Rousseau's most virulent critics: he wrote professors and doctors deriding this assassin of morals and called for his imprisonment.

Bonnet insisted that rational knowledge was not revelation and the soul's material functions were not its God-like essence. Little Émile, Bonnet reminded others, built himself block by block through active inner sensibilities and experiences. His inner life was predicated on things like the quality of his mother's milk and the kindness shown him by others. How could an immortal soul depend on the quality of breast milk? And besides, anything that could grow must surely die. Call it what you want—Émile, Bonnet was sure, possessed a mind made of flesh.

Meanwhile, Rousseau's daily existence became a nightmare. Always quick to take offense, and easily irritated—a police report called him "prickly"—he now had legions of critics, detractors, and haters. Long afraid of being persecuted, he had incited a mob of persecutors. Worried about having no home, he was now unwelcome in his own country. The writer couldn't sleep and often became intensely agitated. He swooned into delirium and black despair. His nerves were fraying. Finally, like many other sufferers, Rousseau wrote a letter to ask for help from the author of that medical self-help book, *Advice to the People*.

It had been three years since Rousseau had met Tissot, and during that time they had struck up a bit of a friendship. After their initial meeting, Tissot sent Rousseau his books. The famed writer confessed that while he no longer read medical books, he had read Tissot's and was troubled to discover the medical effects of masturbation. It was a habit, he told the doctor, that he suffered from himself. Tissot's claims about the pathology associated with overstimulated sensibilities would find their way into Rousseau's *Confessions*, where he highlighted his onanism and events like being spanked at an early age to help make sense of his later proclivities.

On March 16 of 1765, Rousseau now called upon this trusted physician in a crisis. The *philosophe* had taken refuge in Môtiers, a village of 400 in the Swiss canton of Neuchâtel, where the governor, a representative of Frederick the Great, agreed to protect him. An intimate friend of the writer, Isabelle Guyenet, had grown dangerously ill after giving birth. Rousseau called on Tissot to save her. The physician diverted his travels to go to Môtiers, where he discovered more than one *malade* awaiting him. Madame Guyenet had gone mad after giving birth, and Rousseau was in despair over his own plight. His misfortunes had taken him to a breaking point. "Love me, feel sorry for me, reassure me," he begged the physician.

Afterward, Tissot wrote the Russian count Alexandre de Golowkin to report on the two hours he spent with their illustrious friend. The trip only deepened his affection for the man and doubled his sadness over his current state. Tormented more cruelly than anyone on earth, Tissot wrote, Jean-Jacques Rousseau was not equipped to abide such harassment. While for others such threats might be minor, for this sensitive being, the impact was terrific. Now the author was beginning to search for enemies where there were none. At that moment, he was worried about a saboteur, who he believed had published a vile pamphlet under his name so as to discredit him.

If indeed he was becoming paranoid, Rousseau also had a great deal to fear. On March 19th, the Parlement of Paris condemned another of his works, *Letters Written from the Mountains*, as false philosophy that led to depravity. Four days later, Tissot sent a letter to his new patient. The present crisis required action; Rousseau must be freed from the material causes of irritation to his nerves. Change your surroundings, Tissot advised, change not only the air, but everything. A new chain of associations was required to break the hold of that net of ideas that contained his illness. These sick impressions affected his nerves and would provoke the same erroneous emotions inside him and feed his melancholia.

Following the Montpellier model, Tissot sought to rebalance Rousseau's moral and physical being. The doctor firmly addressed the possibility that Rousseau's sensitivity was accentuating, even perhaps creating, more ills. If all that his friend Jean-Jacques feared was so, he wrote, his doctor would be deeply worried, but he was not. Thus, Dr. Tissot tried to console this man who had become a lightning rod for hatred. The doctor believed these attacks were making his patient sink into unremitting agitation, hypochondrical fears, and yes, delusion.

On April 1, Rousseau wrote with the happy news that one of the *malades* in Môtiers was nearly cured: to the delight of all, after closely following Dr. Tissot's recommendations, Isabelle Guyenet had recovered. Tissot had brought health, reason, and consolation to *her*. The results of his own treatment were, however, less admirable. When Tissot argued that Rousseau's psychic suffering increased his physical ills, his patient recoiled. The doctor labored under his own illusions, Rousseau snapped: "All your reasons are weak against the force of sentiment." Dr. Tissot failed to recognize the depths of his suffering. Physical illness was nothing; it came and went. However, the deepest suffering came from the evils of the soul. Those didn't let up. Book burnings, conspiracies, and attacks had not harmed him. No, Rousseau pointedly concluded, his greatest suffering had come from his grave disappointment in his friends.

Rousseau concluded his letter with a paean to the Swiss doctor:

"How often during my last sickness would I have not wished for a Tissot at my bedside, so that when there was no more to do for the body, he could be the doctor of my soul!" A demoralized Tissot sullenly wrote his famed colleague, Bordeu: "There is none among us who does strongly wish to cure J. J. Rousseau, and to give him as much health as had his Émile."

Word had begun to leak out that the once-eccentric Rousseau was now insane. On April 9, d'Alembert send Voltaire a note: "Poor Jean-Jacques is mad." This did little to soften Voltaire's heart. A year earlier, he had stuck his knife in as far as it could go: under the guise of being a Genevan preacher, he had published an eight-page pamphlet that accused Rousseau of having syphilis, of killing his mother-in-law, and one terrible truth among these lies; he revealed the author of Émile's dark secret of having abandoned his own children.

On April 20, 1765, Rousseau wrote to Dr. Tissot to let him know that Isabelle was entirely cured and that Tissot's work had made Jean-Jacques believe in two things he once doubted, miracles and medicine. In May, Tissot wrote Comte Golowkin and informed him that their illustrious friend was more tranquil and restored to some gaiety. This peace would not last.

On the night of September 6, 1765, a mob from Môtiers congregated around Rousseau's home and stoned it. Fearing for his life, the writer fled. Under threat from many directions, without a home, his suspicious nature went wild as he imagined cabals and conspiracies. Persecuted, maligned, accused of great crimes, Rousseau took it upon himself to do what others could not. He would use his powers of understanding and self-reflection to make sense of his life and heal his troubled mind. Thus, the orphan-turned-outcast began his writing cure, his attempt to know and thereby have sway over his fragile sensibility. He left unpublished a short, dry run that revealed his method; he would proceed as an observer, a "botanist" of his own inner flora. And he would leave it to the doctors to figure out how to make use of these insights. His would be a starkly honest, secular work of remembrance, truth-telling, and self-comprehension that commenced with his first memories and led up to the disastrous days of 1765, that year when he reached out to Dr. Tissot, that year when the little peace he could muster in Neuchâtel ended in a hail of stones.

⁓

THE CONFESSIONS, Rousseau's self-portrait, made a show of its nakedness. The book was a breathtaking account of things typically secret, unspoken, unobserved, and even shameful. The title forcefully proposed a secular alternative to the services offered by the Church through its confessional. While always a believer in God and Heaven, Rousseau's worldly torment was not much helped by his time in either the Calvinist or the Catholic church. He would say little about his soul, as instead he strove to understand his inner inclinations, sensitivities, fears, rages, joys, as well as their resultant virtues and vices, reasons and choices.

The result was a revelation. *The Confessions* perfected a voice, an intimate manner of confiding, pleading, and exposing the author's life to his readers, so that soon readers would commonly refer to Rousseau in the first person, as if he were their friend. That authorial voice, Rousseau himself boldly declared in the book's first sentence, never had been heard before. He detailed the losses and passions that launched the mind of "poor Jean-Jacques" (as he often referred to himself) into life's storm, emboldened by his belief that self-knowledge would come through understanding his feelings, his sensible experience, and his pains and failings. With a clinical rigor, he refused to be discreet about his precocious masturbation, his sexual desire, his exposing himself to young women, and more. While published only after his death, Rousseau even dared to mount a stage and give public readings of excerpts of this memoir. Never before had the private sphere so boldly entered the public square.

As for Tissot, his failure to aid Rousseau made its way into his next book on the diseases of writers. The doctor quoted Rousseau on the way intense cogitation weakened the mind and body: "Scholarly work makes men delicate, weakens their temperament, and while the soul retains its vigor with difficulty, the body loses its own. Study wears out the machine." Tissot pointed to Geneva's illustrious exile as an example of such excess, as evidenced by his chronic urinary troubles. Privately, Tissot noted the more disturbing outcome of a taxed imagination: Rousseau, who continued to correspond with the doctor, remained pursued by phantoms of his own making.

In 1766, seeking asylum, Rousseau sailed for England and took refuge with the kindly David Hume, who encouraged him to write his memoirs and lobbied the King of England to grant "our modern Socrates" a pension. However, the mild-mannered Hume was shocked by the intrigue Rousseau soon concocted and glumly concluded: "he is plainly mad, after having long been maddish." The foremost philosopher of sensibility had succumbed to an illness in that domain. While Rousseau had become a beacon who lit the way forward for a new, more equitable society, his alter ego, poor Jean-Jacques, had come to a ruinous end.

Rousseau recognized some of his own folly. He moved back to France and on January 5, 1769, wrote Dr. Tissot to congratulate him for his professorship at the Academy of Lausanne. Then he shared his latest troubles. He was feverish, colicky, riddled by insomnia, and persecuted by others. His person was disfigured in the eyes of the public. What was he to do? An admirer recommended other doctors, but Rousseau replied, "The place that I inhabit caused all the evil and it will be another destination that will heal me."

In Rousseau's last letter to Tissot, he spoke not as a patient, but as an old friend. This "grande malade" now believed that the problem was in his liver, and he thanked the physician for helping him feel better. He accepted Tissot's suggestion to move somewhere with better air and water; he would eat carefully and walk regularly. As for the cream of tartar, he decided against that and assured the doctor that if he was meant to die, Nature knew best. Finally, he ended with a warm goodbye. Tissot, he hoped, would be remembered for his good works. And if his famous patient had never been allowed the honor to speak of this doctor's excellence in public, Rousseau would not forget the sentiments that this doctor had inspired.

IN THE SECOND half of the 18th century, *médecins-philosophes* engaged in critical dialogues on the mind. In Scotland, England, France, and Switzerland, tandems of philosophers and doctors conducted dialogues—Diderot and Bordeu, Rousseau and Tissot, d'Alembert and Barthez—and shared common concerns that no longer belonged in any one intellectual domain. At stake was something urgent and explosive, the building of a natural foundation for individuals in a secular and modern society. Like workers digging a tunnel, the doctors of *le moral* and the philosophers of *esprit* shoved off from their respective shores and, as they neared the center, they tried to join, and thereby create a new ethics and science of man that placed that seemingly unique quality, the willing and creative mind, front and center.

The Montpellier school developed a model in which the realm of mind and meaning might be linked to the body, its passions, fevers, ills, and actions. Their holistic approach made sense, thanks to Haller's nervous physiology, which became an organizing analogy. Humans were first and foremost sensate, not rational or soulful or even moral. While that struck some as Lucretius dressed up in modern garb, these doctors had some scientific evidence to validate their views. And so they pushed their way into the middle of debates on body and soul and offered a third path. Rousseau called it the wise man's materialism, one in which matter was not made of tubes or gears, but was alive with feeling and thought.

As followers of the Montpellier school sought to leave behind the dichotomies of body and soul favored by Cartesians, they applied this new perspective to a host of questions. The overly sensitive were potentially gifted and cursed. Through their receptive nervous systems, these individuals—soon linked to women, children, geniuses and artists—were the antennae of society. They could recognize, feel, and respond to subtle cues that most did not feel. However, the same beings suffered from disorders once called nervous, moral, or mental. Unlike Lockean doctors in England who tried to correct madness through the force of reason, physicians that followed Bordeu and Tissot treated the mentally ill in a manner that mirrored Rousseau's ethos. Reason was a house built on the ground of sensibility. Irritable rage could not be quelled by logic. Interventions to restore health and moral well-being should aim at imbalanced sensibilities.

After 1770, the *médicins-philosophes* rose to prominence. A generation of French doctors followed Bordeu, Barthez, and Tissot, and a line of philosophers sprang up who sought to link physical and moral life in a way that promised to alter political and social beliefs. Metaphysical and ethical questions would find answers thanks to models of an embodied mind that could be known, stabilized, restored, directed, and, when necessary, policed.

While this dialogue began between *philosophes* and physicians, the medical men sought to claim it as their own. Ethics were not for philosophers or theologians, some dared to say. Dr. J. F. Dufour insisted that the effort to link the operations of the mind, its illnesses, and the rules for society must be taken *only* by doctors. In England, a disreputable, half-trained physician who had been run out of Paris, Jean-Paul Marat, insisted that the division of knowledge between *philosophes* and anatomists only meant that there could never be a science of man. These artificially split pursuits should be bridged by doctors who alone witnessed man's suffering in its whole. Bienville, the Montpellier expert on nymphomania, argued that physicians should be entrusted with public morality.

Ironically, this expansion of medical power had no greater

prophet than the often antimedical Rousseau. Men and women were not thinking things, not reasoning machines, and certainly not split between a mechanical body and a soul. They were feeling, sensitive creatures, whose moral and physical lives were deeply intertwined. Through his profoundly influential books, *Julie, or the New Heloise*, *Émile*, and then *The Confessions*, this startling writer bucked many rationalist assumptions and laid out new guidelines for love, childhood development, and the ethics of the self based on mental and emotional sensibility.

Around Europe, a generation of avid Rousseauians popped up, dedicated followers who took that writer as a reflection of what they, in their deepest essence, were and should be. The old order had been not just a politicotheological world, but a full worldview, and its fall offered the opportunities for other modes of self-conceptualization to emerge. Rousseau in his writings had provided such a new conception, one rooted in a unified notion of mind and body, based on a concept that three decades earlier referred to twitching muscles and nerves. Readers began to fall in love à la *Jean-Jacques*, commune with Nature in his fashion, search for authenticity in a solitary life, consider their inalienable political rights in democracy, embrace the truth of passions and sentiments, imitate his ethic of individuality and his ideal of an utterly honest self. A cult grew up around this celebrity. Fans acted as if they knew this recluse and considered him close to their heart—*l'ami Jean-Jacques*, as utter strangers called him. His belief that alienated man must be brought back into harmony with Nature became guidelines for his readers. And smuggled into their new worldview, whether they knew it or not, was a generative model of physiology and psychology based on a vital sensibility.

The young Maximilien de Robespierre soon penned passionate letters after Rousseau's *Nouvelle Héloïse*, and a twenty-two-year-old Napoleon Bonaparte extolled the Rousseauian virtues and reveled in his own authentic aloneness. The grandfather of a young Marie-Henri Beyle, later known as Stendhal, read the works of Jean-Jacques, that honest soul. And the elderly Charlotte-Sophie von d'Aldenburg told her young granddaughter who had become smitten with Rousseau that she would have preferred that the girl choose the Grand Mogul as her godfather. But yet, she had to admitt that *Émile* had created a "revolution in our minds."

After his death, this persecuted and paranoid exile, attacked by the standard-bearers of the *ancien régime* as well as its critics like Voltaire and Diderot, became increasingly cherished by his vast readership. As the novelist George Sand would aptly note, Rousseau's enemies and advocates, his maladies and failures, all faded away, but what remained was that voice of Jean-Jacques, stuck in one's head. He had put forward a new vision of the self, one filled with faults and yet, in its authenticity, noble. And he had unabashedly extolled new ways of considering those great Enlightenment pursuits, human happiness and psychic health. His ethics focused not so much on consciousness and reason, John Locke's rudders, but rather the primacy of the sensitive self. Freed from the corruptions of civilization, an *amour de soi*—self-love—emerged from biological sensibility. In the ethics displayed in *Émile* and the revision of political life in *The Social Contract,* Rousseau built on notions of inner sensibility to unite men and woman in a common sympathy. For some historians, the remaining years of that century in Europe would pivot on these two classic works that Rousseau published in 1762.

"Jean-Jacques," the writer said of himself, was *sui generis,* unlike anyone else on earth, and yet after the 1770s, this became the furthest thing from the truth. Alongside Locke's conscious self, the Swiss writer had created a new model: *le vrai homme, l'honnête homme,* the being born true, honest, sensitive, good, and free, yet everywhere perverted, falsified, and enchained. Perhaps, it was his projection, his fantasy, or perhaps it was a brilliant illumination. Either way, as Jean-Jacques' followers swelled in number, they longed to share his unique identity and soon could declare with him: either I am nobody, or the beginnings of a new nation.

Dr. Mesmer's Invisible Fire

A MORE EXTREME version of Enlightenment materialism, one that went much further than the "wise materialism" of Rousseau and dispensed with *both* the soul and the mind, rolled into Paris with the person of Franz Anton Mesmer. A doctor who had been hounded out of his native Vienna, Mesmer promoted discoveries that, if true, would wipe away the philosophical underpinnings for little Émile, not to mention the Cartesian Cogito and the Galenic humors. His proposals were deeply radical, sealing his fate in his hometown, where he was denounced as an atheist and a fraud. However, this same thinker would be welcomed in a Paris that was transforming under a new king.

Louis XVI had ascended to the throne in 1774. Shy and withdrawn as a child, he had been orphaned like Rousseau and so many others. After his father passed away in 1765, this bookish, diffident heir to the monarchy was provided with a classical education that did not neglect advice from *Émile* and therefore included the pursuit of a practical trade. Married at the age of fifteen to his Habsburg bride, the fourteen-year-old Marie-Antoinette, he took the throne four years later. Quickly, the teenager became the focus of obscene and cruel libels, a genre that flourished during his grandfather's reign. A focus of public fascination was the new king's seeming inability to conceive a child with his wife. The problem was attributed, perhaps not without reason, to the young man's terror of sexual intercourse.

However, the young king had other pressing troubles to keep him up at night, including his country's gargantuan debt, which grew thanks to his decision to support the American colonists, enemies of his enemies, the British. The alliance with the American colonists not only threatened France's financial stability, but also brought home a corps of radicalized soldier-aristocrats. Utopian claims penned by Thomas Jefferson that extolled universal equality, individual liberty, and democratic self-government had been fought for by French troops, who returned home to an absolute monarchy. General Lafayette and his *confrères* had risked their lives for rights that were unimaginable in their own land.

While tentative and at times torn, young King Louis recognized that his reign must be a time of change. The older rebels of the Enlightenment were dying off, often not as outcasts, but as pillars of a new era. A rail-thin Voltaire—that exiled scourge of the Catholic Church—was treated to a hero's return in 1778, when he entered Paris and was fêted at the Academy of Sciences. Jean-Jacques Rousseau died that year, and Condillac, d'Alembert, and Diderot all passed away between 1780 and 1784. Thus, the vanguard of the mid-century *lumières* were buried. Under Louis XVI, a new generation of reformers emerged to take up their spirit of change.

Under Louis XVI, reform spread to different corners of French society, including medicine. For example, the hidebound Paris Faculty of Medicine had long regulated medical practice: they alone were authorized to dispense licenses necessary for practice in their city. Two years after ascending to the throne, Louis XVI shook up that monopoly when he founded the Royal Society of Medicine, a competing body that would focus on science and public health. The Society's very existence implied that the sclerotic Faculty had been so busy resisting change that they had neglected scientific advances and the public welfare. In 1780, this new group snatched up the authority to regulate new medicines and protect patients from quacks. Predicated on the belief that an elite group of doctors could use the rules of evidence and experimentation to determine which cures were scientifically sound, the French Royal Society of Medicine stood in contrast to the free-market ethos that prevailed in England, where it was the buyer's responsibility to beware.

In addition, Louis XVI made some efforts to reform decayed French hospitals, something demanded by advocates since his rise to the throne. Dr. Jacques Tenon, the doctor entrusted with a survey of present conditions, made it clear that hospitals could be seen as "the measure of a civilization, a people." By that standard, he concluded, French civilization was a shambles. And nothing symbolized this failure more than the Hôtel-Dieu.

A hulking, cold, and dank medieval building on the Seine near the Cathedral of Nôtre-Dame, this church-run hospital considered its mission to be the spiritual comfort of the sick as they faced disease and the inevitability of death. The inscription over the hospital's doors inadvertently conveyed some black humor: "Here is the Home of God and the Door to Heaven." Indeed. Visitors were right to believe that one foot inside this hospital would hurry them up to the Hereafter. Wards were staffed by Augustine sisters who tended to a moaning, screaming, human pile. Their focus and training was for the care of souls, so they battled the devil more than fevers. And the nuns' extreme devotion did not include abiding by the suggestions of doctors or surgeons. At the top of the hierarchy, seven dignified administrators that included the Archevêque de Paris, appointed for life terms, ran the institution as they pleased.

And as Tenon documented, what pleased them was appalling. Patients of all sorts not only shared the same ward, but were crammed, up to eight at a time, into the same bed. Epileptics, foaming victims of rabies, the oozing, wounded, and infected, as well as the recently deceased, lay together awaiting their Lord. Twenty-five hundred patients and 300 servants made do in accommodations intended for

less than half that number. The likelihood of death was estimated
to be four times greater than in a provincial French hospital. Simply
put, the Hôtel-Dieu was a hellhole.

In 1786, Louis XVI invited the Academy of Sciences to take up
hospital reform. Dr. Tenon put years of labor into his account, *Rec-
ollections of the Hospitals of Paris*. In the Hôtel-Dieu, Tenon claimed
that there was only one-eighth to one-sixth the amount of air
needed for the inmates to breathe. The 144 barrels of water a day
fell far short of the amount required for patients and staff. Pollution
made the place a disease-ridden cesspool that risked spilling over
into the Seine and contaminating the whole city.

Tenon took special care to note the terrible conditions for those
considered to be maniacs, epileptics, and imbeciles, a long-standing
matter of concern for the government. Still, they had done little to
ameliorate this situation. His survey determined that out of the 20,341
patients in France, 1,331 were insane and were housed in everything
from tiny, private maisons like the Pension du St. Carnillieux (census
of 1) to large poorhouses like the Salpêtrière (census of 600). All the
public facilities were for incurables except for one. Rather horrify-
ingly, the sole treatment facility for the mentally ill who were poor,
the one that supposedly held out hope for their recovery, was none
other than the Hôtel-Dieu.

There, the impoverished sufferers received the standard array of
baths, opiates, bleedings, and purgings. Those who managed to survive but not recover were certified to be beyond hope. They were
carted off to a Hôpital général, which was nothing more than a
warehouse. The men's facility was called the Bicêtre and contained
3,000 inhabitants, of which 220 were mad. Young boys and elderly
men camped together; criminals mingled with the febrile, epileptic,
and orphaned. Women would be sent to the even larger Salpêtrière:
6,000 females, of whom approximately 550 were considered mentally ill. For problematic inmates, there were isolation "loges," two-
meter-square rooms with small windows, straw on the floor, and an

iron ring on the wall for chains. As with London's Bedlam, weekend visitors came to gawk at this misery.

The number of the mad in these poorhouses was dwarfed by thousands of beggars, hundreds of homeless elderly, as well as criminals and hordes of abandoned children. The collapse of French society was nowhere more obvious than in Tenon's figures for the rise of homeless, uncared-for youth. While an average of 1,900 children were abandoned each decade between 1670 and 1740, ensuing decades saw a huge rise. Between 1771 and 1782 alone, 76,735 infants were left to their fate. Given that the total population of Paris was 660,000, this was a staggering figure.

Of course, better facilities were available for Frenchmen of means. Eighteen private establishments, called *maisons de santé* or *pensions bourgeoises* existed around Paris. These private establishments, such as the Pension du St. Belhomme on the Rue Charonne were run by businessmen. They housed a third of all inmates in France. Of the care in these facilities, one doctor quipped that the proprietor was not only indifferent to effective remedies, but unabashedly opposed to them. While the public institutions reeked of massive neglect, the private ones stank of corruption.

Central to this interconnected system of hospitals, jails, poorhouses, and private establishments, was the dreaded *lettres de cachet*. These royal decrees allowed for the detainment and hospitalization or imprisonment of individuals without any evidence. On the authority of the king, the *lettre de cachet* took away one's freedom by administrative fiat. It was an order for imprisonment legitimized by the desire of the police and the king. Criminals, madmen, libertines, truants, weirdos, and troublemakers were all potentially subject to this legal writ, as were disobedient children and wives, relatives who stood in the way of inherited riches, and detested spouses. *Correctionaires*—men and women who needed to be corrected—were confined to restrictive institutions. There was no attempt to treat them, but a *lettre de cachet* kept them in a cell. When they would be freed was anybody's guess.

⸙

AS ENLIGHTENED REFORM efforts for French hospitals and medicine commenced, Mesmer arrived in Paris. Influenced by Newton and possessed of a new medical method, this Austrian doctor claimed to have discovered the source of life in matter that was merely theorized about in Montpellier. Machine-man was lit up not by nervous sensibility or an unknowable "x" factor, but by a kind of magnetism found in all living beings. In February of 1778, when Mesmer arrived in the French capital, an eager populace awaited him.

The French had become fascinated by scientific innovations, unimaginable feats of modern existence such as the astonishing flight of hot air balloons. Gentlemen-scientists played with magnets, while others stunned friends with chemical reactions. Scientific novelty was in the air, quite literally, for one of the most astonishing developments was the attempt to corral the terrifying force of lightning. In the 1740s, lightning bolts were shown by the brilliant Benjamin Franklin to be made of an electrical "fluid," which the jovial American colonist would use to set his brandy on fire. This led to international celebrity. Franklin was, in the words of the German philosopher Immanuel Kant, the new Prometheus. Techniques to capture this mighty heavenly power followed, as Franklin's lightning rods popped up all over France.

Electrical machines also were invented; this new technology gave experimenters the capacity to jolt subjects and, inadvertently, themselves. Around 1750, traveling performers dazzled their audiences with tricks like the teeth-chattering "electric kiss." Simultaneously, doctors began to experiment with electrical charges from one of these devices, known as the Leyden jar. In the view of

Franklin and others, one of the most promising uses of such bottled electricity might be the treatment of nervous ills, things like palsies, convulsions, paralyses, melancholias, and hysterias. By the 1770s, claims for electrical cures for nervous ills were growing, especially in less regulated England, German-speaking principalities, and the outer provinces of France. While the pain of such treatments could be excruciating, electrical enthusiasts like the Halle doctor Christian Kratzenstein persisted. For doctors, the notion that this wild force from the sky might cure cohered with beliefs in the importance of natural forces like climate and air quality. And given the way electricity threw a man to the ground, it was inevitable that some would consider this mighty force the long-sought élan vital, the factor that gave life to the body, and therefore might also possess restorative powers.

The logic for electrical treatments of nervous conditions was simple. If nerves were animated by a vital fluid, then perhaps like eels, humans were electrical beings. While it was understood that illness might arise from structural damage to the nerves, it might also be the result of a stoppage of this nervous fluid's flow. Electrical shocks might clear the blockage.

Manufacturers began to produce cheap electrical devices, and laymen in Britain like John Wesley promoted electrical cures for the masses. In France, Boissier de Sauvages introduced electrical treatments in Montpellier, and Dr. P. J. C. Mauduyt de la Varenne championed electrical therapies in Paris, along with a shady practitioner named Le Dru, who performed his cabinet show under the stage name of "Comus." By 1776, the Royal Society of Medicine was tasked with evaluating whether or not this was a dangerous fad. Doctors conducted experiments that proved the human pulse was affected by small electric shocks. Soon, devotees like Dr. Mauduyt and Le Dru were allowed into the Paris medical establishment. Le Dru not only won approval from the Faculty, but was put in charge of a charity hospital, in which he employed his sizzling therapies.

And so, when Mesmer arrived with claims for a similar force two years later, the ground in Paris had been readied. Montpellier vitalists posited an active force, and doctors wielding portable electrical devices claimed they had isolated that natural force, which if marshaled could revolutionize medicine. The Viennese doctor's theories of an animal magnetic force seemed, like Franklin's electrical fluid, to be the fruit of Enlightenment reason. Mesmer posited a soulless, material cure for moral and physical ills. And his universal fluid put humankind back in direct touch with the planets and the cosmos, not through superstitions and rituals, but with a scientific force that regulated everything in Nature from the stars to the human body.

Born on May 23, 1734, near Lake Constance, in Swabia, Franz Anton Mesmer attended Jesuit universities before studying medicine at the University of Vienna, where he graduated in 1766. His medical school teachers were mostly mechanists influenced by Boerhaave, and his dissertation displayed an ambition to push their assumptions further. Celestial bodies like the stars and the moon exerted force on human bodies, as was obvious in the case of lunatics, whose cycles of madness followed the revolution of the moon. Therefore, a physical force, an "animal gravity" linked the astral and human planes, and should be studied for its effects on health.

Two years later, Mesmer married a rich widow and settled in at a magnificent estate frequented by illustrious friends like the Mozart family. He opened a medical practice and discovered that a Jesuit astronomer from the university, Maximilian Hell, used magnets to treat medical ills like stomach cramps. Mesmer was delighted when Hell agreed to fashion special body magnets for the doctor to clamp onto a patient's feet and abdomen. If celestial bodies moved fluids like the sea, perhaps these magnets could alter pathological tides in the body.

When Mesmer announced the results of his own clinical experiments, he did not mince words. In 1773, he had treated a woman who suffered from convulsions. After he had her swallow iron filings, he employed magnets which produced great pain, a crisis, and then relief. Mesmer believed he had discovered a cure for nervous diseases; his discovery would, he believed, sweep away orthodox medicine and usher in a golden age. So he excitedly informed the president of the Vienna Faculty of Medicine, his old teacher Baron Anton von Störck.

Using the language and logic of physics, starting with the assumption that humans were simply matter in motion, Mesmer announced that he had discovered a universal physical force that acted on nerves, which he called "animal gravity." The true source of sympathy described by Scottish doctors and philosophers, the sen-

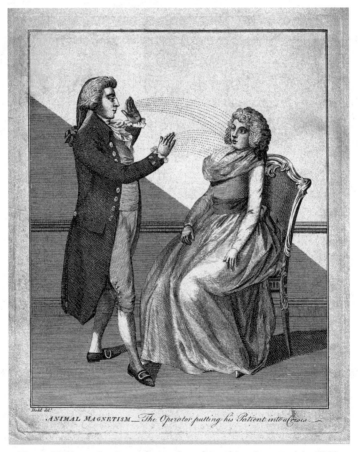

ANIMAL MAGNETISM—The Operator putting his Patient into a crisis.

Figure 30. An animal magnetist places his subject into a crisis, 1802.

sibility of Haller and the Montpellier vitalists, was now revealed as a Newtonian-like force that could be mobilized to treat melancholia, mania, hysteria, and convulsions, not to mention a host of other ills that resulted from nervous dysfunction.

Magnetism with the use of minerals was only half of the story. Mesmer concluded that many things could be magnetized, including bread, trees, and, most important, the human body, which he believed had a special capacity to hold a charge. Therefore, to create an artificial tide in a body, Mesmer stopped using magnets and began to rely on his own natural magnetism: he made twirling "passes" with his hands. And he experimented with his own version of the Leyden jar, which were large baths that supposedly concentrated magnetic force.

In 1775, Mesmer announced these stunning discoveries to academies of sciences across Europe. He waited expectantly. Only the Academy in Berlin bothered to reply; they informed the doctor that he was dreaming. However, word of his efforts reached the Bavarian Academy of Sciences, so the doctor was invited to weigh in on a controversy that had thrown into question the boundaries of science and belief.

A renegade Catholic priest named Father Johann Joseph Gassner had captivated audiences with his capacity to cure convulsions and melancholia through exorcism. While Catholics had used exorcism as a tool to pry believers away from Protestant pastors a century before, times had changed. Even the Pope was now prepared to condemn Gassner for his unorthodox techniques. Using methods that were standard a century earlier, Gassner carefully sought to segregate supernatural torment from natural disease and to claim power over the former. Chanting in Latin and speaking Jesus's name would pain a person whose soul was possessed, while those who did not react to his incantations were sent to a doctor.

In 1775, Dr. Mesmer came to Munich to evaluate Father Gassner's cures, and with their encounter, two worlds collided. Notions of the soul confronted radical materialism. For the savants of the Academy, it was no contest. Dr. Mesmer examined Gassner's sufferers and showed he too could provoke the same torments, not by chanting the name of God, but by manipulating the flow of nervous fluid through animal magnetism. Mesmer's triumphant conclusion: Gassner employed animal magnetism for his cures but didn't know it.

A radical Enlightenment vision had won the day. The torments of the soul were due to nervous energies; in this translation of soul to nerves, there was no need to invoke that third element, the mind. The mind did nothing. Mesmer would continue to elaborate this over the years: spirits, evil charms, and soul possession were the result of nervous forces and magnetism. God's holy powers, he seemed to imply, were actually magnetic.

A victorious Mesmer returned to Vienna, where his work was gathering momentum. He had taken up the treatment of a blind pianist and soon, word of her miraculous cure brought crowds to his door. The woman, Maria Theresia von Paradis, had been unable to see since the age of four. Thanks to well-connected parents, all advantages had been lavished upon her, including embossed maps and learning automata. She developed into a talented pianist and won the support of Queen Maria Theresa. Yet she continued to be tormented by intense eye spasms, melancholia, and fitful rages. Mesmer's former teacher and the queen's chief physician, Dr. Störck, attempted to use electricity to shock the girl's troubles away. Thousands of excruciating jolts to her eyes were to no avail. Uncured, the young woman entered into the care of Mesmer, who denounced this torture, and claimed to manipulate similar nervous energies without more than his own prancing and gesticulating being.

Fraulein Paradis moved into Mesmer's house, where he worked on her with his hands and a short, cone-shaped wand. Incredibly, the girl began to say she could see. Mesmer's face was the first she ever visualized: his nose struck her as a grotesque bit of absurdity. The parents were ecstatic; her father wrote a worshipful testimonial. As for the doctor, he must have known that the cure of such an illustrious person would cement his reputation and give him the recognition he yearned for. The intense treatment continued. At times, however, Fräulein Paradis seemed to be only able to see when Dr. Mesmer was by her side. Conflicts began to emerge with Paradis's parents. Mesmer accused them of wanting to protect their daughter's pension, which was predicated on her disability.

Soon, Dr. Störck and others intervened in what they began to consider immoral activity, perhaps even madness. When the girl's parents came to forcibly retrieve their daughter, Maria clung to Mesmer like a lover. According to Mesmer's own account, the girl's mother threw her daughter headfirst into a wall, while her father charged at him with a sword. When the ugly scene was over, the girl was back home, stone-blind. Dr. Störck concluded that his once-promising medical student was insane.

Furious and publicly humiliated, with little professional future left in Vienna, Mesmer fled. He not only left behind his practice, but also his wife, perhaps as a consequence of his intense engagement with the blind pianist. After a period of wandering, Mesmer resurfaced in Paris. With only an assistant, he settled into a modest apartment on the Place Vendôme and began to see patients. His expectations of world fame seemed dead.

However, in Paris this Viennese doctor became all the rage. There, electrical doctors and their stunned clientele, vitalists from Montpellier, and radical materialists schooled on d'Holbach were all eager to seriously consider his theories. Perhaps this was the long-awaited active force in human bodies. A material nervous force had emerged where once the soul had reigned. Here was the long-sought Newtonian Science of Man. Mesmer seemed to have discovered the physics that determined nervous life. Animal magnetism was the source of what Thomas Willis and others searched for, that "invisible fire" inside.

Dr. Mesmer's reputation grew as he manipulated inner tides. His patients shrieked, laughed, stripped off their clothes, fell into crises, and healed their nervous ills. Inner tides seemed to control their choices and actions. There was never a more powerful spectacle to demonstrate that matter controlled man. Both the torments of the soul and the troubles of the mind, it now seemed, could be explained by magnetic energies.

Mesmer moved into opulently furbished rooms on Rue Coq-Héron, which he filled with tapestries and mirrors. Visitors reported that the space was always animated with the sound of a glass harmonica or piano. As this apartment filled with seekers, Mesmer's technique evolved. Dr. Mesmer commanded center stage, as an imposing healer, who manipulated magnetic energies with his hands, legs, and eyes. Knees touching, he pressed the sick with his thumbs and warned of a coming crisis. Are you feeling sick, are you about to vomit? He moved his hands to what he determined were the north and south poles of the human body. His stare deployed a prodigious amount of animal magnetism directly into the sufferer's being.

Such a treatment was quite labor-intensive, and so to meet the great demand for his services, the doctor increasingly relied on *baquets,* big wooden tubs filled with iron filings that had bars, which projected outward. Patients sat by these tubs holding the bars so as to concentrate the magnetic fluid. As the magnetic forces built, patients fell into a crisis. The idea of a crisis mirrored the vitalist theories of Bordeu, who believed dynamic forces must be provoked into a storm before they would break and be cured.

However, Mesmer's crises were high drama. Patients went into convulsions and rages, they shouted and laughed and writhed in pain, and then would be spirited off to specially designated *chambres des crises,* padded with mattresses. When they emerged from this room, they would be healed.

All of Paris was abuzz. But while his practice boomed, the discoverer of animal magnetism was not content. He sought recognition for his brilliant synthesis of physics and medicine. And so he set himself the task of winning over the authorities in France. He began with the

Academy of Sciences, where he demonstrated how he fixed his gaze on another, not unlike the English doctors Pargeter and Willis. The Academy members were unmoved. He turned to the Royal Society of Medicine. They dryly noted that Mesmer's animal magnetism, unlike electricity, remained a totally unproven force. Finally, thanks to one of Mesmer's most ardent new recruits, Charles Deslon, his work was presented to the conservative Faculty of Medicine. Deslon was the physician to the Comte d'Artois, brother of the king, and so he received the chance to argue for animal magnetism. The Faculty remained unimpressed.

Stymied by these scientific elites, Mesmer turned to the reading public. His 1779 *Memoir on the Discovery of Animal Magnetism* included twenty-seven scientific propositions for a new Newtonian-like force. The first proposition began with the celestial bodies and then zoomed in on the human body. Mesmer did not hold back: The medicine of yore was useless. In Nature, there was one illness, blockages of magnetism, and one cure, his own.

French response was split. In 1780, the Faculty of Paris condemned the doctor as a charlatan. However, as he was about to leave Paris, Marie-Antoinette guaranteed him an annual stipend and a school of his own if he allowed for some oversight. Displaying vanity and a temper that would repeatedly flare, Mesmer slapped away this beneficence not just in private, but in an indignant letter to the public. The doctor proclaimed himself a man of the people, and he doused the queen with contempt. Mesmer again took up his pen to explain his discoveries to the guardians of science. His new book listed each of the forty-seven scientific and medical societies from Cracow to Martinique that received free copies of this work. He even bothered to note how many copies—six to twenty—that he sent each group.

Meanwhile, Mesmer was finding it hard to control his hodge-podge of followers. Animal magnetism was growing from a medical specialty to something bigger. It offered secret knowledge that could not just cure illness, but also create well-being. Thus, as with Rousseau's philosophy of sensibility, it stood as an alternative vision of what might guide a woman's or man's life. However, the growing number of animal magnetists in France constantly infuriated Mesmer, whose demands for power and secrecy were absolute. He grew suspicious of Dr. Deslon's thriving practice and accused him of betraying his master. Thus, Mesmer lost his most esteemed medical follower. In the wake of this conflict, two of Mesmer's lay followers, Nicolas Bergasse and Guillaume Kornman, suggested that a tightly controlled organization of dues-paying followers be created to reign in wild magnetists.

The first Society of Harmony was founded with forty-eight members, only six of whom were doctors or surgeons. The rest were grand bourgeoisie and aristocrats who forked over a small fortune and agreed to follow autocratic rules, which included a restriction on their teaching or practicing animal magnetism without Mesmer's consent. Societies of Harmony sprang up in Lyon, Strasbourg, and elsewhere, making Mesmer wealthy, though these societies did not display much harmony. In 1785, the irascible founder again broke ties, this time with both Bergasse and Kornman, but still the Societies continued to multiply.

For anyone who feared that Dr. Mesmer had scary abilities to command other human beings, there was an obvious irony. The founder of animal magnetism had rather quickly lost control over his own troops. Then one former follower, the repudiated Dr. Deslon, precipitated a defining battle for this community. Despite being disowned by the master, Deslon had continued to agitate for an official evaluation from the authorities. With his powerful connections in the king's court, Deslon got his wish. In March 1784, an official commission was established to investigate animal magnetism. The king appointed five members from the Academy of Sciences, including the celebrated discoverer of electrical fluid, Benjamin Franklin, along with four members from the Faculty of Medicine, including Dr. Joseph-Ignace Guillotin, inventor of a more humanitarian tool for executions. A second commission from the Royal Society of Medicine, which included the electrical doctor Mauduyt, also convened to determine the usefulness of this treatment.

While electrical medicine held promise, Benjamin Franklin was dubious about animal magnetism. "I cannot but fear that the Expectation of great Advantage from the new method of treating Diseases, will prove a great Delusion," wrote the sage from the New World. Drolly, he added, "That Delusion may however, in some cases be of use while it lasts." This was not simply a clever quip, for long ago Franklin had come to recognize the mind's suggestive power over bodily ills. In 1757, approached by patients who heard of miraculous electrical cures for paralysis that had occurred in Germany and Italy, Franklin had begun to shock immobilized arms and legs. For the first five days of these treatments, he noticed minor improvements which then vanished. Franklin wrote a friend, Dr. John Pringle, and confessed that the improvements could have come either from the electricity or from the uplift in spirits that came with the hope of success. He would bring this same critical question to Mesmerism.

The Commission organized a series of experiments. Members subjected themselves to Deslon's powers and felt nothing. At Franklin's estate, a blindfolded twelve-year-old, said to be an adept who could sense magnetized energy, was asked to pick the tree in the garden that had been supercharged by Dr. Deslon, who watched from a distance. The boy strolled past the tree that Deslon had worked on, arrived at another, and fell into a furious fit.

And so, in 1784, a series of devastating reports to the king were published. The Commission of the Academy and the Faculty both concluded that animal magnetism was the result of three things: nervous irritation, a manipulated imagination, and imitation. There was no proof of an animal magnetic fluid. Whatever physical effects occurred were mental, "affectations of the *esprit*." Evidence showed that the imagination could produce sensations like heat and pain in the body. That was the source of Mesmer's cures.

When the report of the Royal Society of Medicine appeared, it added to the Commission's damning report. However, one Royal Society doctor refused to sign on to the report, due to its association with Dr. Mauduyt, the electrical physician. Dr. Antoine Laurent de Jussieu filed his own separate report and claimed both animal magnetism *and* electrical cures were false. While these treatments claimed to directly affect the body and mind through physical forces, they were in fact all due to nervous irritation and the mind's powers.

And so, Mesmerism had sparked a battle between the competing paradigms of soul, brain, and mind. Mersenne and Descartes knew that passive machinery alone could not account for consciousness and its seeming capacity for direct volition: for them a soul was required. In cities like Edinburgh, Montpellier, and Paris, secularizing moderns tried to construct a body driven by a natural, vital force, thereby accounting for a mind with causal power and mentally caused illness. Debates over animal magnetism added a new twist to these debates.

Father Gassner's soul cures had been refuted by Mesmer; they were reframed as physiological. Cosmic magnetism impacted the nerves and controlled volition. Mesmer made passes over magnetized patients, and in the process they lost control of their own subjectivity. They danced or cried or winced because of the flow of magnetic fluid, not because they desired to do so. Their nerves overrode both their minds and souls.

Couched in scientific rhetoric, animal magnetism seemed to be the heir to gravity, or perhaps Newton's theory of ether, which while difficult to prove, seemed like a necessary postulate. For those eager to see science replace superstitious belief, this might be seen as a breakthrough. Natural matter and the rules of motion and energy had taken over the soul. Or so it seemed.

However, in the same way that Mesmer reframed Father Gassner's soul cures as nervous ones, Franklin and his colleagues reframed Mesmer's nervous cures as in fact mental ones. The Viennese doctor's belief in invisible energies had led him to ignore the influence of ideas. His patients were not acting as magnetic machines; rather, they had imitated Mesmer and followed him into some strange, waking reverie. The cause was not magnetic, nor spiritual, but the way ideas could surreptitiously pass from mind to mind.

Franklin's Commission also produced a secret report for the police that accused animal magnetists of posing another risk. The stoking of imaginations between the male magnetist, cozied up against the often female patient, touching her and staring deeply into her eyes, waiting for her to fall into a spasm of eye rolling, cramping, panting and then relief—all this was a sexual pantomime. No doubt, the theatrics were a prelude to the real thing. Though this additional report remained confidential, the word was already out. French readers had already been encouraged to imagine the magnetic encounter as not science, but rather seduction.

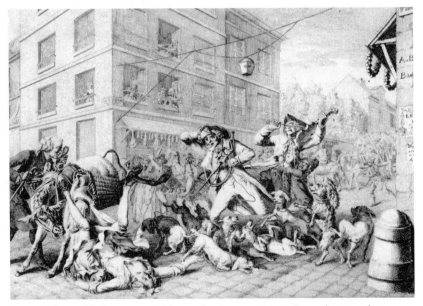

Figure 31. A cartoon satirizes animal magnetists as dogs who provoke sexual and social mayhem.

THE 1784 ROYAL Commission on animal magnetism initiated a furious struggle that revealed deep divisions in French society. Raucous
choruses rose up to applaud or mock the Commission and their official condemnation of Mesmerism. A pamphlet war commenced.

For traditional Parisian doctors, the Commission's report was
gratifying. A threat had been removed. Galenists and iatromechanists
could take solace in the conclusion that Mesmer's cures were imaginary. However, if Mesmer had in fact cured his sufferers through
their imaginations, how was that possible? Dualists could only shrug
their shoulders. Those aligned with Montpellier were better positioned; in 1782, Dr. Pierre Pomme argued that the effects of animal magnetism arose from irritation on a preexisting increased nerve
sensibility. Tissot and the Royal Commission adopted a similar line
of thought: the rubbing and touching of the skin during the séance
aroused nervous sensibilities that effected the imagination and provoked a crisis.

Electrical physicians also scrambled to deal with animal magnetism. One enthusiast, an aristocrat who opened his own electrical
hospital on his estate, sought to co-opt Mesmer. In his account, *The
Friend of Nature, or the Way to Treat Maladies by the Supposed Animal
Magnetism*, he proposed that electrical forces were the true source of
Mesmer's cures. Others tried to make certain that the two approaches
were not linked, an effort that proved futile despite the stark fact
that electricity was a proven force while animal magnetism was not.
After the royal condemnation of animal magnetism in 1784, Parisian
medical authorities, who six years earlier had encouraged electrical
treatments, abruptly did an about-face. Le Dru was reduced to filling
beds in his electrical hospital with poor creatures forced into his care
by *lettres de cachet*.

To further delegitimize animal magnetism, the Commission

created a counternarrative. This Viennese doctor was not a New-ton, but rather one of those discredited misteriosos like Paracelsus. Animal magnetism was a throw back to the occult and alchemical. Despite Mesmer's scientific logic and staunch materialism, his secret methods gave the Commission a chance to link him to a long line of frauds. One well-known advocate of modern medicine, Dr. Michel-Augustin Thouret, devoted 250 pages to that effort, ironically situ-ating Franz Mesmer alongside of Father Gassner. Mesmer was but a new kind of enthusiast, one whose inspired delusions came not from God, but rather from a credulous approach to science.

This effort to crush Mesmer was not left unanswered. His fol-lowers unleashed a flood of first-person testimonials, challenges, and rebuttals. Some lauded this doctor as a working-class hero, unjustly banished by the king. Others accused the Commission of corruption in their "scientific" evaluation. *Letter on Animal Magnetism* by Galart de Montjoye asked how could the great Franklin, known to be too ill to travel to Paris, possibly have examined anything? (He seemed to be unaware that some of the experiments were carried out on Franklin's estate.) Montjoye then gave what seemed to be a firsthand account of the proceedings, in which corrupt commissioners flit-ted about, chatting and laughing, not seriously evaluating anything. While these representatives of the king might say what they will, the public would decide animal magnetism's fate, he declared.

This appeal to the rights of the public became a refrain. Scientific models of truth, established by elites, were pitted against popular will and freedom of choice. For Montjoye and others, the public was endowed with reason and could determine the truth of Mesmerism. It didn't require the gamesmanship of corrupt commissions. If the French public wanted animal magnetism, they should have it. How-ever, *savants* considered science the arbiter of truth, and surely did not trust a poorly educated populace. And, the Franklin Commission had added a disturbing new wrinkle: Mesmerism, they concluded, easily fooled the more educated members of society. It was a form of faith healing that played to their beliefs in the illuminating power of science. In trying to rid the world of superstition, the demystifiers of the Enlightenment had created their own illusions! The imagination of the Enlightenment subject, schooled to accept invisible forces that lifted hot-air balloons into the air and held planets in orbit, had developed into a credulity for unseen material forces.

If this wasn't the end of the Enlightenment, it was the clear demonstration of its limits: a growing cadre of experts and authorities demanded belief in science from the masses, though science itself was dependent on skepticism and checking for oneself. And yet few aside from gentlemen of leisure and doctors had the capacity to check for themselves. The rest would have to take it on faith that a lightning rod would save their home or that Franz Anton Mesmer was a fraud. By 1784, many in France questioned the authority of the scientific *grands hommes*, whose claims to truth only stoked long-simmering class resentment. Testimonials, often signed and listed in groups, portrayed Mesmerism as an easy, cheap remedy outlawed by elites interested in maintaining corporate monopolies and protecting their pocketbooks.

The political aspirations of animal magnetism were openly revealed when the first sanctioned practitioner in England, John Bell, a member of the Society of Harmony in Paris, returned home to spread the word. His *New System of the World* began with Newton's gravity, moved to a universal magnetic fluid, and then continued on to a utopian society that existed in harmony. Energies freely flowed in bodies, and affections united men in a social equilibrium. Animal magnetism brought humans toward that ideal of togetherness and communal peace. Blockages of magnetic flow led to illness, while the disruption of the mind's magnetic flow led to an insular, selfish wickedness. No priests or ministers were needed. Physical harmony was the job of magnetic doctors, Bell declared, while the search for a moral harmony must be the object of government.

Others grasped the radical possibilities of magnetism. In *The*

Mesmerian Moralist, the writer Jean-Baptiste Salaville used this materialist science to rethink sex, love, and morality. In twelve letters, the
author advised an unnamed female correspondent to forget religion,
which only tyrannized her. Sex was a natural force: Mesmer was its
Newton. He was the genius who discovered the true energy behind
sexual attraction. Magnetic connections between people, the *rapport*,
allowed one human to influence the will of another, through invisible energies. Animal magnetism led all men and women to act like
magnets and join in love.

This magnetizer's belief in natural sexual forces and the new
materialist rules for sexual desire found an appreciative audience in
France, where readers gobbled up libertine literature. If once a libertine was an often anticlerical freethinker, by Mesmer's time the term
had come to connote those commited to free love, sexual license, and
seduction. In 1777, Vivant Denon published his novel *No Tomorrow*,
a tale of a naïf who entered a world of aristocratic seduction and cruelty. In 1782, Pierre Choderlos de Laclos published *Dangerous Liaisons*, a disturbing epistolary novel that depicted hedonists, in thrall
to a cult of sensibility, engaged in sexual games of seduction and
betrayal, all with the belief that Nature commanded them. As one
vicious rake repeated, if I must do these things, it is not my fault. The
staging of Beaumarchais's *The Marriage of Figaro* in 1784 encouraged
the audience to similarly question conventional sexual morality.

The king and the Catholic Church leaned on each other: assaults
on the theological order were attacks on the political order. Both of
these pillars were threatened by the Society of Harmony. For Guillaume Kornman and Nicolas Bergasse, like their student John Bell,
animal magnetism held utopian possibilities. This new physics could
help liberate people and restore their natural magnetic bonds. Through
mesmeric séances, individuals could be returned to a natural harmony
with themselves and others. Healing for individuals, families, and
societies would come through the magnetizing tub. Rousseau's natural man could be freed of corruption through that pool.

Such curative powers were required to combat perverse forces in French society, in which immorality destroyed the magnetic ties of a family, as highlighted in the notorious case of Guillaume Kornman himself. Kornman's faithless wife had been a source of torment to him for years; in part, this was what led him to Dr. Mesmer. In 1787, a public scandal ensued when this aggrieved husband pressed an adultery suit against her. His ally from the Society of Harmony, Nicolas Bergasse rose to his friend's defense and described the disruption of this family due to venal libertines from the court. Old lechers had ruined the rapport between Kornman and his wife. Her persistent adultery was not just a crime, but a magnetic sickness. Kornman's wife was defended by Beaumarchais, whose scorn for fidelity was well known. The real-life drama played out in the newspapers and was probably a source for Mozart's *Così fan tutte*, in which the Viennese composer ridiculed the notion that physical rapports could force lovers to switch partners, as if they were a bunch of magnets.

If some envisioned a Mesmeric utopia, others scorned this as a fad. During the 1784 pamphlet wars, mocking reports, pornographic cartoons, racy ballads, bawdy jokes and numerous satires churned forth from the press. One of the most biting tracts, *Mesmer Justified* ridiculed the Viennese doctor as a little god in his "Temple of Divinity." On the stage, *The Modern Doctors* and *The Health Tub* took up the rich comic possibilities afforded by Mesmer and his swooning patients. For others, the plush setting of Mesmer's clinic could not help but recall the libertine's *petite maison*, that love nest, in which seduction was hurried along thanks to *coup d'oeil* paintings, candles, and erotic sculptures that were so enticing even the most careful virgin could not resist.

Alongside the first-person accounts of cures, there were also a number of testimonials by those who had faked illnesses that were not detected and others who attended séances and left uncured. Of these, the most damaging was unintended. Antoine Court de Gébelin penned a glowing account of his magnetic cure, then promptly died in Mesmer's own home. The Viennese doctor's humiliation was only exacerbated shortly thereafter when a pianist arrived in Paris for a month of performances. Well-informed music lovers tittered as Dr. Mesmer attended a performance of the talented Maria Theresia von Paradis from Vienna, a brilliant musician he once had treated, who was perfectly, completely blind.

MESMERISM SHOULD HAVE died. Its founder had lost control of his own movement and, despite clear, scientific logic, his claims for a neurophysics that eliminated the soul and the mind had been roundly rejected by elites around Europe. The undeniable effects of his energies on patients were reinterpreted by the Commission to be, not magnetism's effect on the nerves, but rather mostly the result of an entity Mesmer had bypassed completely, the mind's faculty of imagination. Angry and proud, Mesmer fled Paris and spent much of the rest of his life in bitter isolation. However, the movement he started did not perish, thanks to a reconceptualization that transformed the Viennese doctor's debunked tidal energies into something else.

Franklin's report heaped scorn on the magnetic force Mesmer hypothesized, but it also generated widespread curiosity about the Viennese doctor's undeniable effect on patients. If there was no magnetic fluid, what powers resided in this charismatic man? How could he get so many to contort, grimace, and convulse on cue? Could the imagination alone create all that? In America, John Adams and Dr. Benjamin Rush were delighted by Franklin's exposé, but both men agreed that the Commission raised an important issue when they granted such power to the irrational imagination. What did that mean about human reason, will, and autonomy? If such a formidable force existed in the mind, the Americans urged doctors to harness it. In fact, a new theory based on irrational mental phenomena already had been created by one of Mesmer's followers.

Like a number of aimless aristocrats in France, the three Puységur brothers fell hard for Mesmer. From an august line, these young men held the titles of viscount, count, and marquis. The viscount and count were among the first dozen to register for the Paris Society of Harmony. The marquis, though late to the party, changed the course of animal magnetism.

In 1784, the peak year of the Mesmer craze, the marquis began to take the health of the peasants on his estate into his own hands. One of his first cases was a stableboy, the twenty-three-year-old Victor Race, who was in bed for four days with pains and fever. Victor suffered from lung congestion, for which the marquis employed Mesmer's technique. To Puységur's astonishment, the young man fell into a waking sleep—"magnetic sleep," the marquis would later call it. The normally taciturn, obedient peasant, though clearly not awake, spoke candidly of his private life and its miseries. The marquis instinctively took it upon himself to combat these negative thoughts with more joyful ones: Victor had won a prize! He was dancing at a fair! He was singing! When Race awoke, he remembered nothing. Soon, his health returned.

What had transpired? Mesmer had no interest in talk; he placed no power in words, ideas, imagination, and reason. He would have been offended by the notion that his cures worked on anything but the nerves. For Mesmer, the magnetizer exerted his will as a conductor of a force that linked two nervous systems into one. For a short while, their animal machines were wired together. However, the Marquis de Puységur was confronted not with two magnets in movement, but two subjects controlled by one will, his own. Victor absorbed the marquis's ideas without any hint of his own likes and dislikes. He had surrendered his ability to choose, want, or freely act. In magnetic sleep, his mind lost one of its most distinguishing features: intentional volition. In this weird state, the mind did not just become will-less but, according to the marquis, it became clairvoyant. Magnetized humans could gaze into the past and future, as well as peer through clothing and inside bodies.

To make matters even more astonishing, Puységur found that he did not even need to speak to convey his thoughts to Victor. Thoughts simply transferred from one mind to the other. He could arrest Victor's associations, change and rearrange them: he had complete control over the peasant's inner life. As lord of the estate, he already exercised a great deal of command over his peasants, but now the marquis could tell them how and what to think. He paused, however, when he considered the danger of this power falling into the wrong hands. An evil magnetizer could penetrate the secrets of others, abuse their confidence, and wreak havoc.

Magnetic sleep, he concluded, was some previously unknown form of somnambulism, one that could now be artificially invoked. With this, the marquis discovered another Victor inside Victor Race, and perhaps another self inside all selves. The hidden Victor was none of the things John Locke proposed: he was not conscious, not rational, and not autonomous. In fact, his mind was deeply vulnerable to others through that domain that Lockeans had no use for, the imagination. Victor's associations did not arise from sensation or reflection, but rather a dreamy intersubjective existence. Through establishing a deep rapport with his magnetist, the two could be one, master and slave, suggester and magnetized. Although no philosopher, Puységur could not help but recognize that his discovery raised profound questions, which he confined to a series of endnotes. However, he dared to say that animal magnetism proved what great physiologists and doctors had long labored to demonstrate, namely that spiritual life was dependent on material existence. Though their ultimate origin remained mysterious, thought and will were both part of material life, part of the mind.

When in 1786 the marquis published his account of magnetic sleep, the response from Mesmer was swift. Magnetic sleep did not exist in *sane* people; it was a symptom of mental illness. Dreams were a nocturnal kind of insanity, and waking dreams due to dysregulated sleep were the source of this Victor's madness. However, the marquis did not recant. Instead, the rift between Mesmer and Puységur split this already fragmented movement.

After 1786, the Societies of Harmony were divided. Some stubbornly defended animal magnetism and stuck to their founder's physics. Others adopted Puységur's mentalist model; for them, the cures of animal magnetism were due to acts of verbal and nonverbal suggestions made in rapport. And finally, a third group—to the horror of Mesmer—argued that magnetic sleep demonstrated supernatural powers. Artificial somnambulism placed one man's spirit in contact with another's. Puységur's *somnambule* displayed the unnatural powers of the immortal soul.

Neurophysics, mental suggestion, and soul travel jostled for a place in the splintered movement. In the Societies of Harmony in Strasbourg and in Lyon, mystics listening for secret messages took over what had once been a radically materialist movement. For them, the marquis had discovered a vessel for voyages into eternity. Harmonic Societies spread and mingled with Freemasonry, Rousseauian advocates of the return to Nature, and spiritualists interested in Emanuel Swedenborg. All over Europe, Victor Race's voice in his state of magnetized sleep became the secret song buried in the mind, or was it perhaps the sound of angels?

ANIMAL MAGNETISM AND magnetic somnambulism were not easy to dismiss. For no matter which explanation was proffered, there was the stunning demonstration of a hidden being within the self, and of beings who lost their will to another. Locke's thinking matter now seemed to possess multiple persons that could agitate, remember, and act. In this way, animal magnetism and somnambulism became fault lines that could shake notions of the rational self and the reliability of the mind. And that made these phenomena dangerous.

After all, as most *philosophes* knew, enlightenment was a state of mind. It depended on one's capacity to know truth from error, fact from belief, knowledge from ignorance, and science from superstition. The center of this universe was human intellect and its capacities for understanding, powers once attributed to the supernatural but increasingly given over to a thinking thing in the human head. The mind's faculties were central to the construction of new but legitimate authority in a world where Church, monarch, and soul were placed on the defensive. When that common denominator, the mind, wobbled, so did the social, political, and moral case of the Illuminati. And wobble it did. For this natural entity was prone to all of the misfortunes of the material world. By the late 18th century, the list of troubles that might undercut the mind's stability had grown: in addition to classical concerns of being overwhelmed by the passions, Lockean cognitive misassociations, and imbalances based on sensibility, there was now this bizarre, unconscious, *other* self.

Animal magnetism raised the possibility of a mind alienated from itself. The Marquis de Puységur proclaimed that to put someone under magnetic sleep required only two things: belief and will. If the mind could be so easily turned into a passive vehicle for others, how could one trust it to guide a life, a family, or a nation?

These debates did not go gently away. In England, Lockean pedagogues and moralists were thrilled to see Mesmer debunked. In their primers, they had stressed proper rational conduct and rules of behavior as prisons built to contain the passions. However, they could not be fully content, for the 1784 Commission still pointed to the faculty of imagination as a source of blind volition that emerged as reason helplessly stood by. This threatened notions of *self-*

governance, as well as moral and legal systems predicated on the rule of reason. Meanwhile, in the Societies of Harmony, utopians saw magnetism as a path to social equality, based on collectivism and the abdication of individual will.

A Plain and Rational Account of the Nature and Effects of Animal Magnetism by John Pearson mocked those innocents who advocated such irrationalism. He drew portraits—meant to be hilarious—of magnetized valets telling their lords to bugger off. He imagined some wide-eyed devil that threw whole legislatures into disarray, and took revenge on preachers by pushing them into a magnetic crisis. Not sure his readers would get the joke, Pearson added a blunt addendum to make it clear that this was all hogwash.

In fact, fears of magnetism's demagogic potential would not abate. Five years later, one of England's great poets, Samuel Taylor Coleridge was not joking when he wrote:

> William Pitt, the political Animal Magnetist . . . has most foully worked on the diseased fancy of Englishmen . . . thrown the nation into a feverish slumber, and is now bringing it to a crisis which may convulse mortality!

For Coleridge, Pitt's power lay not in a vital fluid, but rather in the realm of the psyche. Desperate, uneducated, and helpless worshipers yearned for answers. With these as his eager audience, this wizard swooped in. Political self-rule was predicated on a self that could command control over its own agency. If a whole nation could be entranced, and if enlightened self-interest could turn to blind obedience, what was the future of representative forms of governance?

Coleridge was not alone in believing that Mesmer explained a demagogue's power. The poet Robert Southey saw animal magnetism at the heart of the fanaticism that drove revolutionary movements. James Tilly Matthews accused Prime Minister Pitt of using magnetic spies to entrance the nation. He announced these charges at the House of Commons, where he was not laughed out of the chamber, but rather locked up in Bedlam.

These threats of Mesmerists having their way with the body politic were not just hypothetical. In fact, such a revolt had already taken place thanks to the Marquis de Puységur's brother, Antoine-Hyacinth-Anne de Chastenet de Puységur, the Comte de Chastenet. The first Puységur to be enthralled with Mesmerism, this naval officer employed its powers on board his ship. For a few months in 1784, he demonstrated animal magnetism while docked in the French colony of Saint-Domingue in what is now Haiti. The count installed magnetic tubs in poorhouses; a Society of Harmony was established, and, as the count sailed off, colonialism, slavery, and Mesmerism began to mix.

Class assumptions in Mesmeric discourse were generally quite clear. Aristocrats placed spells on their peasants and never were mesmerized in return. Some memoirs displayed an anxiety about the tables turning, and the potential leveling effects of this technique, which intrinsically held no preference for master or slave. Others calmed themselves by highlighting the absurdity of a situation in which a common footman could see through the clothes of the lady of the house. Racial questions also emerged. Would Native Americans be immune to animal magnetism? Coleridge wondered. If this was Enlightenment faith healing, as the Franklin Commission seemed to say, shouldn't it require a subject who had been inculcated with the beliefs of the *lumières*?

Apparently not. In Saint-Domingue, the French colonists found their African slaves were not immune to animal magnetism. Plantation owners began to entrance their slaves, so as to preserve their strength and increase their production. While traditional African medicine and sorcery were forbidden, Mesmeric rituals were fostered by slave owners, and eventually the slaves quietly incorporated Mesmer into their voodoo rituals. In 1791, the first slave revolt occurred, and far away from Saint-Domingue, a smug Franz Anton Mesmer took credit: the African slaves, made more aware of their natural harmonies, had risen up in the first magnetic revolution.

By the time these slaves revolted, Mesmer might have more modestly noted, there were other powerful models of rebellion that may have also inspired them. Two years earlier in France, a revolution had commenced. Amid the many cataclysmic changes that followed, the Societies for Harmony were disbanded and many aristocratic magnetists, including the Marquis de Puységur landed in prison. After 1789, animal magnetism, artificial somnambulism, and magnetic sleep, these nearly unfathomable matters of nerve, mind, or soul, would be chased from the great cities, the medical schools, and the academies of science. However, they would not be completely forgotten. Instead, these practices and theories were kept alive by a handful of disreputable provincial doctors and country healers, who quietly kept at it for the next half-century until their moment came again and their challenge to the rational self and the conscious subject burst forth again in Paris under the new name of hypnotism.

Journey to the End of Reason

PIERRE-JEAN-GEORGES CABANIS WAS hungry for something new. Like much of Paris, he hurried to witness the exploits of Franz Anton Mesmer, eager for not just a new kind of medicine, but a thoroughly scientific vision of humanity. Perhaps we were walking, talking, nervous magnets? In 1783, Cabanis, a medical student, neglected preparations for an upcoming exam in order to witness Mesmer's wild show. He left unimpressed. Soon, the Faculty condemned Mesmer and threatened to expel any doctors who showed interest in this fraud. Devoted magnetists and their adherents slipped away. The young Cabanis returned to his home, a villa so thick with visiting dignitaries and thinkers dedicated to rational progress that it would later seem to be a government in waiting.

Situated on two acres on the outskirts of Paris, Auteuil was the estate of Madame Helvétius, the widow of the famed author of *On the Spirit*. Her husband's naturalization of the spirit had drawn bitter attacks from Jesuits, who were in turn blamed for his heresies by more extreme Jansenists. By taking sensationalism to its natural conclusion, Helvétius had not only questioned conventional religious notions of being, but also challenged gender, racial, and class prejudices, including those held by many moderns. For example, unlike Rousseau, he insisted that the intellect of a woman would be no different than that of a man if both were granted the same education. The same could be said for the poor, foreigners, even savages. In line with Montesquieu's views, he posited that the mind had no inherent racial, sexual, or class essence, but was wholly made up of external influences. Distinctions based on such essences were sought out by those who would justify slavery, discrimination against Moslems, Hindus, and Jews, and the subjugation of women. All this was nothing more than a masquerade of self-interest.

Before the publication of his book in 1751, Helvétius had married Anne-Catherine de Ligniville. The niece of a famed salonist, Madame de Graffigny, Anne became a master at curating her own dazzling evenings, bringing together a who's who of cutting-edge writers, artists, and politicians. One wit called her salon the "Estates General of the Human Mind." However, after the publication of *On the Spirit*, the couples' life was thrown into turmoil. The Catholic Church sought to make an example out of this well-connected philosopher and pressed their case against Helvétius, so that even his friendship with Malesherbes could not prevent his exile. Those with a relationship to preserve with the king turned their backs on him, including former allies like the naturalist Buffon and the duplicitous Friedrich Melchior Grimm. Both denounced *On the Spirit*. And yet, while many scrambled away from their one-time friend, the now nearly blind Marquise du Deffand spoke for many when she wearily proclaimed, "They make so much ado about Helvétius because he has revealed everybody's secret." For a widening circle of the salon elite, it was no news that man's *esprit* was a natural mind and that pleasure and pain dictated human actions.

When her husband died in 1771, Anne sold their luxurious apartment on the Rue Sainte-Anne, and on July 26, 1773, she purchased a small retreat on the city's outskirts in Auteuil. However, this vibrant, intelligent woman discovered she was not quite ready for retirement. Auteuil was too quiet. She began to populate her estate—first with eighteen cats, three dogs, and countless chickens, canaries, and pigeons. Then she added a stunning menagerie of brilliant men—it was said she enjoyed brilliant women less. Anne sat at the center of a network of like-minded thinkers. Her home became the meeting place for poets, dramatists, economists, social reformers, scientists, and technocrats, all in some way in league with her husband's views, all somehow in on the Marquise du Deffand's secret.

An invitation to Auteuil was coveted, for it could change a man's life. Celebrities retreated to her estate to get away from the glare of public life. Government power brokers came to hobnob, brainstorm, negotiate, and be amused. Some adored this coterie so much that they purchased properties nearby, just to be close to the action. A favored few moved onto the grounds. Martin Lefebvre de La Roche, known as the Abbé de La Roche, after abandoning the Church,

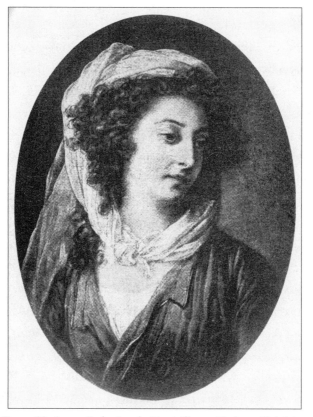

Figure 32. Anne-Catherine de Ligniville, or Madame Helvétius.

became a dedicated acolyte of Helvétius. When the *philosophe* died, he left the abbé a substantial sum of money and made him his literary executor, leaving him responsible for a mass of material that had been withheld from publication. The abbé fervently took up the work of bringing out these remaining works, alongside Madame Helvétius, as a resident of Auteuil.

Pierre Jean-Georges Cabanis was another of the full-time residents. Born in Brive, Cabanis had lost his mother when he was young, and he grew into a rebellious troublemaker. Expelled from his local school, the fourteen-year old was packed off to Paris by his exasperated father. Armed with a letter from the government minister Turgot, the boy was scheduled to stay for a while in the capital under the care of a poet, Antoine Roucher. However, once Cabanis tasted Parisian literary life, he never looked back. He began to write poetry and made an impression in Roucher's salon. After Turgot's ministry collapsed in 1776, Cabanis decided to study medicine, perhaps spurred by the recognition that this influential family friend would no longer be able to open doors for him. In 1778, Turgot and Roucher introduced the teenager to Madame Helvétius, who was captivated. Having lost a son of the same age, Anne grew attached to the boy and asked him to move in.

Among the regular visitors at Auteuil, one luminary shined brighter than the rest. Madame Helvétius regularly hosted the "Electrical Minister" from America, that paragon of Enlightenment possibility, Benjamin Franklin. While fashionable Paris fell hard for the large American, he himself fell for, among others, Anne. Franklin's affection for ladies was well known. When one flirt asked if he desired her most of all, the *savant* declared that by the laws of attraction, as long as she stood *that* close to him, he did. Though ever on the prowl, Franklin grew close to Helvétius' widow. From his home in neighboring Passy, he would walk to Auteuil every Wednesday and Saturday to visit; she returned the favor by visiting his home once a week.

Auteuil was worth the walk. The place buzzed with brilliant and witty conversation and the avid pursuit of innovation and reform. For Helvétius's conception of the mind not only led to a critique of traditions and conventions; it also led to great optimism about the possibilities of human progress. If the mind was built only through external nurturance, then the improvement of education and environment could lead to not just betterment, but something close to perfection. A mind, unburdened by superstition and lifted up by logic, could take flight. At Auteuil, avatars of progress contemplated the beneficial impact of land ownership, new economic models of wealth creation, Deism and atheism, civil projects, and constitutional monarchy. Following Helvétius himself, they touted gender equality, the end of slavery, the abolition of feudal rights, and the suppression of corporate privileges. Auteuil became a think tank for what might emerge out of the rotting feudal order.

But Auteuil was not all business. Serious contemplation alternated with raillery, coquetries, song, and bons mots. Franklin wrote to Cabanis that he would not easily forget Anne, that sweet matron who, when displeased, languorously extended her "long, handsome arm and whispered, 'there, kiss my hand: I forgive you.'" Franklin even published a *bagatelle* that purported to reveal a spurned marriage proposal to Anne. In it, the American Prometheus returned home from this rejection and proceeded to dream that he had gone to Heaven, where he discovered Monsieur Helvétius and Mrs. Franklin joined in a celestial tryst. He awoke and urged Anne to reconsider his proposal as an act of vengeance on their deceased spouses.

Optimism flowered in Madame Helvétius's garden, but there were a few thorns. The dour playwright and moralist Sébastien-Roch Nicolas, known as "Chamfort," a regular at Auteuil, was deeply skeptical of many of these reforms. Influenced by Rousseau, this one-time libertine had made his name with *The Young Indian*, a drama of civilization's corruption and the noble savage's purity. Chamfort never wavered from this view; at his death, he left behind biting aphorisms with a sarcastic working title: *Products of a Perfected Civilization*. The pure products of French culture, he believed, went a bit crazy. Their fate was artificial character, false reason, immorality, and hideous deceit. Chamfort's negativity was eccentric at Auteuil. One regular noted that a morning spent in conversation with him was like attending an execution.

There were other dissidents. The Montpellier expert on woman-kind, Pierre Roussel, spent hours at Auteuil working on his political journalism and a follow-up to his book on woman's sensibility—naturally, a companion work on men. Roussel deeply admired the brilliance of Madame Helvétius, despite the fact that his views of womankind held that her gender was fundamentally inferior. It was a view that was tolerated, although it was diametrically opposed to the protofeminist views of the widow's husband.

Architects of progress visited Auteuil from Louis XVI's government, including Anne-Robert-Jacques Turgot. An old friend of Madame Helvétius who also had asked for the widow's hand, Turgot invited a stream of his powerful friends to visit her retreat, many of whom became members of this unofficial club. Having begun his career as an encyclopedist, Turgot moved into administrative positions where he sought to actualize progressive goals. An advocate for tax reform, liberal economics, and free trade, he secured the appointment of controller general for Louis XVI. Thus, he faced mountainous deficits, the real possibility of national bankruptcy, and entrenched interests among the aristocracy and the guilds that rejected any proposals for austerity. His refusal to support the American colonists was strictly economic; his attempts to control spending and his loss of support from the queen led to his being sacked after only twenty months in office.

However, Turgot's influence did not disappear. His opposition to the heavy hand of the state, his belief in liberal economics, and radical democracy—he was gravely disappointed that the Americans refused to outlaw slavery—influenced his student, another regular at

Auteuil, Nicolas de Condorcet. A talented math student who won the support of d'Alembert, Condorcet met Turgot and began to consider how science, statistics, and probability could improve public policy. Like his mentor, he became an advocate for free trade, universal public education, and the abolition of slavery. And unlike his mentor, Condorcet managed to maintain his position in the government after Turgot's meteoric rise and fall.

Condorcet believed facts and increased knowledge would sweep away ignorance and lead toward a better future. In his posthumous work, *Sketch for a Historical Picture of the Progress of the Human Mind*, he hoped that certainty in the natural sciences would result in an irrefutable science of morals and behavior. With such a science, debates over values could be put aside for rational action and clear-eyed justice. Another Auteuil regular, the Comte de Volney, agreed: a mathematics of morality would change politics into law-based, universal science. Evil and sin would be reframed as medical illnesses and statistical deviations.

WHILE THEY ENVISIONED a quantifiable science of behavior that would stabilize a secular political order, these would-be architects of the future were not planning revolution. However, after the American uprising in 1776, revolts against the old order broke out all around Europe. Upheavals took place in Ireland, Geneva, Belgium, and Poland, as well as parts of Russia, Bohemia, and Hungary. In 1787, the Dutch erected a Temple of Liberty and claimed liberty was an inalienable right of all citizens. However, with the sole exception of the New World colonists, none of these uprisings succeeded.

Then on May 1, 1789, the calling of the Estates-General in France for the first time since 1615 initiated a series of events that led to the destruction of the Bourbon monarchy. Royal authority gradually broke down. On April 11, 1788, the Parlement dared to tell the king that his will alone was not enough to make law. These reformers still considered Louis the father of the nation, but many dreamt of a constitutional monarchy.

France's king remained convinced that public order emanated from his being. However, belief in Louis XVI's supernaturally based authority had eroded. The British rabble-rouser Thomas Paine, in his wildly successful 1776 pamphlet *Common Sense*, denounced the supposedly elevated souls of princes and kings:

> Male and female are the distinctions of nature, good and bad the distinctions of heaven, but how a race of men came into the world so exalted above the rest, and distinguished like some new species, is worth inquiring into, and whether they are the means of happiness or of misery to mankind.

An alternative notion of state power began to be heard, one proposed by Rousseau. Marie-Antoinette herself took a pilgrimage to Rousseau's tomb. Did she know this thinker claimed all legitimate sovereignty stemmed from the *volonté générale*—general will—a term once used by Pascal to refer to the will of God, but which Jean-Jacques considered the will of the people? This political philosophy directly contradicted the king's authority, and it became central to the Estates-General. Another of the disgruntled men held back by the *ancien régime*, the Abbé Sieyès, explicitly employed Rousseau to argue that the Third Estate alone represented the people and their will.

While the king's authority was challenged, the other central source of authority of the regime, the protectors of French souls, the Catholic Church, began to splinter. Parish priests began to look with a jaundiced eye at the bishops and archbishops of their own church. While a local priest often barely scraped by, elite churchmen lived in opulent splendor. That cheerful hypocrite, Charles-Maurice de Talleyrand-Périgord, the Bishop of Autun, commanded a massive income, flaunted his fine robes, freely consorted with his mistress, and at times could barely get through a service without losing his place or cracking up.

When the Third Estate convened, bourgeois merchants, lawyers, government officials, writers, and doctors flooded into French political life. In 40,000 separate assemblies throughout France, these men giddily employed their logic and power of argument to exercise some modicum of power and self-governance. Before long, a thousand different minds pursuing different aims had been engaged. The demands were quite disparate, but a number united for a while under a leader who had been imprisoned frequently as an incorrigible brute. Honoré-Gabriel de Riqueti, the Count of Mirabeau, channeled their voices through his own.

The son of a tyrannical father who considered him to be a demon, the young Mirabeau did his best to meet his father's expectations. He became a dedicated rake who specialized in scandal and wasted his family's money. His father used the *lettre de cachet* to forcibly lock the boy away again and again. At seventeen, this savage was sent to the Isle of Rhé for two years. After a terrible trick played on an aristocrat's daughter, he was imprisoned again. Finally, this inmate landed in the Chateau de Vincennes, where another locked-away libertine, the Marquis de Sade, spat on him.

While imprisoned, Mirabeau, like some notable prisoners before and since, became literary. He read Rousseau and penned pornographic novels such as *The Lifted Curtain, or the Education of Laura* and *My Conversion, or the Libertine of Quality*. He conjured up fantasies of utter freedom, void of the normal restraints of morality; in his mind, all pleasurable excesses were allowed. Locked away by his father, living under an absolute monarchy in a barely lit dungeon, he needed only to close his eyes to make the world explode.

With his wildness, cruelty, and relentlessly stoked passions, Mirabeau was susceptible to the claim, offered by a critic years later, that he had the "spice of insanity." If so, all it took was a revolution to

cure him. Released from Vincennes after three years of imprisonment, Mirabeau sailed to England, grew disappointed with that
country, and returned to France to discover his calling. With the
convening of the Third Estate, each province required its own fighters for freedom. He was happy to become one. A believer in constitutional monarchy, Mirabeau impressed others with his impassioned,
thoughtful declarations. Locked away so often, he had had a good
deal of time to consider the precious value of liberty.

In June of 1789, the Third Estate declared itself the National
Assembly, after a motion by Mirabeau nullified all taxes not approved
by that body. On June 17, this swell of small-time notables dared to
invite nobles and ecclesiastical leaders of the other two orders to join
them. As the Comte d'Antraigues would declare, "The Third Estate
is not an order, it is the nation itself." The Tennis Court Oath established that the sole source of legitimate authority was the general will
of the people.

All this intoxicating liberty, however, could not fill the stomachs
of the poor. Famine drove homeless and hungry masses into Paris,
where riot and revolt began to explode. Rumor had it that the king
would send troops in to slaughter the troublemakers. Panic propelled
a fateful cascade of events: a huge cache of 30,000 muskets were
taken from the Hôpital des Invalides and distributed in the streets for
self-defense. Then, one of the great symbolic moments in modernity took place, thanks to an irrefutable bit of logic: what use were
guns without gunpowder? Powder was stored in one of the regime's
dreaded fortresses, one that like the Hôtel-Dieu reeked of cruelty and
death: the Bastille.

The conditions at the Bastille were bad, but not the worst. For
example, within the fortress walls lived Mirabeau's one-time nemesis, Donatien-Alphonse-François de Sade. The immoralist who gave
his name to sexual cruelty had been transferred from cell number 6
at Vincennes to a private chamber at the Bastille, where he was com-
fortably surrounded by a private library of six hundred works, fine

furniture, and precious portraits. Not considered mad but rather evil, he was able to smoke and drink at his leisure.

As crowds grew around the Bastille, Sade tried to incite them by screaming that the prisoners inside were being slaughtered. These lies were not appreciated by his jailers. On July 4, 1789, Sade was whisked away from the Bastille to the Charenton, the lunatic asylum run by the Brothers of Charity. This sudden transfer forced him to leave behind his valuable possessions, as well as a hidden scroll that contained a novel called the *120 Days of Sodom*. It was intended to be the most horrifying tale ever told, and now its proud author believed it was lost. At Charenton, the marquis found himself among the mentally ill. He took bitter exception to being told his aggressively immoral philosophy was an illness. And he feared his imprisonment with lunatics was intended to make him lose his mind.

This sudden transfer also meant that on the fateful day of July 14, 1789, the marquis was not among those liberated from the Bastille when a mob stormed the fortress in search of gunpowder. Almost immediately, their pragmatic purpose faded and the symbolism of their actions gripped the country's imagination. The people had pushed their way into one of the king's fortresses. They had liberated long-enchained victims of arbitrary authority. For all the poor and starving, all the beaten-down workers and angry artisans, this liberation was touted as theirs as well.

Tabloid accounts went to work creating a mythology in which it might seem that all of France had been liberated on that fateful day. The motley mob that pushed their way forward—in the eyes of one royalist observer, drunken "heroes of the tavern"—were soon replaced, as impromptu cafés were set up before the Bastille walls. Everyone came to take in the extraordinary events; orators mixed with well-dressed ladies, fashionable men, dancers, actors and actresses, and men of letters. They had come to watch the Old France die or perhaps, wait for a new France to be born.

In the end, the storming of the Bastille freed a total of seven pris-

oners, four forgers, one libertine, and two men who suffered from
mental illness. Of those last two, an elderly white-bearded fellow
imprisoned for many years seemed most serene about the explosive,
unprecedented events of the day. He calmly reveled in the crowd's
adulation, something he assumed was his right as Emperor Julius
Caesar.

⁓

THE SHIFTING FATES of Mirabeau, the soon-to-be-liberated Marquis
de Sade, and the deluded "Julius Caesar" made it clear that the old
walls that once separated the sane from the immoral and the mad
were coming down. The joyous liberation of the Bastille reinforced
the belief that the ethical order of French society had changed. On
August 26, 1789, the Marquis de Lafayette, with some consultation
from his friend Thomas Jefferson, proposed the Declaration of the
Rights of Man. Modeled on the American Declaration of Independence, this document asserted that men were born free and equal,
and that law was an expression of the general will. That powerful
symbol of arbitrary power, the detested *lettre de cachet*, was abolished
for everything except sedition or family delinquency. The French,
who had so recently created huge circles around magnetized trees,
now proudly planted Trees of Liberty.

In Britain, the French Revolution was initially greeted by many
as an extension of their own Glorious Revolution a century earlier.
However, rather quickly, Edmund Burke became frightened, then
angered, by the proceedings. His *Reflections on the Revolution in France*
decried the disruption of the nobility and clergy as a kind of collective insanity. The past was being despoiled, and by whom? Illiberal men who touted liberty, ignoramuses who yelled about science,
and savages who destroyed humanity. "We are not the converts of
Rousseau; we are not the disciples of Voltaire. Helvétius has made
no progress amongst us," he seethed. "Atheists are not our preach-

ers, madmen are not our lawgivers." France had gone insane, Burke repeated over and over. Were Britons supposed to congratulate this maniac who had escaped the "protective restraint of his cell" and now stood squinting in the sunlight?

Burke found few readers, but he engendered an indignant reply that spread like wildfire. After America, Thomas Paine had shipped off to France, stalking revolution. Paine's reply to Burke, *Rights of Man,* countered that author's befuddlement over the chaos in Paris, suggesting that a "mental revolution" had taken place in the French nation prior to the outbreak of violence. The sudden political eruptions were no more than a consequence of that prior psychological transformation: "The mind of the nation had changed. . . ."

Certainly, there was unprecedented change. The National Assembly transformed itself into the Constituent Assembly, and in that guise, over the next two years, remade much of French life. They created a new taxation system, abolished titles and ranks, and swept away guilds and old economic regulations. They erased old geographic divisions and established 83 *départments.* In November 1789, all church property, some 10 percent of French land, was confiscated. A Civil Constitution of the Clergy was declared in which French priests proclaimed themselves independent of the Pope. Whole religious orders were outlawed. Education was secularized; children would be brought up based on the theories of the mind put forward by Locke, Helvétius, Condillac, and Bonnet.

All this was met with enthusiasm in Auteuil. Cabanis joined the crowd at the Bastille soon after July 14, and was introduced to Mirabeau. As Mirabeau rose in prominence, Cabanis became his personal doctor and speechwriter. Condorcet also quickly jumped into the middle of the fray. The changes Turgot had advocated were now enacted and more. Guilds weren't reformed, they were eliminated. Aristocrats did not have to give ground toward the goal of economic liberalization; their titles were abolished. Nobles now lost their lineages and remerged into the new order with new identities, often as lawyers. On March 13, 1790, *lettres de cachet* were restricted to prisoners condemned to death and the insane. Libertines and outcasts, including the Marquis de Sade, returned to freedom. It was a new dawn, and the bourgeois technocrats and intellectuals of Auteuil had reason to believe that the coming day would belong to them. They built an altar to the *patrie* with busts of Voltaire, Rousseau, Franklin, Helvétius, and Mirabeau.

Marie-Antoinette's brother and the leaders of Prussia watched the fall of the Bourbons in horror and considered taking up arms. Across France, peasants, artisans, and rebels prepared for the worst. Having just acted in a vertiginously free manner, common people began to fear massive reprisals. Rumors swirled about approaching marauders from Austria, Sardinia, Spain, or elsewhere. A "Great Fear" banded citizens together. Brothers and sisters in arms, they commandeered castles, formed militias, and prepared for a still-invisible foe.

Mirabeau and other leaders of the uprising had no intention of replacing the king. They hoped for a constitutional monarchy and saw popular democracy as no different from allowing the passionate excesses of the body to dwarf reason. It was a problem Mirabeau knew well; he had matured out of his wild youth and sought the same moderation for his nation. He even lectured the National Assembly on its "irritability," as if it were a nervous, sick body. Meanwhile, he himself was ill. Mirabeau's failing health, his doctor believed, was due to the pressures of the dramatic times. To write eloquent protests, in which reason took on the voice of passion, meant Mirabeau spent many nights working without sleep. He spent his days arguing, debating, negotiating, and planning, and was barely able to contain the impact such excitement made on his body. Eye problems preceded colic, then breathing difficulties and rheumatic complaints.

For Cabanis, the mental had clearly dysregulated the physical. This leader's excessive work, contentious intellectual exertion, and intense emotions shredded the sensible fibers of his body and led this strong-willed man to have the nervous system of a delicate woman. He fell prey to terrible anxiety, in which he would tremble and sink to the ground. The passionate orator who publicly cried "To arms! To arms!" in the quiet of his own chambers, came apart. On April 2, 1791, Mirabeau whispered his last words to Cabanis, who in this treacherous atmosphere was promptly accused of murder.

Soon afterward, Mirabeau's dreams for France also passed away. The secular modernists and constitutional monarchists were suddenly undermined by the disastrous attempt of the king to flee his own capital. After June 21, when the king and his family were stopped and returned to Paris, there could be no doubt that he had hoped to rally a Royalist army and invade. Radicals who had called for the end of monarchy, constitutional or otherwise, now held the upper hand. France was ruled by a traitorous king. Revolutionary fervor was stoked in pamphlets, cartoons, and short-lived newspapers, 184 of which were launched in 1789 alone. Marat, the failed electrical doctor, now became reincarnated as a journalist and publisher of *Friend of the People*. Jacques Hébert, under the pseudonym Le Père Duchesne, greeted his readers with today's great outrage in publications that reached over a million Frenchmen. A Royalist until the king's flight to Varennes, Le Père Duchesne now turned his rage on the "fat pig" who was France's monarch. His trademark was a linguistic tick that signaled his disgust with the reigning moral order: he used the word "fuck" insistently, at times almost as a point of punctuation. For example, he wrote, "I confess, fuck, that the misery of the people is disgusting," or "Me, fuck, I am a bête noire," or "Marat is dead, fuck."

Passion for revolution was cultivated in mass gatherings and small clubs. Radicals of different stripes met in the Feuillants Club and in the Cordeliers Club, where members called for "tyrannicide." Others such as the Society of Revolutionary Republican Women sought to find a place for those quite obviously ignored by this fraternity, women. Of these clubs, the most powerful became the Jacobins, a group that first espoused brotherly solidarity and equality. In the months after the king's dash away from Paris, the Jacobins grew more powerful, led by Maximilien Robespierre, a minor deputy in the Estates-General who had imbibed a major dose of Rousseau. In over 150 electrifying speeches, injected with Jean-Jacques's combination of openhearted sympathy, moral politics, and self-pity, Robespierre called for a cleansing of France, the emancipation of the Jews and slaves, and—in what would prove deeply ironic—the abolition of the death penalty.

Surrounded by belligerent enemies, the French army initiated an offensive on April 20, 1792. Rather vertiginously, the country was at war with countries that sought to save *their* king from his people. Marat, the proud and angry *sans-culottes*, the implacable *enragés*, and Robespierre all called for Louis' dethronement. And as chaos rose, the libertarian and rationalist ideals of the Revolution came up against the brute logic of violence. The symbol of this descent was a progressive, utilitarian invention now put to depraved use. Dr. Joseph-Ignace Guillotin, who sat on the Franklin Commission that judged Mesmer, had created a means by which executions could be quick and surgical, freed from the barbaric trappings of the hangman. In the spring of 1792, his razorous machine was put to work. Militants who once called for the end of the death penalty and rejoiced over the elimination of *lettres de cachet*, now chopped off heads and employed arbitrary arrest. Implacable priests were guillotined and imprisoned en masse, as were draft dodgers, those accused of the crime of moderation, and peasants suspected of Royalist beliefs. Old feuds between neighbors now could be settled by the nod of a Jacobin head.

Robespierre called for true patriots to rise up against "moderate" traitors, backstabbing outsiders, foreigners, nobles, and unrepentant priests. In the fall of 1792, this blood lust could be contained no more. Widespread massacres by bands of armed men took place in prisons, poorhouses, and churches. The September massacres left

1,400 dead, including churchmen, prostitutes, the mentally ill, criminals, and court sycophants, all Frenchmen deemed beyond moral regeneration. Moderates of the Jacobin party, the Girondins, tried to protest, but they were silenced with threats of retribution.

France had become a battleground with many fronts. Attacking perceived enemies only heightened fear that bloody revenge would pop out from around the next corner. Paranoia and violence begat more paranoia and more violence. High ideals nurtured by a century of virtuosi and *lumières*, dreams of liberty, the rule of reason, equality, and fraternity, had come down to this: kill or be killed.

When Louis XVI was put on trial, that sly advocate of the encyclopedists, Malesherbes, volunteered to defend the monarch in court. While the vote was close, the king was condemned to die. Louis XVI, once believed to rule thanks to divine authority, now simply became Louis Capet. On January 21, 1793, his hair was cut and at 10:22 in the morning, his head was placed under the guillotine's blade. The execution of the king signaled the beginning of an all-out war with European powers led by royals, some related to Louis, who could easily imagine their own heads placed under that blade.

The guillotining of the king also horrified many Frenchmen. It caused spontaneous protests and prompted a crackdown on internal enemies by the Jacobin regime. The Committee of Public Safety was founded on April 6 with nine members. From its name, the committee would have seemed to be an innocuous bureaucratic endeavor, like one of those committees formed during the last years of the king's reign, perhaps focused on sanitation. In fact, its mission was cleansing of a different sort: the Committee became the violent arm of radicals who sought to rid France of its illnesses. Enemies were dehumanized and reduced to cancers, bizarre growths, cloacae, diseases, all *things* that needed to be surgically removed to keep the Revolution alive.

After the moderates were overrun by radicals, the radicals were overrun by ultraradicals. In this atmosphere, the Auteuil group were in danger. Roucher, the poet who introduced Cabanis to Madame Helvétius, was beheaded. Volney was imprisoned. In December of 1792, the Jacobins ordered the destruction of the Auteuil bust of Helvétius—hated by Robespierre as the enemy of poor Jean-Jacques—as well as that of Mirabeau, who had been transformed from hero to goat when it was revealed that he had taken money from the king. Condorcet, a leader of the moderate Girondist branch of the Jacobins, became a wanted man. When the Committee called for his arrest, Cabanis flew into action and hid his friend and brother-in-law at the home of Madame Helvétius. When that hiding place became unsafe, Condorcet was spirited away to a secret house by Cabanis and his medical friend, Philippe Pinel. The wanted man survived for a year in hiding, but eventually died, probably due to self-administered poison after a failed escape. In mourning, his wife threw herself into translating Adam Smith's *Theory of Moral Sentiments* and writing *Letters on Sympathy*, as if this was still a war of ideas and words.

LONG SHUNNED, DEMEANED, and marginalized French citizens now assumed power. Of the many astonishing rebirths ushered in by this radicalized revolution, none was more shocking than that of Citizen Sade. Imprisoned much of his life for the rape, drugging, and sexual abuse of prostitutes, servants, and others, the marquis shed his title and joined a radical group, the Piques Section. As a connoisseur of the horrors offered up at Vincennes, the Bastille, and the Charenton, he was placed on a citizen's commission to inspect the hospitals. The author of still-unpublished dramas of necrophilia, incest, pedophilia, and the delights of murder and torture was almost made a magistrate. Sade himself could hardly believe it.

The inmates had taken over, and immoralists were now in charge of reforming the law.

As reprisals, accusations, and violence escalated, Cabanis refused to abandon the elderly Madame Helvétius, despite strident attacks by Robespierre against her husband and other *philosophes* who defamed Rousseau. Mysteriously, Cabanis's own political credibility remained intact. Despite his association with Mirabeau and the Auteuil group, he was considered loyal enough to be appointed as one of twelve jurors on the Extraordinary Criminal Court for political crimes, which later became the Revolutionary Tribunal.

With Girondin leaders in hiding or under house arrest, and with opposition presses closed down, Jacobins now pursued a cutthroat path. By July 1793, the Committee on Public Safety and the Revolutionary Tribunal were killing machines that sought to terrorize the country into submission. With the Terror, Robespierre believed, virtue would return to France. This was far from the path of reason, and for Marat that was a good thing. The revolution had almost been destroyed by those who believed arid reason should guide it.

For Robespierre, France was to be remade not by encyclopedists, not by Diderot, science, and truth, but by Rousseauian honest men filled with deep sentiments and sincere feelings. The passions of the *honnête homme*, the authentic sensibilities of the inner man, that natural nobility in each breast, these were the only sure guides for the Revolution. However, as the bloodshed continued, such nobility seemed rare indeed.

Tyranny bred zealous freedom fighters, whose quest for freedom turned into licenses to kill. Sade himself became an exemplar of this transformation. "Fanaticism in me," he observed, "is the product of the persecutions I have endured from my tyrants." Jailers had hoped to break Sade of his beliefs. They tried to force the prisoner in cell number 6 to abstain from his carnal philosophy, and as they did, phantoms more blasphemous than ever rose up in his head. Sade himself wondered if more indulgence á la Émile would not have led him to change his ways. However, after years of imprisonment, Sade considered himself a hardened zealot, a man whose shocking principles had become his sole means of emotional survival.

In 1795, Citizen Sade published *Philosophy in the Bedroom*, in which he called for a new ethic to preserve republican liberty. Libertinism was not immoral, but rather should be the new morality, one that broke decisively with the lies of organized religions. These irrational tales corrupted men and forced them from the path dictated by Nature: "No voice save that of the passions can conduct you to happiness," he wrote, sounding like Rousseau, one of his inspirations. Chop down the tree of superstition, liberate Europe from censor and scepter! Morals must be rewritten so that private sexual lusts are allowed—there can be no evil in Nature's promptings—while public corruption is forbidden. Sodomy, incest, infidelity, even murder might be justified under the laws of Nature, but theft, lies, and breach of civic duty could not be. Atheism and Lucretian hedonism should guide France forward.

In his desire for a new ethical contract, Citizen Sade was not alone. Having temporarily quieted the opposition, the National Convention took up the dechristianization of France. After routing the preachers, the Jacobins sought to establish a culture with secular morality based on reason. Right and wrong would be determined without Heaven and Hell. However, eradicating the vestiges of Christianity required much more than that. Dechristianization meant nothing less than a reconfiguration of time and space, meanings, names, symbols, and myths. If the National Convention wanted to root out centuries of Christian culture, it would have to dig deeply.

In October of 1793, they began: a new calendar rid France of Gregorian time and restarted world history. Year I would commence along with the birth of the French Republic, on what was once known as September 22, 1792. The twelve months would all be renamed after Nature: November 21 to December 20 would be Frimaire, while August 18 to September 16 would become Fructidor. Each month would consist of three ten-day periods (Primidi, Duodi, Tridi . . .), with the tenth day being a day of rest. Days themselves would now consist of 10 hours, made up of 100 minutes, each of which held 100 seconds. Sundays, religious holidays, and saints' days were erased.

Churches would ring their bells and pay homage to the mind, not the soul. This would be a new "Cult of Reason." It was a deistic or atheistic alternative to Catholicism, as pushed by Père Duchesne and other radicals. On November 10, 1793, an inaugural Festival of Liberty took place at the Temple of Reason, formerly the Cathedral of Nôtre Dame. The Temple was outfitted with an altar to Truth, effigies of Voltaire, Rousseau, and the now-deceased Franklin, and a massive, artificial mountain signifying Robespierre's Montagnard group of Jacobins. The apotheosis of the revelry was an operatic song performed by Liberty, a voluptuous opera singer, who bowed to the flame of Reason.

The former physician and ultraradical Pierre-Gaspard Chaumette had organized this spectacle and delivered a speech that asserted the equality of all races; therefore, he called for the abolition of slavery in the colonies. His commitment to the eradication of Christianity led him to change his first name to the dechristianized, if unwieldy, Anaxagoras. Churches around France became Temples of Reason that offered praises to Truth and Philosophy; to mark this shift, such temples were set up in the former site of royal coronations, the cathedral in Reims, and the burial place of French kings, the Basilica of Saint-Denis.

However, by late 1793, the Temple for Reason stood in a pool of blood. Reasonable minds had long been overrun by fear, rage, and a lust for domination: everywhere passions were in charge. And in fact, the effort to create a new Cult of Reason split the Jacobins. Robespierre considered it a farce. Like Jean-Jacques who attacked Diderot and Helvétius for their rationalism and atheism, Robespierre had no sympathy for nonbelievers. Having amassed near-dictatorial powers, in May of 1794, this menacing patriot decreed atheism to be aristocratic. The Convention announced that the French nation believed in the immortality of the soul, and officially recognized a Supreme Being. It may have seemed that Robespierre had recognized a country after slaughtering its ambassadors, but nonetheless, festivals on June 8 designated France's return to the Supreme Being; Robespierre himself stepped forward to burn a statue of Atheism.

In July of 1794, or the 9th of Thermidor, the Terror ended. Robespierre and 83 of his followers were executed and the Jacobin club was dissolved. The Terror murdered perhaps 250,000 Frenchmen. Primary among them were aristocrats and clergy. The dead included Marie-Antoinette, long prepared for her death by being reduced in the press to a traitorous whore. Brought to court, she was subjected to accusations that seemed to be dreamed up by Citizen Sade. It was claimed that she masturbated and seduced her own son to ruin his body and mind, as per the doctrines of Dr. Samuel Tissot. The seven-year-old was made to sign a document attesting to these outrages before being returned to a cage, where he soon perished.

Even that ardent advocate of the Revolution Thomas Paine

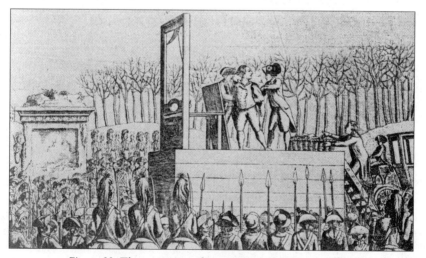

Figure 33. The execution of Louis XVI by guillotine, 1793.

was stunned by the horrifying turn of events. After having justified the Revolution so powerfully in 1791, he had joined the Convention despite not speaking a word of French, for the ideals of universal brotherhood prevailed within him. However, the Terror soon came after Paine's friends, and then in 1793, the Committee of Public Safety locked him up. The author of *The Rights of Man* barely survived. Two years later, he rose up to denounce the corruption of the revolution's principles. The intolerant persecutions of the Church, so long drummed into the populace, had been reborn in secular form. The Inquisition had changed its name to the Revolutionary Tribunal, and witch burnings had transformed into political beheadings.

THE THERMIDORIAN REACTION ended the Terror and returned to power the stunned, moderate reformers such as those associated with Auteuil. They now stepped forward into a transformed world. Utopians once in search of perfectability, optimistic believers in mankind's capacity for reason and progress, they had encountered something inside their fellow humans that had roared like a beast. As they sought to remake the ravaged institutions of France, they could not forget the spasms of passion that swept up their countrymen. And, these survivors had to acknowledge that reason alone had not only not prevailed, it had been shouted down and routed. Old Malesherbes told a friend, "In times of violent passions, one must surely keep from speaking reason. (Otherwise) one may even harm reason, for enthusiasts will excite people against the same truths that, in another time, would be received with general approbation."

What had happened? For many, like Edmund Burke, the answer was simple: sinners and atheists, having already overthrown all vestiges of Christian morality, had run riot. Religion once held back the baser impulses of mankind. If its barriers to disorder were dismissed as superstitions, if heavenly reward and hellish torment for the ever-lasting soul were all dismissed as delusions, then humans would turn on each other like animals. Royalists and followers of Hobbes might have agreed.

Still, the Thermidorian Reaction in France would not turn back to either kings or priests. Instead, these reformers insisted that the tools of reason could be employed to protect the public from collective violence and madness. In this way, a once hushed-up idea boldly entered the public square. For over a century, a hidden anti-Cartesian, mentalist tradition in France had been constructed, one that rivaled the rational soul or the immaterial Cogito. It included ancient forefathers like Lucretius and Epicurus, as well as Gassendi, Willis, Hobbes, and Locke, the English doctors of the mind, Montesquieu, Helvétius, Condillac, and the Montpellier medical philosophers, Tissot, and even the Marquis de Puységur. There were important differences among these thinkers, but they all contended that at the core of human beings was an embodied, natural mind that was fragile and could easily become influenced, deluded, or ill.

Without fear of the censors, a science and medicine of the *esprit* could step forward from its hiding places and take up its pressing tasks, one of which was to respond to the chaos of the recent past. Thomas Paine believed that years of chipping away at the old *mentalité* had changed the French nation and created a revolution from within. When the Bastille was stormed, he had argued, a new order of thought pressed forward its own logic. However, if this new mode of thought embraced individual freedom, autonomous choice, and the search for happiness, did it also countenance summary executions, parading heads on poles, and rampaging fury?

Pierre Bayle scandalized many when he argued that a modern society of atheists could be moral. A century later, the first European experiment with secular ethics looked to many as if it had turned into a catastrophe. Reason had stood helplessly aside as fear, swift violence, and massacres provoked retribution and a near-continuous cycle of murder. Of course, Bayle's experiment had been conducted during a war for survival, hardly a conducive atmosphere for civility. Yet it forced the scattered and stunned secularists to rethink their views. If a society would be predicated on autonomous individuals who pursued happiness, it required stable and reasonable citizens, and it needed an authority to restrict and contain those whose search for happiness made them villains. If priests no longer shepherded their flocks away from temptations, a secular society based on empowered, free citizenry needed to protect itself against Sades and Robespierres. It required forces of secular control to block unreason from filling the streets with blood.

Citizens and Alienists

T HE REVOLUTION RID France of old institutions before it
built new ones. In medicine, the immediate result was disaster. After 1791, there was no medical guild, and a year later all the
medical faculties were abolished. Religious orders and feudal powers
that once supported hospices and hospitals were routed, and financial
support for these institutions disappeared. The Grey Sisters, an order
of nuns who functioned as nurses, were chased from the wards. They
were not replaced.

In 1792, a five-person Hospital Committee was finally appointed
to rebuild and reform Paris's hospitals. Since the fall of the Bastille,
this job was now freighted with symbolic weight. Hospital and prison
reform went hand in hand, since the imprisoned, the poor, and the
sick were often housed *en masse* in the king's institutions. The new
order would be different.

Nearly a decade earlier, a Royal Commission had asked Dr. Jean
Colombier to institute reform. Colombier was a maverick who after
graduating from medical school attempted to open a practice based
on annual patient subscriptions, an innovation rapidly shut down by
the Faculty. In 1780, this upstart gave up his practice and officially
became the inspector of all hospitals, prisons, and private *maisons de
force* in France.

In 1764, a royal decree on vagabonds had established the right
to arrest beggars and place them in *dépôts de mendicité*, privately contracted prisons often with horrible conditions. Colombier began with
these institutions, stipulating some basic health provisions. In 1785,
he joined with another hospital inspector, Dr. François Doublet, to
publish guidelines for the care of *insensés*, madmen who required special considerations and segregation. In addition to basic health provisions and the need to abolish cruelty by attendants, these authors,
likely influenced by the debates about animal magnetism, asked caretakers to beware. Through imitation and the imagination, madness
might be passed on to them.

Colombier and Doublet's recommendations were distributed
throughout the kingdom. And they were echoed by another pre-
revolutionary reformer, Jacques Tenon. He too dwelled on the need
to reinvent hospitals and create specialized ones for the mentally ill.
After traveling through France and England for two years, Tenon
discovered encouraging examples in Lyon and Rouen. He stressed
that hospitals for the mad must be thought of as qualitatively different: unlike other hospitals, these institutions *were* the very instruments of cure:

> They are themselves the means of healing. It must be that the
> madman, during the course of treatment not be antagonized,
> that he be able to, in the moments when he is under surveil-
> lance, go out of his room, run about the gallery, go to the
> promenading area, and do exercise that dissipates him and that
> nature commands.

If the treatment for madness was the mad hospital, Tenon continued, then the two best examples were London's St. Luke's and
Bethlem. Tenon cautioned that little was known about what kinds of
madness would be cured by immersion in these new environments.
However, following the sensationalists and post-Lockeans, a growing

consensus had emerged that environments could both cure and create murderers and maniacs. In 1787, the progressive Royal Academy
of Sciences ratified Tenon's plan, but typically, nothing came of it.

Tenon was not the only one who had noticed what had transpired in the British Isles. In the late 18th century, hospital reform for
the mad had taken root in scattered outposts throughout Europe. In
Florence in 1788, supported by Grand Duke Leopold, Dr. Vincenzo
Chiarugi opened the newly constructed Bonifazio Hospital, built for
125 insane patients. Impressed by Locke, Voltaire, and the philosophes, Chiarugi was nonetheless a Catholic committed to Cartesian
dualism. While he discounted theories of possession and witchcraft
as almost universally fabricated, he held the belief that souls were
immune from mortal decay. Still, brains, nervous systems, and lower
faculties, such as the imagination, might be affected by illness, and
for these sufferers, his new hospital would be the cure.

While most of his treatments centered upon the use of seda-
tives and stimulants, Chiarugi also sought to create emotional coun-
terbalances to manage unruly passions, and demanded that doctors
calibrate their own passions so as to meet the needs of the patient.
Chiarugi asked his staff to treat the mad with respect, and forbade
threats and blows as useless and counterproductive.

Dr. Chiarugi was one of a number of physicians and laymen
who simultaneously began to use more humanitarian methods with
the mentally ill in Europe. However, the motives of these doctors
were not simply humanitarian. After all, the kindest doctor had been
trained to carve a stone out from a writhing patient's innards if that
mauling would save a life. Physicians were trained to perform ghastly
tasks, like cutting off a leg, in the service of a cure. What distinguished an act of torture from heroism rested in good part on the
action's rationale and efficacy.

Thus, while discourses on political liberty helped spur change,
humanitarian attitudes toward the mentally ill were greatly aided by
theories of a sensationalist mind exquisitely responsive to the envi-

ronment, and notions of mental illnesses as dysregulated nervous sensibility. Chaining the enraged now took on new meaning. After the work of Haller, a few doctors began to use soothing, gentler treatments, rather like gardeners trying to tend to a wilting plant. Rousseau wrote about his attempts to heal his frayed nerves through a calming retreat to Nature. A hospital, some began to imagine, could do the same: it could provide asylum. Even if the results were not always clearly efficacious, they made sense with the rising cult of sensibility and were embraced by patients who flocked to these less brutal regimes.

Before the Revolution, the bureaucrats at Auteuil often voiced recommendations for medical change. Colombier spent time there along with the hospital reformer from Montpellier, Jean-Antoine Chaptal, Cabanis's friend. When the old order fell, Cabanis and his Auteuil friend, Dr. Michel-Augustin Thouret, were named to the Hospital Committee and given the opportunity to reconceive the entire system. As optimistic progressives, their hopes were high. In 1790, a young Cabanis had already written his own *Observations on Hospitals*, an essay heavily reliant on Tenon. However, as a mark of the changing times, Cabanis's opening premise differed: while Tenon argued that good hospitals were the mark of beneficent civilization, Cabanis proposed that their existence was a necessary evil, implying that someday such institutions might no longer be needed.

The 1792 Hospital Commission confronted a situation that had only deteriorated since the time of Colombier and Tenon. Cabanis and his allies thought it best to break up the huge, monolithic institutions and found smaller, specialized facilities as well as two large teaching hospitals. They proposed that infectious and insane patients be moved to separate quarters, that the poor be distinguished from the insane, and, at places like Bicêtre, the criminals be segregated from the ill. Confinement should be temporary, medical, and only as needed, for the mad were not felons. Chains should be abolished; order could be maintained with the newly invented straightjacket.

Liberty should be curtailed only temporarily, and only for the protection of individuals and the public.

None of these plans came to anything, as the Committee was
disbanded. However before its demise, the Hospital Committee was
able to make a fateful political appointment; Cabanis and Thouret
handed the leadership of the Bicêtre to their friend, an Auteuil regular Philippe Pinel. This failed doctor was handed a hornet's nest and
he eagerly grabbed it.

BORN INTO A family of doctors in 1745, Philippe Pinel was raised
in a small village in the southwestern Tarn region. Schooled first
by the rigorous Doctrinaires of Lavaur, the pious boy received his
degree after completing his final interrogation on the immortality of the soul. At the age of seventeen, he traveled to Toulouse to
continue his studies, decided to abandon theology, and discovered
a talent for mathematics. He studied with Jean-Baptiste Gardeil, a
friend of Diderot and d'Alembert, and imbibed Locke and Condillac,
Rousseau and Voltaire. In 1766, Pinel made his way to the Mecca of
medicine, Montpellier, to follow his father into that profession. He
studied with the systematizer Boissier de Sauvages and the vitalist
Barthez. His friend, a medical student but soon minister of internal affairs under Napoleon, Jean-Antoine Chaptal, described their
education in the animal economy, monistic vitalism, and a holism
in which the physical, the psychological, and the social were linked.
The ambitious Chaptal even dared to write a medical thesis that covered that wide range, focusing on the effects of the environment and
education on sensibility, reason, and moral faculties, as well as the
influence of governments on the well-being of a nation. Pinel drank
in the same beliefs, but did not himself write a thesis; instead, he
made some extra money by ghost writing theses for lazy students.

For the next twelve years, Pinel lived in Montpellier, joined the local Royal Society, and sought to apply his mathematical interests to physiology. In a sign of things to come, he tried to cure his friend Chaptal from melancholia using Tissot's mental means, in this case a reading diet of Hippocrates, Plutarch, and Montaigne. Then in 1778, Pinel—like so many ambitious Montpellier graduates—walked to Paris, armed with a letter of recommendation that touted his skills in math. He was accompanied by an English companion, whose tutorials in that language would later prove valuable. In Paris, Pinel met up with his younger brother, Louis, and a cured Chaptal. The young men were in the Jardin du Luxembourg when the news of Rousseau's death arrived. According to family lore, their dedication to Jean-Jacques carried them by foot to Ermenon-Ville, where they spent the day at the tomb with the grieving widow.

Back in Paris, this young doctor hustled to get by as a tutor, a journalist, and an English translator. In 1780, he began to write on public health for the *Journal de Paris*. In 1782, then two more times, Pinel applied for the Deist prize, which paid for impoverished students to study and win admission to the Medical Faculty of Paris. All three times, he was rejected. Records show that his second attempt in 1784 provoked especially caustic commentary. The applicant's knowledge was deemed insufficient in nearly everything—anatomy, physiology, chemistry, and pharmacy. Friends would later attribute this calamitous showing to the doctor's timidity and his stutter. Pinel considered abandoning medicine.

In 1784, he landed a job that allowed him to make an "honest living," unlike those Parisian doctors that he scorned for leeching off rich patrons. He was appointed editor of the *Gazette de santé*, a small medical journal. Excited by intellectual life in Paris, he spent his evenings rapt in studies. As an editor, Pinel began to turn his attention to matters of the moral and mental. However, his interest was also compelled by tragedy. A close friend, twenty-four years old and gifted, had come to Paris in search of glory. Constant scholarship and rigorous asceticism had transformed this never-named, but never-forgotten friend into a sufferer of crippling headaches, nose-bleeds, body aches, and a highly wound-up sensibility. At times jubilant, this man would suddenly plunge into blackness. At one point, he asked Philippe to end his misery and shoot him.

Pinel sprang into action. However, his friend resisted his advice and continued to deteriorate, descending further into despair until his parents sent him to the grim Hôtel-Dieu. They recommended relocation to a rural village in the Pyrenees, presumably for a change in climate. This broken man returned from the mountains unchanged. He refused to eat and finally ran away from his parents' home. When his dead body was found in the woods, he was clutching a copy of Plato's work on the immortality of the soul.

This tragedy pulled Pinel into the controversies over mental therapies, just as Dr. Mesmer had become the talk of *tout Paris*. During the year of 1784, one could hardly be an editor of a medical journal and not become immersed in the fascinating claims and counterclaims surrounding Mesmer. Pinel spent some two months with Mesmer's advocate, Deslon, and his first editorial on the subject was not unsympathetic. For a student of vitalists like Barthez and Bordeu, the notion of a subtle energy whose movements dictated health and illness was not hard to imagine. Mesmer had created a reasonable theory, Pinel concluded. But was it true? Animal magnetism, he concluded, would either usher in an amazing new chapter in medicine or go down in history as an extraordinary fraud.

Once the Royal Committees produced their damning reports, the *Gazette de santé* promptly fell in line. Imitation, touch, and the imagination were proven to be the only causes at work in Mesmer's passes and his *baquet*. Mesmerism for Pinel was now a closed case. The editor became fed up with incessant accusations and counteraccusations; he announced the *Gazette* would no longer dwell on this delusion, this stain on the century of the *philosophes*. If the man was timid when speaking in public, he was not so with his pen. When challenged in a letter from a magnetist named Father Hervier, Pinel lost his cool and accused Mesmer's followers of not being deluded, but rather thieves.

The idea that imitation, touch, and the imagination had very significant power to influence the sick stimulated Pinel to consider the way spiritual and religious consolation might work. Haunted by his friend's suicide, Pinel grew curious about cures that might restore a depressed sensibility. An ancient Egyptian ritual from priests in a Temple of Saturn used sexual pleasure to cure melancholia, Pinel noted. He discussed the case of a suicidal melancholic who was attacked by brigands, and in the course of fending them off was cured. Reading great writers, having sex, and being offered warm consolation all seemed to realign the animal economy.

As hopes for Mesmerism plummeted, Pinel threw himself into the work of the Scottish inventor of neurosis, William Cullen. Like Robert Whytt, Cullen was a natural for Montpellier doctors, for he too looked to integrate external and internal influences as they affected sympathies and sensitivities in the nervous system. Pinel translated Cullen's work, but unfortunately for the luckless doctor, his work appeared side by side with another translation by Éduoard Bosquillon, a distinguished doctor who was also a professor of Greek at the Collège de France. In the *Journal de Paris*, Bosquillon trashed Pinel's translation; Pinel returned fire from the *Gazette de santé*, but the academic disparity between the two men made the battle no contest. Philippe fell into a state of despair. He refused to leave his bedroom for days until a friend came over with translations of Sappho, which apparently helped him shake off his despondency.

A year later, the hapless man's prospects improved a bit. Pinel had been illegally practicing medicine at private *maisons de santé* for at least two years, and now he landed a similar job at the posh Pension Belhomme on the Rue de Charonne. For seven years, Pinel tended to rich sufferers of senility, childlike "idiots," and *maladies d'esprit*. Despite all of the Belhomme's finery, Pinel grew uncomfortable. His boss showed a distinct proclivity for failed treatments, which kept his beds and coffers filled. Adding to the impression that this was a luxurious holding pen were regular visits by, not medical consultants, but the police.

While at the Belhomme, Pinel's *Gazette* increased its coverage of mental maladies. Then in 1789, the astonishing news of King George's cure filtered into France. In the *Gazette de santé*, Pinel tried to take in this unbelievable fact. In an essay on moral treatment, he hurried from ancient philosophers to this breakthrough. Armed with anecdotes of Dr. Willis staring down the monarch and bringing him to his senses, Pinel noted that Willis expressed "an air of importance, an inflexible firmness, the rare talent to grasp the incoherent and absurd perceptions of maniacs and to bring them back to ideas that are more piously distinguished." And using such techniques, St. Luke's in London, an envious Pinel announced, maintained a 10-out-of-12 cure rate for maniacs. Mental illnesses were curable in England.

The news of George's recovery arrived as the Bastille was liberated and the Revolution commenced. Over the next years, these two watershed events combined to offer Philippe Pinel great possibilities. Just as an incorrigible Don Juan locked up by his father became the great orator of liberty, and a small-time lawyer obsessed with Rousseau grabbed the reins of the radical Jacobins, this stuttering, medical reject would seize the day and become the self-appointed founder of French mental medicine.

By 1785, thanks to his journalism, the middle-aged Pinel began to receive some recognition. He scored an invitation to Auteuil, where he befriended those with common roots in medicine, especially Cabanis. In addition, he rubbed shoulders with Condorcet and was flattered to have Franklin urge him to immigrate to America. When the Bastille fell, Pinel's support for the Revolution was unequivocal. After July 14, he jumped into debates on postrevolutionary medicine and drafted a plan for "Reform in the Method of Teaching the Healing Art." His conclusions were not subtle: freedom was the cure for all ills. It had a healthy effect not just on the body politic, but also on individuals.

During Year II of the Revolution, as Robespierre and the Committee for Public Safety menaced and murdered those with any hint of Royalist sympathies, Cabanis and Thouret managed to appoint Pinel superintendent of the Bicêtre, a sprawling snake pit that made the Bastille seem quaint. In September of 1793, Citizen Pinel jumped into his work with all the pent-up energy of someone who had spent too long on the outside looking in.

As the Terror raged, Citizen Pinel's political bona fides remained unquestionable. He had even stood guard with his citizen's brigade, as the drums rolled and the king was beheaded. The spectacle, however, sickened him. In a letter describing that fateful day to his brother, Philippe confessed that he was tormented by his participation. He recalled the haunting, last words of the king: "I forgive all my enemies," and how the rest of his speech was drowned out by drums. A colossal injustice had been done, Philippe concluded, though he assured his brother that he was no Royalist.

When Pinel arrived at the Bicêtre, it badly needed a new start. A disgrace for decades, the institution was also the recent site of a slaughter. A year earlier, during the September massacres, members of the Commune, intoxicated with fear that prisoners were in revolt, moved in and systematically murdered helpless and unarmed detainees. In the end, 162 men were killed, including many boys. The director of the Bicêtre, far from protecting those in his charge, lustily participated in the killing. Pinel was his replacement.

Despite his credibility as a revolutionary, it was not a bad time for Pinel to leave one aspect of his own history behind. After the fall of the Bastille and the rise of the Jacobins, his former employer, Jacques Belhomme, discovered a lucrative, new market: aristocrats willing to pay anything to be declared mad so as to be tucked away at the Pension Belhomme. The Duchess of Orleans, the comtes de Roure, de Breteuil, Talleyrand, and Volney, all entered Belhomme's facility for "treatment." However, woe unto those who ran out of money. Once squeezed dry, they would be tossed over to the Jacobins and their fate. Belhomme's cruel game eventually came apart. Two months after Pinel entered the sprawling Bicêtre, his scandalous former employer was arrested.

And so, with the Terror in scarlet bloom, on September 11, 1793, this forty-eight-year-old doctor arrived at a massive hospital and surprisingly found this institution was already in the process of reforming itself. The engineer of these changes was Jean-Baptiste Pussin. Pussin was not a doctor, but he had served as governor of the Bicêtre for eight years. In the egalitarian spirit of the times, these two citizens met and it quickly became clear that the doctor had a great deal to learn.

Admitted to the Bicêtre for scrofula, Pussin, then a tanner, had remained on as a caretaker after his cure. First assigned to children, by 1785 the thirty-nine-year-old Pussin had been transferred to the 7th Ward, which housed 200 insane men. Thirteen years later, while trying to advocate for funds and recognition, Pussin claimed that upon taking up this post, he was nearly pummeled to death by a manic priest, an experience that made him seek change. Instead of calling for more restraints, he concluded that fewer were needed. If beating an animal cowed it for a while, eventually it only fueled more rage. It was a logic that former patients like Pussin and prisoners like Sade immediately saw, but one their jailers mostly did not. Like Rousseau, Pussin believed his charges would be less volatile if attendants met fury with a firm kindness. And this softer approach was aided by a new invention: Guilleret, the in-house *tapissier* at the Bicêtre, had created a waistcoat that wrapped one's arms helplessly behind the back. In 1790, Pussin began to employ the *camisole de force* or straitjacket instead of chains.

Pussin's innovations would become a source of contention, as others lined up to take credit for these more humane advances. For example, the hospital in Avignon had a superintendent named Brouet

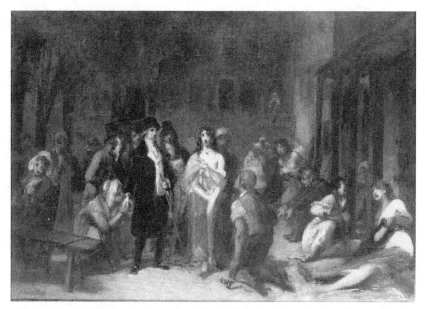

Figure 34. *Pinel Freeing the Insane from Their Chains*, by Tony Robert-Fleury (1876).

and a Dr. Joseph Gastaldy: inspired by the English, they too had instituted a brand of psychic treatment. A smattering of others in France could also make a case for bringing mental treatment to their country. In 1791, a civil servant from the Var wrote a pamphlet in which a Rousseauian wise man cured the mad by becoming a repository of their pains, and searching their histories for the source of their ills, so as to break their spell. Along with the pioneering efforts of Chiarugi, the Turin doctor Joseph Daquin, influenced by the cure rates reported in England, initiated moral treatments in the hospitals of Chambery and published his *Philosophy of Madness* in 1791. He too would claim to have preceded the others.

While each of these individuals seem to have adopted the British modes of mind management, Pussin and Pinel were different precisely because of where they stood—at the center of the revolution. Pussin insisted that he had reformed his ward *prior* to the fall of the Bastille, but still these innovations would be co-opted by the anti-Royalists, as a symbol of their promise for a more humane society. And the disbanding of the conservative Paris Faculty made resistance to these innovations minimal.

The political conditions were ripe for a reform that institutionalized the medicine of *l'esprit*, one that harmonized with nationalistic and political imperatives. However, it was not at all clear that those hopes would be invested in the timid Pinel, the tanner Pussin, and an inferno called the Bicêtre. In Year III, the Charenton, formerly run by the Brothers of St. Jean de Dieu and tainted by its history of acting as a Royalist penal institution, was closed by the Jacobins, then reopened two years later, after the rise of the Directory, as a fully secularized, progressive hospital for the mad. It would replace the Hôtel-Dieu—now called the Grand Hospice d'Humanité—as the center for the active treatment of the mentally ill. For this purpose, the institution would be run by another *médecin-philosophe*, Citizen Gastaldy of Avignon. This doctor and the new Charenton claimed that they would restore France's honor and do what the British already could do: cure those afflicted by insanity.

At first, Pinel made no such promises. During his eighteen months at the Bicêtre, he closely observed Pussin's methods and kept his head down as his friends in the Girondin were hunted and on the run. Pussin had pulled together a dossier for his new boss on admissions, death rates, and discharges. Pinel began to study the men locked up in this penal colony, while outside the long-oppressed ran wild with their new freedoms.

IN 1794, the fall of Robespierre and the Jacobin dictatorship and the rise of the Thermidorian Reaction brought Philippe Pinel's reforming allies back into power, but they had been changed. Their bright hopes of reason, liberty, and equality had been dimmed. Old ideals had not been violated, as Thomas Paine would write; they were abandoned. Francisco de Goya, the masterful Spanish printmaker and painter, captured the frailty of Enlightenment hopes in his print called *The Sleep of Reason Produces Monsters*. The engraving, begun around 1797, depicts the artist asleep on his drafting table, his head nestled in his arms as owls and bats accost him. "Fantasy abandoned by reason produces impossible monsters . . . ," he wrote beneath the image.

In December 1794, Philippe Pinel scheduled a talk before the Society for Natural History on these same beasts of unreason. The timing of the event was political. Thanks to his pull, Pinel had just been appointed Chair of Medical Hygiene at the newly formed medical school, the École de Santé; this was an opportunity to prove his worth. And the locale was also no accident. Even during the Terror, the Society for Natural History was a safe haven for science, for

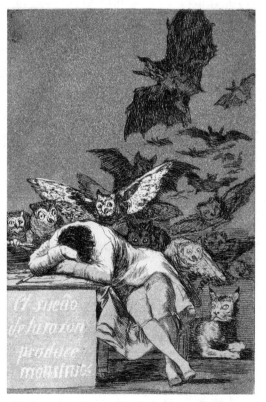

Figure 35. Francisco Goya, *The Sleep of Reason Produces Monsters*, from *Los Caprichos* (1797–1799).

somehow the Jacobin revolutionaries had been convinced that this body differed from other elitist institutions. While the Academy of Sciences and the Academy of Medicine were shuttered, the Society for Natural History's doors remained open.

Natural history had been a passion for Pinel. Quiet and observant, he had joined others who took up the encyclopedist zeal for classification, including doctors like Félix Vicq d'Azyr and naturalists like Jean-Baptiste de Lamarck. Pinel helped write an appeal to preserve a state-run menagerie to replace the king's, and shared his studies on the skull of an elephant and the brain of a cow. On this wintery day in December, Pinel's talk would be on madness, seen through the lens of natural history. It was Citizen Pinel's first exegesis on what he called "mania" and "alienated reason."

The novice shed little new light on these subjects; however, he showcased his rhetorical skill by weaving the fate of the mentally ill into the pressing concerns of his audience. Pinel insisted the mad should engender tenderness, since their condition stemmed from a too-vibrant sensitivity, dignified qualities we might otherwise value. The exalted sensitivity of the orator, engineer, or painter, and the mournful despair of those whose losses had overwhelmed them, were easily imaginable: they were the troubles of our sisters and brothers. Out of love for France, Dr. Pinel revealed that he had been forced to hospitalize a famed sculptor, a reminder that confinement could be patriotic and that mad citizens could also be great ones. Citizen Pinel thus sought to harmonize a redefined notion of medical confinement with the ideals of the Revolution.

Under the *ancien régime*, Pinel contended, the Bicêtre had been nothing more than a prison. No one paid any attention to treating deranged reason. That had changed, thanks to a novel therapeutic ethos, one that didn't so much imprison as cure.

Of course, Pinel knew all this was a fairy tale. While the previous director may have been a brute, Pussin had instituted humanitarian reforms without the help of the Revolution. But such inconvenient facts were swept away in the service of a greater goal, which was justifying the confinement of citizens who were mentally ill. While modern means of curing the mentally ill in asylums had gone nowhere in Germany or Spain, Pinel informed his listeners, in England such innovations had flourished. "Why does that haughty and self-righteous nation spoil such a great gift to humanity by keeping a mysterious silence and guiltily casting a veil over its skill to restore distracted reason?" he demanded. The French must make efforts to right this wrong.

And so, this political appointee in his inaugural talk on mental illness framed his work as that of a dedicated revolutionary, an egalitarian, and a patriot. There was little natural history and a great deal of posturing, all of which led to Pinel's peroration, which included a desperate appeal for funds. Madness did not obliterate the entire mind and was potentially curable; the secret of English moral management must be discovered anew by the French, and it would be if monies were made available. A more terrible truth was then revealed: the mad in Paris's hospitals had been starving to death in shocking numbers. In one year alone, 95 of 151 mentally ill men at Pinel's facility perished from hunger. Friends of humanity should blanch at such a horror, he declared.

After the fall of the Bastille, liberty had been the rallying cry of the French. Unjustly locked away for years, those like Mirabeau hoped to liberate the others who had been chained to a wall by heartless tyrants. The great author once quipped that while he knew the poorhouses were to punish lawbreakers and restrain the insane, he only later learned that they were to transform men into criminals and make them mad. Those unjustly chained and locked away through *lettres de cachet* were a potent symbol of the arbitrary authority and repression of the king. Now that France had won its freedom, some asked, why should there be such places?

However, after the Terror, the Girondists were not eager to embrace unrestrained, Jacobin polemics on liberation. They had seen enough to know where that could lead. The first ideal of the Revolution, liberty, had become both a joy and a danger. It had led to happiness and rampaging riot. Freedom and social stability could coexist only if citizens controlled themselves. Just as a century earlier in England, religious tolerance required a line beyond which individuals could not go. France's newly acquired liberties forced forward the question: where does individual freedom end? This new republic required the creation of boundaries, to mark those who were not simply freely acting beings, but rather pathologically out of control. Otherwise, Girondists like Pinel and Cabanis feared, the goals of the Revolution would come undone thanks to the frenzy of citizen-maniacs.

Pinel had seen such chaos firsthand. During the Terror, an armed throng invaded the Bicêtre. The liberators went from cell to cell, interviewed the inmates, and offered to release them. The armed men reached a seemingly well-behaved fellow, who politely requested his liberty. With a saber pushed up against his chest, Pussin freed this citizen. Liberty, equality, and fraternity danced together as the mob disappeared. Later that day, the same angry band hustled the maniac back to his cell. He had rewarded his emancipators by filching one of their swords and swinging it wildly into them.

Before the Society for Natural History, Citizen Pinel revealed that he strove to avoid chains—those dark symbols of the old order—and when possible, used mental management. His understanding of such psychological means was still rather crude and, ironically, involved a good deal of brute authority and psychic terror. The fear of force made inmates control themselves. Quiet intimidation, he believed, would break the will of the furious without leaving a scar.

Words and reason were hardly force enough when the Jacobins rampaged. Some of the rioters, ultraradicals to the left of Robespierre's Montagnards, defined themselves by their distaste for such talk: they were the *enragés*. Père Duchesne's essays stoked their anger;

eager readers awaited for today's Great Rage or Great Indignation. He himself believed the Revolution should follow its heart: "Brave sans-culottes, why have you had this revolution? Isn't it to be happy, fuck?!" For Hébert, Marat, and Robespierre, the Revolution came to usher in a joyous, pure society, which would rise from the fire of their passions.

However, those filled with such emotion were at risk, according to some doctors, of developing a kind of madness called revolutionary fever. Such was the fate of Théroigne de Méricourt, the so-called Fury of the Gironde. She was not the only one upended by the emotional tumult. The very stages of the Revolution were at times named by an overwhelming passion: thus, the Great Fear preceded the Terror and the emergence of the enraged ones. The citizens of France swung between raucous celebrations, wrath, and quivering fear.

Philippe Pinel positioned himself as an enlightened voice that might tend to a manic nation. Armed with mental models of treatment, he framed the plight of the mad in terms that cohered with the original ideals of the Revolution, and yet seemed to offer the hope that a man might stabilize his own freedom with internal restraints that modulated emotion.

Pinel's influence spread. In 1795, he left Pussin behind and moved on to another massive mess, the female equivalent of the Bicêtre, the Salpêtrière. As he did this, he was promoted to Professor of Pathological Medicine, another step up the ladder for which Citizen Pinel had almost no qualifications. Nonetheless, this patronage appointment had a salutary effect: it encouraged Pinel to justify himself. He sat down to try his hand at medical classification. Before such a tall task, Pinel seemed poorly equipped, but the time was right. Medicine was up for grabs. The Paris Faculty had been disbanded; licensing had been suspended. Where there once was an entrenched orthodoxy, there now was a vacuum. Power came from political sway, which Pinel, thanks to his Auteuil friends, possessed.

And so he began to dream up a medicine for a novel era in history. Many of his notions were not clear improvements, but they fell on burnt-over soil.

In 1798, after three years of labor, Pinel published *Philosophical Nosography, or the Method of Applied Analysis*, which showed off an understanding of statistics, the study of natural history, and a logical rigor that could not have been predicted. Prerevolutionary medicine was a vain mockery, he announced, but a new medicine would rest solidly on the conceptual tool of *analysis*. Analysis came from Condillac, whose sensationalist epistemology encouraged very close attention to the parts that made up more complex wholes. Pinel would present a naturalistic account of the parts that made up more complex, discrete disease categories. True to his Montpellier roots, he announced that the foundation for all such classification was the essential properties of sensibility and irritability.

Pinel's taxonomy of disease sought to distinguish four coherent classes, each of which contained orders, genera, and species. The fourth class was called "Névroses" after neurosis, the term used by William Cullen, the Scottish doctor Pinel had translated. Nervous troubles were divided into four. The first, "Vesanies," a Latin word for madness, included hypochondria, melancholia, mania, and hysteria. Pinel opined that these *aliénations d'esprit* were not just "Locke and Condillac's" disruption of cognitive understanding, but for now did not elaborate.

While Plutarch once called for a reciprocal dependence between moral philosophy and medicine, Pinel went further and called for *le moral* to become medical. Years of cultivation by medically oriented *lumières*, he asserted, were now ready for harvest. Small experiments in mental medicine had been started in England, but now these tenuous studies could bloom in a land unencumbered by censorship from the Church. A new field of mental medicine could flourish in the liberated, secular land of France.

Pinel's *Nosography* was seen as a breakthrough for French medicine, though after the Revolution there was little left to break. This call for reform went through six editions in the next twenty years; it cast aside weary notions and offered a fresh, logical method for distinguishing illnesses, a matter critical to rational medical practice. Many were inspired by this approach, including Pinel's patron and friend, Pierre-Jean-Georges Cabanis.

The politically nimble Cabanis had managed to survive the many turns of the Revolution, no mean feat. He had tied his fate to Mirabeau, then repositioned himself when the Orator of Liberty was denounced as a traitor. He whisked Condorcet to a safe house and sympathized with the Girondins, but presented himself to the radical Montagnards in a manner that won him a seat on the Revolutionary Tribunal. After Robespierre's demise, Cabanis scrambled back to the center and, with the new government, wielded significant political power. However, Cabanis's ambition was far more than that: if Pinel was attempting to re-create medicine and the treatment of the mind, Cabanis threw himself into making a human science that could establish natural laws to govern ethics, law, and social policy.

This ambitious effort began by looking backward. In the winter of Year III, the Commissioner of Public Instruction, another dedicated follower of Madame Helvétius, Dominique-Joseph Garat, planned to revamp French education, a critical project for the secularization of the country. To further this project, he encouraged Cabanis to write a history of medicine that would act as a road map for that field's teachers. Cabanis's own medical training was laughably scant. He had studied privately with a student of the Montpellier school, then traveled to Reims, where in a single year he procured his medical degree and license, probably by buying them. Amid the heady atmosphere at Auteuil, however, this novice had grown confident enough to propose reforms. In 1788, he published his fascinating *Certainty in Medicine*, in which he rejected the reduction of his field to chemistry or physics, and called for medicine to establish its own logic and epistemology.

After Garat's invitation, on July 6, 1795, Cabanis produced *General Considerations on the Revolutions in the Art of Healing*. This was a time of renewal, he wrote, a time to institutionalize the advances inaugurated by isolated freethinkers. To unify and synthesize this past, medical knowledge required a strenuous analysis à la Condillac, with logical study of identities and differences, compositions and decompositions. Medicine could then create a new chain of being in which the inert became organized into the vegetable kingdom, which, when endowed with sensitivity, led to animal life. Living beings through increasingly complex organization produced all qualities of man, including reason.

This final link between physiology and the mind was critical for Cabanis's larger purpose. Morals and medicine were two branches of a "science of man," what the Germans called anthropology. Such a science should guide moralists and legislators toward the goal of perfectibility. Oppression, vice, and misery could be transformed by science into liberty, virtue, and happiness.

In Paris, Montpellier, and Auteuil, such speculations had been tossed about, but Cabanis was now in a position to actualize such hopes. In December of 1795, he had his chance. The newly formed National Institute of Sciences and Arts opened its doors. It would be egalitarian, with no officers and leaders. Its members took an oath against royalty, and an unspoken new elite emerged: those who faithfully served the Revolution. Dr. Cabanis was one. The Institute was divided into three. Physical and Mathematical Sciences was the First Class, while Literature and Fine Arts made up the Third. In between these traditional areas of study was the Second Class of Moral and Political Sciences.

This Second Class, Cabanis hoped, would rationally guide the agendas of the state. As such, Cabanis recognized, it might pose a challenge to political authority; however, only despots need fear. In a republic, objective truths about human behavior would be a welcome source of information that helped ensure political stability. The Second Class would create not just more *médecins-philosophes,* but also a new breed of physician-legislators like Cabanis himself.

The meetings of the Second Class were like reunions of Auteuil; they included Garat, Volney, Victor de Sèze, and the influential Antoine Destutt de Tracy. Members of that group were younger and more radical than colleagues in the two other classes. In their effort to link natural science to ethics and social reform, they pushed forward a secular and naturalized mind, and an empirical science of ideas.

Of the six sections in the Second Class, one particularly focused on this task, the Section on the Analysis of Sensations and Ideas. Members of this group could not just follow the path cut by Condillac, since for them, the founder of the analytic method had two critical flaws. First, he had rid himself of Locke's theory of active mental reflection and replaced it, nominally at least, with a weak notion of the soul that hovered above the mental faculties. Without fear of retribution, Destutt de Tracy sliced away this remnant of superstition and declared that all the faculties of the so-called soul were actually composed of sensations. Higher-level functions like reflection, intention, and morality were the same.

In a lecture before the Institute on June 20, 1796, Destutt de Tracy framed what he believed was a new tradition, one that took Locke as its Copernicus, and sought to replace metaphysics as first among all sciences. Since metaphysics referred to immaterial matters, this was not simply a new variant of that enterprise, since, as Locke showed, thinking was surely material. To call this new science "psychology" would be misleading, since that term commonly meant the study of the soul, an ethereal object that no one in his audience could pretend to possess. Instead, Destutt de Tracy proposed a new name for this science—"ideology." Ideologists studied ideas, their sources, combinations, and results. This field excluded metaphysicians. Ideas were part of the natural world, and could be seen as a subset of zoology.

The rational soul had traveled a long road, and now in this secular society, its once divine intellectual functions were to be seen as part of animal life. This last claim, which no doubt brought gasps to some of the Cartesians that still remained, also required a second modification of Condillac. That philosopher's ideas and sensations floated about in ether and were not tied to the body. Beginning on February 16, 1796, Dr. Cabanis began a series of lectures that he hoped would integrate consciousness into physiology and anatomy. The result was *On the Relations Between the Physical and the Moral Aspects of Man*. The title echoed four decades of prior works by Lacaze, Bordeu, Barthez, and others; however, like Destutt de Tracy, Cabanis could say out loud what many long had spoken of in private.

As Cabanis lectured, however, this nascent secular order pitched back and forth. Fearful of the *sans-culottes* as well as the resurgent threat of Royalists, the Directory was formed in 1795, and, with the second constitution, it created electoral colleges that sought to ensure that only well-established citizens would be elected. The rise of neo-monarchists elected to the Convention led to the Fructidor coup d'état in the fall of 1797. The army now held back Royalist reaction and militant terror. Meanwhile, revolutionary republics sprouted up around France, as war whipped up new opponents to the feudal order. For believers in the rule of reason, this made the project of creating a stable, legitimizing basis for secular ethics even more pressing.

Festivals and temples of reason, mass celebrations of *la patrie*, nationalism, and the new honorific title of "citizen" were all efforts to deepen commitments to reason and the state. Secular catechisms appeared such as Volney's *Catechism of the French Citizien* and Jean-François Saint-Lambert's catechism for children, which began: "What is a man? A sensible and reasonable being. As a sensible and reasonable being, what must he do? Search for pleasure and avoid pain." Pupils would commit themselves to this pledge, and it was hoped, secure the new order.

In 1797, François-René de Chateaubriand, in a study of revolutions, plaintively asked, "Which will be the religion that replaces Christianity?" To answer this call, a new cult sprang up called Théophilanthropes. Its leader, Jean-Baptiste Chemin-Dupontès, proclaimed that sun worshipers and disciples of Moses, Jesus, and Mohammed were all fundamentally the same. They shared belief in the existence of God and the immortality of the soul. If one accepted those two beliefs, reason could then step in and create a natural ethic. The founder of Théophilanthropie churned out manuals for behavior and didactic tracts. By 1802, Théophilanthropie was practiced in nineteen Parisian venues that had once been Catholic churches.

The Second Class of the National Institute also took up this challenge. In 1797 and then again in 1798, it held contests on the question "What are the most suitable institutions to establish the morality of the people?" Destutt de Tracy explicitly warned that the myth of eternal punishment was not relevant to this question. When the Institute members read through the entries, however, they found that two of the three proposed solutions employed reward in Heaven and damnation in Hell.

Tension between atheists and the believers soon boiled over. One of the judges of the ethics essay contest, the Deist Bernardin de Saint-Pierre, rose before his colleagues to denounce natural principles for morality. He decried the destructive influence of moral relativity and insisted ideas of right and wrong were absolute and did not vary due to sex, religion, or nation. An outraged Volney and Cabanis shouted him down. Saint-Pierre later wrote that Cabanis thundered: "I swear there is no God. I wish that His name never be pronounced within these walls."

However without the fear of divine retribution, how would society ensure the morality of its members? For Cabanis, the answer was clear: France would develop a human science based on pleasure and pain, human sensibility, and reason. In the preface to his *Memoirs*, Dr. Cabanis reminded his reader that the natural claims of virtue were exceedingly powerful. Pleasure paved the road to virtue. Cabanis cited Benjamin Franklin, who once remarked that if rogues knew how much delight resided in virtue, they would roguishly pursue it.

The origins of human science, for Cabanis, began with John Locke. The Frenchman then sketched out recent efforts, including those of Helvétius, Condillac, and Haller. For Cabanis, like many of his colleagues, sensibility remained central to his integration of mind and body. Cabanis spent the second and third lectures detailing his more specific understanding of sensation and sensibility. And he wondered if nervous sensibility might be electrical. In 1791, Luigi Galvani had demonstrated that animals seemed to possess electric properties that they secreted from their nerves. If the nervous system was a kind of Leyden jar, then it made sense that some might have higher voltages than others. With the eyes of the eager social planner, Cabanis advised mating humans much as horses were bred, with an eye toward perfecting imbalances of nervous temperament. Understanding such differences was critical, he continued, for sensibility was the basis of moral sympathy as articulated by Shaftesbury, Adam Smith, and Francis Hutcheson.

Cabanis focused on physiological variables that might alter behavior, morals, and thought. Age was a central consideration, since the inner life of juveniles obviously differed from the elderly. Men differed from women in a manner that, in the author's opinion, showered favors on the former. Different temperaments, diets, and climates led to different ethical and intellectual types. Finally, illnesses could obviously affect one's mentality, but if cured, immoral inclinations, ignorant beliefs, and criminal actions could be eradicated.

During the first ten lectures, the doctor lavished attention on the environmental and physical drivers of inner life while focusing little attention on the mind's power to stir the nervous system into action. Adding to the misperception that Cabanis only believed the causal flow went from body to mind, he employed an analogy that would be much repeated: the brain, he wrote, secreted thought in the way that the stomach churned out its juices. Before publishing these lectures, Cabanis added a bit more on mental influences and was clear that cures for sick thoughts and behaviors could be either physical or mental, since the action of sensibility allowed the body to affect the mind, and the mind to impact the body.

Cabanis hoped his new human science would replace the Church as a legitimate source of secular morality and a compass for social policy. After its publication in 1802, *On the Relations Between the Physical and the Moral Aspects of Man* went through eight editions in the next few years and influenced many readers, including the sixteen-year-old Stendhal, who considered the book to be his Bible.

A new moral rulebook was urgently required. As the calendar was dechristianized, Cabanis and his colleagues sought to replace over a millennia of belief in the soul, the Christian virtues and vices, and Heaven and Hell. Still the future of this program seemed bright, for its leader was a powerhouse. Elected in 1798 to the lower house of the legislature, the Council of 500, Cabanis also accepted a patronage job at the medical school. However, despite the fact that Cabanis, Garat, Volney, and others sat near the pinnacle of power, seismic events kept rumbling from the streets below. In 1797, after the Fructidor Coup purged the government of suspected Royalists, moderates became panicked that the rout of Royalists would lead to a neo-Jacobin uprising. In 1799, Cabanis and others dropped their commitments to liberty and advocated severe restrictions on the rights of assembly.

When General Napoleon Bonaparte returned from his campaign in Italy, he aligned himself with the moderates and the intellectuals of the National Academy. He was elected to the Class of Physical and Mathematical Sciences, and consorted with a number of the Auteuil regulars, who included his brother Lucien. When Bonaparte left for the conquest of Egypt, he brought with him a troop of ideologists and promised to start a journal dedicated to revitalizing Egypt that borrowed the name of the main ideologist journal. When Bonaparte rushed back to Paris and staged a coup, the intellectuals of Auteuil stood behind him. For Cabanis and others, the Coup of 18 Brumaire was a desperate attempt to salvage the liberal gains of the Revolution by fighting off the Royalists on one side and the neo-Jacobins on the other.

Napoleon placed Cabanis, Garat, Volney, and Tracy in the Senate, lucrative positions that paid three times a medical professor's salary. The new savior of France even paid a ceremonial visit to Madame Helvétius in Auteuil, where he marvelled that these few acres had yielded so much. The alignment of the ideologists with the General promised to usher in a new age. Science and power would create a new society that balanced the demands of freedom with social order, the hopes for egalitarianism with a science of human nature.

AS CABANIS LECTURED on human science, Philippe Pinel sometimes stepped away from his overwhelming tasks at the Salpêtrière to speak at the Competitive Medical Society of Paris, a progressive group he helped to found in 1796. In 1797, Pinel gave a lecture—"On Periodic or Intermittent Mania"—which was not without political polemic. One frenzied man, who believed he was the prophet Mohammed and greeted cannon fire with delight, was the prototype for the "supernatural inspiration" of fanatics and the prophets of old. The doctor called for the use of Locke and Condillac to study these sudden manic disturbances and the troubles found among those yearning for glory, the hermits, the unhappy lovers, those called possessed, and those who specialized in illusions like soothsaying, oracles, and spells.

In 1798 and 1799, Pinel returned to this Society to discuss the treatment of madness. Over time, his lectures began to thicken; political asides diminished as his expertise deepened. Pinel brought his prior interests to this project; there were statistics and probability, comparative natural history, anatomy, classification, and much effort devoted to therapies, especially mental treatments. In these lectures, Pinel dismissed the British Battie, Arnold, and Willis, the German Johann Greding, and the Italian Chiaruggi. He acknowledged that some healers empirically discovered restorative methods, like his dear friend Pussin, as well as Willis, John Haslam of Bethlehem Hospital, and others in the Var and Amsterdam, but these honorable efforts fell short of a fully conceptualized mental therapy.

Amid this wholesale dismissal of his predecessors, Pinel's critiques of the British were most strenuous, for they stood most directly in the way of his own claims for priority. One author did receive praise— Alexander Crichton. In 1798, this Westminister doctor published *Inquiry into the Nature and Origin of Mental Derangement*. Crichton shared Pinel's interest in the analytic mehod, and he too began with irritability and sensibility as the building blocks of psychic life. Proficient in German, Crichton also provided Pinel with a summary of German research. Thus, Pinel, though unable to read that language, could make a show of having evaluated German as well as English and French alternatives before coming to his own conclusions.

Pinel understood that to stabilize a field of *médecine mentale*, he needed to do something about the Babel that surrounded strange inner states. In English, general terms like madness, derangement, delirium, lunacy, and insanity mixed promiscuously with more specific names like mania and melancholia; French words for mental derangements were also a mishmash. Writers seemed to choose from a haphazard lexicon that included *folie, fou, délire, insensé*, and *démence*.

Pinel hoped to put an end to that. When his lectures were pulled together and expanded into a book, they constituted his hopes for a new standardized field, mental medicine. Published in Year IX of the new secular calendar, or 1801, *A Medico-Philosophical Treatise on Mental Alienation or Mania* opened grandly, tying itself to the progress of society: "the progressive march of the *lumières* on the character and the treatment of mental alienation is entirely related to . . . the varied degree of advancement of a people's civilization." Pinel promised to employ medicine and philosophy to further this process.

However, the title immediately disoriented readers by equating two things not commonly considered synonymous. While Hippocrates used "mania" as a general word for insanity, Galen had refined that concept to specifically refer to states of delirium without fever, a meaning that stuck. In that way, mania was a narrow, specific subset of madness. Alienation of the mind also had a long history. The notion probably originated with Plotinus, whose radically monistic philosophy began with a principle of universal Oneness, an absolute unity from which humans could become fragmented and thus alienated. The specific phrase—mental alienation—had been used by another classical author that Pinel knew, the Roman physician Caelius Aurelianus, who referred to madness as an *alienatio mentis*. While other doctors had employed the phrase, Pinel now made a great claim for this notion and hence seemed to equate mania, a sickness of the humors, with all mental estrangement.

Even while creating his own confusion, Pinel himself complained about the fog created by ill-defined mental states. Before the "French and English" ideologists, there was no proper language to make critical distinctions. Pinel would rely on the "modern psychologists" like Locke and Condillac, but even that posed a problem, since Locke's "mind" had no exact French equivalent. And so, Pinel proposed "alienation mentale," a slight modification of common phrases like *aliénation de l'esprit* and *aliénation de raison*. Thanks to the spirit of free inquiry encouraged by the Revolution, Citizen Pinel would openly discuss the mind without the old "fetters." He explicitly tied his project to Cabanis's: "The analysis of the functions of human understanding," he wrote, "is without doubt strongly advanced by the compiled work of the Ideologists."

In 1809, when the second edition of the *Treatise* appeared, Pinel dropped "mania" from the title and let his new nomenclature stand alone. Using the method of analysis, those formerly deemed crazy, insensible, and alienated of either spirit or reason, would be reconceived as mentally alienated. The sufferers were *les aliénés*—the alienated, and those who treated them would be called alienists by some.

Pinel's *Treatise* proposed a theory of the origin, development, and effects of mental illness. Doctors long assumed alienation stemmed from incurable brain lesions, he argued; the mad were thus locked away and treated brutally. The cruel treatment of the mentally ill, Pinel added, was akin to the oppression of citizens by a despotic government. That was all wrong. Countless autopsies— Pinel conducted thirty-six himself—turned up nothing special. Meanwhile, moral treatment cured some cases, and if mental interventions could cure, then mental causes must be at play. And so, the lies and tyrannies of the Old Regime were exposed.

The *Treatise* depended on rigorous thought, the cold eye of a naturalist, and not least of all, compelling stories. Pinel told of his own journey, which he imbued with a touch of pathos and heroism. He told of the student who begged Philippe to shoot him and, after returning from the Hôtel-Dieu, committed suicide. The death, Pinel concluded, was an indictment of a callous orthodoxy that refused to try new treatments. He told of the Pension Belhomme, with its infamous, avaricious owner, and then spoke frankly of his own trial by fire at the Bicêtre.

A good deal of this narrative was self-serving. However, Pinel did not hold back from describing cases that ended badly. And he did not hide the appalling fact that many in his charge died. He accused the revolutionary governments of causing many of those deaths by starvation. After intense lobbying, Dr. Pinel had been relieved when the Assembly had increased bread rations to 2 kg a day per man at the Bicêtre, but he recounted his horror when he returned to find that the ration had been cut to a paltry 3.4 ounces. Corpses were everywhere. With the Jacobins now routed, Pinel angrily wrote:

I leave it to the historian of the revolution to paint, in its proper and odious colors, that most barbarous and tyrannical measure which deprived infirmaries and hospitals of their valuable endowments, and abandoned the diseased and the infirm to all the vicissitudes of public fortune.

Pinel moved on to case histories, some of which would become paradigmatic, repeated nearly verbatim in French, German, and English textbooks. Committed to a view of nervous sensibility, in which external stimuli became internalized, Pinel's mentally ill reflected the immense stresses of the time; here were those who quite literally went mad when much of the country was in upheaval. "The storms of revolution stirred up corresponding tempests in the passions of men," he explained, "and overwhelmed not a few in a total ruin of their distinguished birthrights as rational beings."

Pinel's most repeated case was that of a master watchmaker, once obsessed with the possibility of perpetual motion, who in his mind had become convinced he had been guillotined, only to then receive a reprieve after the deed was done. A careless worker, he believed, must have then reached into the pile of heads and grabbed the wrong one to sew it back onto his body, for this was not his face. Tormented by his strange features, the man would beseech those around him: Look at this twisted mouth! Look at these rotten teeth! Mine were so handsome; these are hideous. To counter this man's delusion, Pinel and his attendants devised a plan: the craftsman would be cured of his illness through the intense engagement of his other, still-sane mental faculties. The director set him up with tools and facilities to get back to designing and building a perpetual motion machine. In the end, the patient constructed a beautiful geared device and gave up the idea that his head was not his own.

The case of the watchmaker, Pinel wrote, demolished thousands of metaphysical books on the supposed unity of the mind or soul. This starkly insane man easily summoned up enough reason to build an engineering marvel. Mental diseases were partial, Pinel asserted with Locke. The mad were not wholly lost to reason.

Others under Pinel's care also had illnesses that mirrored the events in France. A religious enthusiast became mad when the Catholic Church was abolished. Devoted stewards and valets from the household of aristocrats and princes fell into melancholia. A gentleman who lost everything now declared he was Mohammed. A ruined denizen of Versailles announced he was King of the World. At the Bicêtre, he shared quarters with the three kings of France. There were also two Austrian prisoners with a delusional fear of the guillotine. Sadly, they turned out to be sane and were beheaded.

The case of the Austrians highlighted the difficulty of judging different beliefs based on subjective reports. Pinel's work, however, would not rely on case histories alone. It would be the first true natural history of madness that used analysis and statistics. Condorcet and other Auteuil technocrats had embraced the mathematical study of patterns and probabilities, and Pinel adopted their approach. Statistics showed that alienation was provoked by domestic misfortune, obstacles to marriage, stressors related to the Revolution, and, lastly, religious fanaticism. Of two hundred maniacs, the doctor counted 59 that cycled in and out of sanity, 53 had irregular paroxysms, while only 6 were regular in their furies. These periods ranged from every fifteen days to every three months, a simple observation that utterly undermined those who would only follow Locke and Condillac. Delusions among these patients would come and go, while Locke's cognitive disorder should have had no means of intermittently curing itself.

So while adopting the post-Lockean ideologist framework, Pinel also complicated that cogntive model by pointing to the disruptive role of the passions. Rational beings could be overrun by "ungovernable" fury, a notion whose political significance could not have been lost on his readers. These furious beings, between episodes, were the most affectionate husbands and impassioned lovers, the purest patriots and responsible citizens. But when pushed too far, these sensitive citizens flipped into raving mania, or possibly its twin, melancholia. The mad were therefore frequently sane, and the sane potentially mad.

Along with mania and melancholia, Pinel classified dementia and idiocy, two disorders that broadened mental medicine to include anatomical brain disorders. This was a bow to German and Italian doctors who, following Herman Boerhaave, looked for mechanical disruptions in insanity. But what was that anatomical cause? The copious data on skulls and brains pointed every which way. Pinel's autopsies revealed no distinctive brain lesions in mania and melancholia, but he did conclude that distorted skulls existed in cases of idiotism. Dementia had no such stigmata. Still, these two brain illnesses—one of youth and the other of old age—were equally incurable.

For mania and melancholia, Pinel confessed that after much experimentation he had been forced to conclude that pharmaceutical treatments were rubbish. Mental treatment was effective in some cases, an admission that caused Pinel to again vent his anger at the English, who refused to reveal their methods. Their priority in such therapeutics, he huffed, included a good deal of pretension. From his reading, Pinel had decided, the secret to English moral treatment was that there was no secret.

Pinel protested a bit too much. He clearly learned a good deal from his extensive study of English therapists. However, he poured scorn especially on the miraculous Dr. Francis Willis. Willis had cured his king and advertised an astonishing 90 percent cure rate, but he never discussed his failures. No doubt Willis's ostentatious advertisements for himself had been dictated by British empiricism, Pinel added sarcastically, knowing that many of his readers would know that Willis had recently traveled to Portugal to treat the queen for a massive fee and utterly failed. Pinel dismissed the treatments of Arnold and Harper, and reserved faint praise for Crichton. His strategies had not come from them, but rather from that humble tanner, Citizen Pussin.

At the Bicêtre, Pussin had discovered that his attendants, his "interior police," kept the peace with a kind but steely resolve. Pinel concluded that positive and negative rewards could push patients to reassert their own mental self-control over ungovernable emotions. Pinel tailored his treatments; for the religious enthusiast who saw the Devil, there would be isolation, the removal of religious artifacts, the forced reading of antireligious tracts, and relentless argument in which the virtuous Ancients were contrasted with nonsensical saints.

Contrary affects could be mobilized to restore balance. Consolation helped melancholics. Diversion could be effective, as demonstrated by the watchmaker. Theatrical manipulation could be used: when three maniacs, all of whom claimed to be Louis XVI, fell into a dark dispute, Pussin's wife pulled aside one of the kings and persuaded him not to debase himself by holding direct discussions with such rabble. He lifted his nose and walked away.

Finally, the asylum would be a therapeutic tool. By extracting patients from their environments, this enclosed world offered these *aliénés* a chance to rebalance their inner worlds. A policeman within those walls would become internalized in the mind and thus help reestablish the rule of reason within. The doctor and staff must be the model of balance, their passions controlled by reason, their demeanor intimidating but never violent. They must respect the ill as citizens and mirror an enlightened government's approach to its people.

During Robert Burton's time, melancholia had been the catchall term for mental ills. Philippe Pinel's *Treatise* moved mania closer to the center. This illness, with its periodic frenzy and furor, made sense in a world where liberty came suddenly and the unfettered masses erupted into violence. Mania, the furious exuberance that leads a man or woman to break all boundaries, and throws reason over in a burst of passion, was the madness of the day. For Pinel and his followers, it would be the test case for their new mental medicine.

Pinel's work was heralded as a great advance and applauded by his ideologist friends like Cabanis, Maine de Biran, and Destutt de

Tracy. Immediately translated into German in 1801, his book caught the attention of doctors, as well as philosophers like G. W. F. Hegel, who was impressed by the notion of alienation. In 1804, Pinel's book appeared in Spanish, and two years later it reached British shores.

Moral and psychic treatments were a half-century old by the time Pinel embraced them. Humanitarian care of the confined was hardly new. However, in the wake of the Revolution, Citizen Pinel pulled these together with other strands to argue for a new field that would use case histories, statistics, analysis, and the observation of brains and minds to treat the mad citizens of France. In the conclusion of his *Treatise*, he expressed the hope that these fundamental principles of mental medicine would encourage the government to create a "superstructure" for mental treatment superior to any in the world.

WHEN THE FRENCH Revolution drove out the Church and the protectors of the soul, a fully formed secular, modern lineage of the mind was waiting, ready to emerge. Constructed by doctors and philosophers like Locke, Helvétius, Condillac, Bordeu, Diderot, Haller, Barthez, and others, it had been mostly made in the shadows. Almost all these thinkers had twisted themselves to somehow accommodate some aspect of the soul, but now that effort could be left aside by secular naturalists who embraced an embodied mind as the essence of being, and sought to synthesize, institutionalize, and disseminate human science and mental medicine. However, as this post-Revolutionary project began to take off, its two wings came apart. In a rapidly shifting political climate, the fate of Cabanis's science would differ greatly from Pinel's medicine.

Once Napoleon was installed as First Consul, Royalist exiles began to filter back into France, looking to reclaim what was left of their land and fortunes. Almost immediately, a chorus of Christians took aim at the so-called science that claimed to prove there was no soul. Returning from England, Chateaubriand repented for his atheist ways and pressed his eloquence into the service of restoring the intellectual respectability of Christianity. After a century of attacks by *philosophes*, he now sang of the beauty and power of Christ. A sufferer of melancholia who tried to commit suicide in his youth, Chateaubriand had watched from afar as his elderly mother and other relatives were imprisoned by the Jacobins. When his mother died, the young man returned to his faith, the one force that could counter his despair. In 1802, he published *The Genius of Christianity*, which bitterly attacked atheistic natural historians and mocked "our recent Ideologues" who dared separate the human mind from the Divine one.

With Napoleon's rise, Cabanis and the ideologists began to bear the brunt of attacks from other quarters. In 1800, the press began to use the term "ideologue" derisively. To make matters worse, the ideologists split within their ranks. In the Analysis subsection, the medical doctors tended to follow Cabanis in pursing physiological ideology, while philosophers like Tracy focused on philosophical ideology. Still, none of this would have been catastrophic, had there not been a shift in French politics.

As Bonaparte began to be criticized by liberals, moderates, and intellectuals for consolidating too much power, he soured on those thinkers who once embraced him as one of their own. First came the censorship of the press. Any doubt about where the First Consul stood regarding the advocates of human science was dispelled in February of 1801 when he contemptuously referred to them as miserable materialists.

As Cabanis knew, human science posed a direct challenge to the Church, but it would not bother any political power, save for the despot. Unfortunately, despotism was in the offing. In 1802, Bonaparte completed his transformation when he signed the Concordat with the Pope. Soon appointed First Consul for Life, Bonaparte concluded his reconciliation with the Catholic Church. It only remained to scatter their opponents. Religions like Théophilanthropie were banned overnight. Next, the intellectual base for the atheistic naturalists would be disbanded.

This unpleasant job fell to Philippe Pinel's old Montpellier friend Chaptal, the minister whose medical dissertation years earlier embodied the hope that one could link physiology and the mind's workings to society and government. Over the years, he had aided his old friend, for instance by transferring Pussin and his wife to the Salpêtrière in 1801, when Pinel badly needed them. Chaptal was now tasked with dismantling—not the whole National Institute—but just the part that linked the mind with the physical world, and hence carried political risk.

On January 23, 1803, the Second Class was disbanded. The natural sciences faculty remained intact, as did the Third Class, which was rededicated to literature and the study of the French language. The ideologues were reassigned to the Third Class and put to work on the politically safe task of studying the French language. Control of the primary schools was returned to the Church.

By the time Cabanis died on May 5, 1808, the ideologues' project was in serious decline. His eulogy was delivered by Destutt de Tracy, whose lament could have been for the dream of creating a natural science of humankind. As a hero of the Revolution, Cabanis was accorded a burial in the Pantheon; however, his heart was not in the proceedings. Someone had absconded with that organ and buried it where it belonged, in Auteuil, the home he had inherited from Madame Helvétius.

The ideologists faded for now, as did their attempt to create a new morality based on science. The contemptuous epithet for advocates of this science of ideas—ideologues—stuck and became synonymous with a hardheaded commitment to a thought system. In a further embarrassment to Cabanis's project, ideology would later be turned inside out by followers of Karl Marx. For them, the term signified a froth of ideas that served to obscure determining material forces.

The fate of the ideologues seemed to augur poorly for its allied field, mental medicine. However, there were also critical distinctions between these endeavors. Alienism posed less of a threat than Cabanis's wider program. For there was also an undeniably conservative element to Pinel's aims. A cynical emperor could not fail but note that mental medicine offered to tame the wilder elements of society; it would neutralize their furor, their violent resistance, and then return them to society as integrated, peaceful citizens. Asylums could be used much as the king had once used *lettres of cachet*; mental medicine could rid Napoleon of rabble-rousers and wild-eyed insurgents. Where doctors saw illness, a ruler would see agitators. Without the brute force of the police, mental medicine could restrain and retrain France's marginal, dangerous citizens.

In 1800, the civilizing and policing possibilities of mental medicine were put on display in a sensational case. In 1797, a feral child straggled into the town of Aveyron, then escaped, only to be recaptured in 1800. Covered in scars, the approximately twelve-year-old animal-child hoofed about like a beast, thoroughly unaware of civilized norms. He was mute and selectively deaf; how he survived in the wild was anybody's guess. In August of 1800, the child was ceremoniously brought to Paris and placed at the National Institution for Deaf-Mutes run by Abbé Roch-Ambroise Sicard. Sicard had impressed Napoleon's brother Lucien, then the Minister of the Interior. He was given free reign to remedy the boy's disabilities through mentalist means.

This task fell to the physician at this institution, a twenty-five-year-old former student of Pinel, Jean-Marc-Gaspard Itard. Itard threw himself into this case, which was closely followed in the press and would come to influence pedagogues as well as those concerned with the rehabilitation for childhood disabilities. The Society of Observers of Mankind, a short-lived anthropological society made up of some sixty ideologues who survived Napoleon's ire a bit longer than the Second Class, appointed a commission that included Pinel to oversee the civilizing of "Victor." Chaptal agreed to have the government subsidize Dr. Itard's intensive therapeutic program to tame this savage. He would use sensationalist psychology and mental treatment to awaken and train the boy's dormant senses and populate his empty mind.

While captivating to the general newspaper reader, Victor's plight also captured the interest of those who struggled to define man's natural state. So when Victor arrived in the French capital, he unwittingly came wrapped in decades of discourse about Locke's tabula rasa, Condillac's statue, and Rousseau's noble savage. Natural scientists, doctors, and the emerging students of human science all saw him as a test case for their ideas. Much hinged on Dr. Itard's treatment.

In May of 1801, less than a year into this experiment, Philippe Pinel publicly announced that his student's treatment of Victor had failed. He told the press that the boy suffered from idiotism and was incapable of developing his mental faculties. This simply may have been sound clinical judgment—in fact, Victor never mastered more than a few phrases of French—but Pinel's proclamation also seemed preemptive. Earlier that year, that doctor published his *Treatise*. Perhaps he feared the wondrous case of Victor, should it fail, would discredit his mental treatment, therapeutics that he had stated clearly were useless with idiots.

Stunned, Dr. Itard insisted that Victor had in fact improved. His first goal had been to help this creature attach to social life, and that had been a success. After devoting five years to the boy's treatment, Itard reported that the one-time savage had transformed into a perfectly decorous, though almost entirely mute, Frenchman. Importantly for imperial technocrats in strange lands, prison reformers, and directors of mental asylums, Itard reported that Victor had developed a capacity for sympathy, thus morality, as well as a capacity to regulate himself within society.

As the Catholic Church moved back to the center of French life,

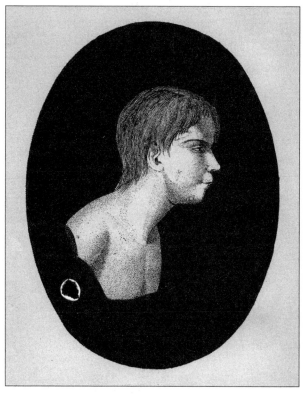

Figure 36. Victor, the wild boy of Aveyron, circa 1800.

mental medicine did not disappear. In 1803, the "immortal" Pinel, as he was sometimes now called, was appointed consultant physician to the emperor and a year later awarded the Legion of Honor. Though not without rivals, his mental medicine had been firmly planted in the Bicêtre and Salpêtrière hospitals, the scientific associations of France, and the École de Santé medical school.

In 1802, Pinel expanded his domain by opening a private treatment facility on 8 Rue Buffon to compete with the slippery Belhomme, who astonishingly had reopened for business. Pinel's private madhouse would be run by a promising thirty-year-old doctor, Jean-Étienne-Dominique Esquirol. Their collaboration would prove fateful as mental medicine moved forward even as political life in France swerved back toward the past.

PART IV

THE SERPENT
THAT ATE
ITS TAIL

Nature should be
visible Mind,
Mind being invisible Nature.

—F. W. J. SCHELLING

16

Kant and the Age of Self-Criticism

AFTER 1800, for decades, France would remain stormy and teeter on the brink of political collapse. Napoleon's Consulate and then the First Empire gave some solidity to the country for fourteen years, but the price was high: a return of absolutism and a retreat from freedoms won in the Revolution. The Catholic Church marched back into schools and villages and remained fierce in its opposition to materialistic ideologies. Radical attempts at dechristianization had utterly failed, but at the same time advocates of secularism were never vanquished. They remained as a persistent, if marginalized, group of anticlerical rebels, social critics, and scientific demystifiers.

However, by the time Napoleon declared the end of the Revolution and made peace with the Catholic Church, a forceful challenge to Enlightenment rationality had emerged from an unlikely venue. Before 1800, all things German were beneath contempt for the European elite; anyone with something serious to say, it was assumed, said it in French. However, a brilliant woman who had been chased out of France by Bonaparte traveled across the Rhine and soon reported that German thinkers had developed a devastating critique of Enlightenment philosophy and its theories of the mind.

Germaine de Staël lived a life of great turbulence. Born in 1766, the daughter of the fabulously wealthy Genevan financier Jacques Necker and a strict Protestant mother, Suzanne Curchod, she was pushed to equal the *philosophes* that populated her mother's dinner table. The young Germaine suffered her first nervous breakdown at age thirteen. It would be the first of many times that she struggled with suicidality and a deep-seated despair.

After he was called to Paris to save Louis XVI's government, Jacques Necker became legendary. The finance minister's twenty-two-year-old daughter quickly made her own mark with a book on Rousseau. And even as the young woman's intellect began to be widely celebrated, her mother remained unimpressed: "That is nothing, absolutely nothing, compared to what I wanted to make of her," she complained.

When the Revolution commenced, the baroness embraced liberal convictions on the equal rights of humankind and advocated for a constitutional monarchy. However, with the rise of the Terror, she was forced to flee first for Switzerland, then England. By then, she recognized that her marriage to Baron Erik de Staël-Holstein, a dissolute gambler and diplomat from Sweden, was a loveless failure. Separated from her husband, she sought out lovers and became an easy target for scandalmongers. She was simply too rich, too smart, and too defiant not to be detested.

Even as she tried to free herself from the traps of convention, Germaine displayed little talent for happiness. Her first choice of a lover was the malicious Talleyrand, who later mocked her. She would have children with four men and suffer greatly with each relationship. Her *Essay on the Passions,* written in 1796, was an openly avowed attempt at self-cure. Impulsive emotions undermined happiness, she argued, and ruined that complex state which was never one simple thing but—for individuals and nations—came from the union of contraries, such as a balance of hope and fear, liberty, and stability.

At the end of the book, the author candidly admitted that she herself remained uncured and unhappy.

With the rise of Bonaparte, Germaine de Staël sailed back to France. However, as the First Consul crept toward dictatorship, she grew critical. Fearful of this woman's sway over a wide network of salon elites, Napoleon declared her to be an enemy of the state. In 1803, she was told to stay a minimum of fifty miles from Paris. Then a hundred miles. Finally, Napoleon dispatched the serpent-tongued Talleyrand, who told Madame de Staël he was *so* delighted to hear she was going away on a long trip. When she curtly replied that in fact she had no such plans, he insisted that he was quite sure that she *did*. The baroness quickly packed and fled for the border.

Her destination was not haphazard. Germaine de Staël would travel to German-speaking cities, where she knew she would encounter the intellectual progeny of a thinker that had captivated her. In 1802, she wrote:

> I am a bad metaphysician and yet I have argued about Kant with all the men of our country. . . . I find the metaphysics of Locke quite compatible with his. Locke has seen very well from where ideas come to us; Kant seeks to discover what faculty in us receives them. To me it is impossible not to have the feeling that a power exists within us, which modifies the feelings which are transmitted to it. But is not that power the soul, is it not the secret which is forbidden us, and can we look at ourselves think, without breaking that unity which truly constitutes intellectual existence!

The Prussian philosopher Immanuel Kant gave a glimpse of what dark depths lay beneath those ideas, and Madame de Staël confessed, "I prefer that glimpse to all material clarity."

ENLIGHTENMENT HAD COME relatively late to the small kingdoms and closed-off principalities that made up the German territories. The decentralization of power into small feudal estates, with independent states and many sovereigns and princes commanding tiny imperial cities, made it impossible for swift change to be mandated from above. In 1800, liberal principalities existed adjacent to ones with no freedom of the press and tight clerical control. Unlike in England, America, and France, no successful revolution in the name of liberty had taken place in the diverse little lands that Madame de Staël would prematurely refer to as Germany.

Still, the Enlightenment commitments to reason, liberty, and individual autonomy, the defeat of superstition, and the truth of science penetrated German-speaking elites. Prominent and influential early 18th-century Enlightenment figures included Gottfried Leibniz and Christian Wolff, both of whom, by 1730, supported natural law and the freedom of thought. However, notions of universal rights, tolerance, and the freedom of conscience did not emerge as social forces until after the 1770s, spurred on in part by the inspiring events in America.

Late to join, Enlightenment thinkers in places like Königsberg, Jena, Vienna, Halle, and Berlin were positioned to critically survey the Age of Reason and pose searching questions regarding conflicts and paradoxes that may have been invisible in the context of creation. If the Age of Reason was engendered by critical thought, the time was now ripe for self-criticism. And so, after 1800, German analyses of liberalism and modernity coalesced into a competing tradition. What Kant called the Age of Criticism would spawn Idealism, Romanticism, and the political theories of the Counter-Enlightenment.

Germanic attacks on assumptions at the core of Enlightenment modernity would focus on the nature and capacities of reason and the mind. In 1784, these discussions grew into a public debate in Prussia over this simple question: what is enlightenment? In Germanic lands, the late 17th century brought forth an offshoot of Lutheranism called Pietism, which had its own answer. As with religious enthusiasts in England and the Jansenists in France, the Pietists believed that enlightenment came from the personal change of heart that took place when the Lord's commandments spoke to one's soul, entered one's heart, and enlightened one's eyes.

In opposition to this spiritual notion of enlightenment, there now stood a century of secular alternatives to this question. And of all Germanic lands, Prussia was perhaps most open to free deliberation on matters that might seem to threaten clerical interests. When Frederick II came to power, he had immediately signaled a clean break with his father and the Pietists who advised him. The early advocate for psychology Christian Wolff, who had been driven from his home thanks to those zealots, was now brought back home. Frederick the Great provided him with refuge alongside scandalous figures like La Mettrie and Voltaire. Prussia became a safe haven for those who questioned religion.

And so in 1784, the Prussian son of Pietists, Immanuel Kant, sought to define enlightenment. Pre-enlightenment man lived by faith like a wide-eyed child, he wrote. Such an immature person depended on writers, priests, and doctors to tell him what to think, how to act, and what to eat. These shackles destroyed the *one* human quality that led to progress: free inquiry. Like Gassendi a century before him, Kant quoted Horace: "Sapere aude"—Dare to know! However, there was a catch. Scholars privately should consider even the most scandalous things, but in the public arena, they must be citizens who paid taxes and officers who followed rules. Priests had every right to privately question doctrines, but no right to sow dissent from the pulpit. Otherwise, society would descend into chaos.

For Kant, enlightenment married liberty of thought with obedient actions. Thus, it promised to create torn citizens, whose conventional behavior was no window into their rebel hearts. While under the rule of Frederick the Great, Kant seemed unperturbed by this prospect. And the professor's division between knowledge and power conveniently mirrored the mandates of his king. Frederick fostered freedom of thought, as long as it did not include critiques of his own absolute power. In 1784, Kant agreed and even went so far as to call the age of Enlightenment the "century of Frederick."

Madame de Staël dryly observed of German intellectuals that "they join the greatest boldness in thought to the most obedient character." In 1784, such was the case of Immanuel Kant, the middle-aged professor who knelt down before his king a mere three years after he had set in motion a revolution so profound that it would indelibly alter the Age of Reason and link it much more to his name than his ruler's.

Born in 1724, the greatest of the late Enlightenment philosophers grew up, studied, worked, and died in Königsberg in East Prussia. He came of age during Frederick's liberalizing reign and enjoyed forty-six years of that king's commitment to freedom. Emanuel's own commitment to freedom manifested itself early. His strict Pietist background encouraged the boy to interpret the Bible literally; after learning Hebrew, he insisted that his studies revealed an error and required him to change his baptized name from Emanuel to Immanuel. At sixteen, the boy entered the university and there encountered the writings of Newton and Wolff. He embraced these new vistas, and after a few years, the young Kant began publishing tracts in a thoroughly unfashionable field.

Metaphysics had fallen on hard times. Attacked for its airy presumptions, this one-time queen of the sciences had lost her crown. In the early decades of the 18th century, German philosophers like Christian Wolff and Gottfried Leibniz tried to salvage philosophical proofs of God's existence, the soul's immortality, and first causes. To

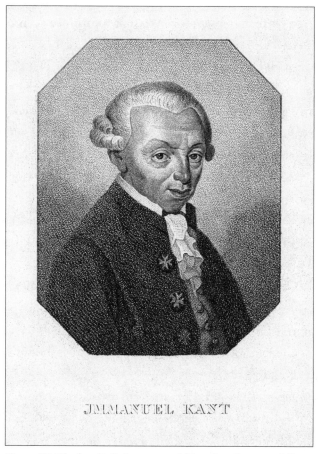

Figure 37. The late Enlightenment philosopher, Immanuel Kant.

do so, Leibniz populated the universe with "monads," spiritual substances with varied degrees of consciousness. This rearguard action
disgusted Pietists, who saw such rationales as nothing more than a
snake's whisper.

The young Kant fell in love with metaphysics. Committed to
natural science, he grew disdainful of Pietist claims of supernatural
events and immersed himself in the frays that centered on Leibniz
and Wolff. Over the next years, he ran through different metaphysical approaches that he hoped would secure knowledge of God and the

soul, while beating back mystical, orthodox Lutherans. Kant hoped
to found a new metaphysics, one that cut a path between occultism
and the mechanization of humanity.

For twenty-five years, he worked on this project. First, he
became a devoted Cartesian rationalist. Disappointed, he turned to
empiricism and immersed himself in Shaftesbury, Hutcheson, and
Locke. For a while, Kant adopted the vitalistic materialism that had
been so generative in France. Around 1765, his hard heart broke
when he read Rousseau, who convinced him that reason did not
lead to morals; Jean-Jacques forced the professor to reflect on the
disdainful manner in which he "despised the common man who
knows nothing." Next, David Hume awoke him from a "dogmatic
slumber" with his insistence that causal connections were nothing
more than sequential associations in time. And yet, despite these
breakthroughs, around 1766, Kant still found himself lost in a forest
of abstractions. He scaled back his hopes. If metaphysics could not
secure knowledge of God and the soul, perhaps he should only seek
the limits of reason.

A fastidious, lifelong bachelor, Kant would later be caricatured
as a Prussian automaton whose afternoon stroll was so precisely
timed that his neighbors set their watches to it. However, during
these decades of struggle, Kant manifested great intellectual flexi-
bility as he immersed himself in the alternatives bequeathed to him
since Descartes. For over two decades, in eleven generally forgotten
works, Kant searched for his own enlightenment. Finally in 1770, at
the relatively advanced age of forty-six, Kant published a dissertation
that sketched out a new set of answers. Eleven years later, he had
worked out those ideas and published his magnum opus, *Critique of
Pure Reason*. It was a masterpiece that instantly recast all of Kant's
prior works as juvenilia, tributes to his own long years of immaturity
before this extraordinary illumination.

At the center of this work was another of Kant's armchair epiphanies. Unlike Locke, who contended that sensations were kinds of

ideas, Kant concluded that human knowledge must be analyzed by separating thought from sensibility. Each adhered to principles of their own. Kant's revelation was not original. Leibniz divided the empirical and rational, and Wolff famously divvied up his study of human understanding into empirical and rational psychology.

However, Kant went further. With rapier-like precision, piercing skepticism, and a logical power that crossed over into genius, Kant took this simple dichotomy and built upon it. He left no prior positions standing before pulling together a synthesis that he hoped would resolve crucial paradoxes that plagued the Age of Reason. After 1781, Kant applied this new model of knowledge to aesthetics, morals, politics, religion, and psychology. He fervently beat back opponents and worked out implications, exceptions, and clarifications of what he hoped would be a broad new Kantian science. When readers complained that his writing was dry, long-winded, and nearly incomprehensible, he dutifully delivered a condensed account for educators who, he uncharitably suggested, had no real business trying to understand the real thing. Kant lent them a hand, since he believed no one could move forward without answering his *Critique*. "To evade it," he wrote with Olympian assurance, "is impossible."

Kant believed that the universe was wholly deterministic but that humans possessed the capacity for free moral choice. He sought to reconcile this old paradox without the aid of the Christian soul. In *Critique of Pure Reason*, Kant immediately swept aside some proposed solutions: he threw scorn on those who believed that they had put an end to metaphysics with a "*physiology* of human understanding—that of the celebrated Locke." At the same time, he attacked those who deluded themselves into believing reason could prove God's existence and the soul's eternal life. The philosopher Moses Mendelssohn, himself a target of some of Kant's ire, referred to these critiques as "world-crushing." Through decimating, scrupulous analysis, Kant seemed to leave no option but to void the claims of radical materialism and dogmatic religion, fatalism and superstition, atheism and spiritual enthusiasm. By demonstrating the limits of reason, he seemed to undermine a good deal that had taken place during the Age of Reason.

Kant began by subjecting one of the central notions of the French Enlightenment—sensibility—to a withering examination from which it would never fully recover. That concept, so crucial to 18th-century physiologists, Montpellier vitalists, Rousseauians, and post-Lockean sensationalists, had become a part of human science, psychology, aesthetics, medicine, and political discourse. For Pinel, it was the bedrock for his mental medicine; for many aesthetes and novelists it represented a new common sense. Sensibility allowed for biological and highly determined bodies to develop emergent structures so that they could also have active minds that could freely choose and act. It linked body and mind.

But what *was* sensibility? Sensations, Kant argued, could not be simply passive imprints of external objects on a passive clay tablet. Rather, these impressions must be transformed by active modes of understanding. It is a testament to Kant's victory over post-Lockean thought that his inaccurate portrayal of the British thinker—who in fact did consider the active power of reflection in the mind—held for the next century. As for vitalists who conceptualized the active, internally structuring force as sensibility, this generative concept could never be proven. Sensibility had become an emperor whose state of undress was quite visible to outsiders. From Prussia, Kant quickly rejected this postulate and looked to metaphysics for answers.

Sensations were predicated on a prior understanding of both space and time. Inner perception was organized by prior active forms in the mind, what he called "transcendental *a prioris*." Because of the given forms of space and time, perception only revealed appearances as always already transformed by those conditions. And so for Kant, outer objects in the world affected our sensibility and led to inner representations, then intuitions and thoughts about these appearances. Nonetheless, the outer object was in itself unknowable.

Empiricism assumed that external sensations translated into reliable and valid representations of the world. Since Bacon, science had been predicated on this belief. Kant threw a wrench into these works. He argued that such perceptions might reflect the phenomena of experience, but they never penetrated into the true nature of things, what Kant called their "noumena." Noumena were unknowable in themselves, beyond the scope of sensation and perception, beyond sensibility. In this way, the *Critique of Pure Reason* disallowed speculative excesses from cocky scientists.

Kant applied the same rationale to the inner world. Human beings never truly knew themselves through introspection. They could never grasp the structures that formed their own perceptions and knowledge. Inner perceptions might lead to intuitions as the basis for psychology, but such knowledge never penetrated into the forces that structured the self. All those who had tried to know the mind rationally, including Descartes and Locke, were imposters. The mind in its essence was a mystery, beyond experience, beyond knowledge.

This was the murky depth inside mental life that Germaine de Staël glimpsed in Kant. However, in discussing the mind, Kant faced a familiar problem. German—like French—possessed clear words for soul (*Seele*) and spirit (*Geist*), but it possessed no derivative of the Latin *mentis*, no word for the mind. Kant employed soul and spirit, even when his intended meanings wildly diverged from theological definitions. As a new German discourse emerged on subjectivity and inner life, it would be plagued by this kind of semantic slippage.

In Kant's case, *Seele* would be defined in a way that allowed for belief but gave no succor to believers. He shot down rational proofs of God's existence and offered unknowingness to believers as their reward. Kant expressed hostility to ecclesiastic authority, openly opposed formal religious ceremonies, and rejected prayer and attempts to elicit divine intervention as superstitions. When Kant used the word "soul" to refer to the noumena of human interior life, he made it clear that his "thinking self (the soul)" was denied its central religious characteristic, permanence. Reason, the philosopher asserted, could only prove that the soul existed *during* life, not afterward.

Introspection allowed for the study of the inner parade of consciousness, but not the active modes by which a person could know. Mental representations were the proper objects of empirical psychology, but inner observation of that sort could never penetrate the underlying essence of selfhood. That "transcendental object of inner sense" could only be reached through a rational doctrine of the "soul."

This was Kant's solution to Mersenne's riddle. Inner life was in part determined, but part unknowable and free. The soul in its essence was not tied to natural constraints and was the hidden source of free will and human morality. To argue for moral freedom in a world of matter, Kant upheld the validity of empiricism for natural phenomena, and did not cross the bounds of reason, as Leibniz did with his monads. Kant simply demarcated the line beyond which reason had no right to go. In that timeless and spaceless world of things-in-themselves, Kant allowed an enlightened rational being to believe that man was more than a machine.

Consciousness along with memory had been the defining characteristic of selfhood for John Locke, but now that seemed superficial. Kant made the self an enduring mystery, a composite of a superficial conscious mental life and an unknowable depth. While the first part of his synthesis would create great excitement among philosophers who took up the study of mental representations and the phenomenology of consciousness, the glimpse of the mysterious essence that so thrilled Madame de Staël would prove irresistible to a young generation who would come to be called the Romantics.

⸜⸝

IMMANUEL KANT BECAME the central figure of the German Enlightenment, the thinker who simultaneously represented its apogee and its end. His analyses, including his *Critique of Pure Reason*, *Critique of Practical Reason*, and *Critique of Judgment,* published between 1781 and 1790, loomed so large that they ushered in a period that could only be called post-Kantian. In the end, the Prussian's penetrating assessment of over a century of debates between empiricists and rationalists undermined both positions. Kant examined each of these buildings and exposed rot in their foundations. His critiques sounded the death knell for exaggeratedly optimistic Enlightenment perspectives that conceived of the individual mind and society as endlessly alterable and ameliorable. Materialistic vitalism was also badly damaged by his strike, for sensibility, its core notion, was found to be an unknowable process, thus eliminating the very naturalism that gave that theory its advantage.

In matters of theology, Kant undercut not only the traditional foes of the enlightened, those who upheld superstition and miraculous beliefs, but also those who dared to use reason to verify God and soul. "Rational religion" had been a critical bridge for those who wanted to abide by science while not losing their souls. Kant demonstrated that this endeavor was held together by an untenable paradox. Its advocates committed themselves to the belief that reason resided in a supernatural home, one that, despite many logical twists and turns, could only be based on faith. Since the late 17th century, in England, Holland, Scotland, and France, philosophers had sought to square this circle. None succeeded. Kant himself came up with complex and differing rationales for faith in God, but none were based on proofs from reason. Efforts to logically comprehend an intuition were false. Before God or the soul, reason must fall silent.

While undermining rational religion, Kant also turned on those like La Mettrie, Diderot, Helvétius, and Cabanis, radical atheists, mechanists, and vitalists of sensibility, who sought to deny God and the soul through science. They were spouting nonsense. When it came to the inner essence of the world or the mind, science could claim no authority. Perception offered no direct knowledge of the transcendent. The mind had no capacity to know such unimaginable things. Neither rational religion nor natural science had any standing regarding the existence of souls. The holders of such beliefs had built castles on thin air.

Professor Kant had labored hard, but was it all to reinvent the wheel? Was this not Descartes's famous solution? He had concluded that we simply live in two worlds, one of soul and the other of Nature. Contrarians like Friedrich Heinrich Jacobi read Kant this way, but such an interpretation was problematic. Descartes's "I think" revealed nothing other than surface appearances for Kant; introspection could not be used to establish a realm outside nature. Kant had actually shown, many agreed, that humans lived in one world, split into two distinct perspectives. Appearances were accessible through our senses, but reason could show things that existed in themselves, apart from the moldings of subjectivity. Objects had an underlying essence; that truth was unavoidable. It was the known unknown of mental life. And so, while perception might give us *a* world, it did not offer us *the* world that existed outside of our senses.

In the last years of the 18th century, it became clear that Immanuel Kant had answered so many hanging questions that he had all but brought an end to the prior debates on the nature of reason that dated back to Descartes, Hobbes, and Gassendi. Kant turned reason onto itself and in the process both legitimized it and limited its range. His critique chopped away at religious claims and unwarranted extensions of natural science. In the end, his critical system retained some place for belief and mystery, while vigorously defending reason's claims for verifiable knowledge.

Kant also sought to alter notions of unreason. Drs. Locke and

Willis had allowed for a reasonable man to be part mad, thanks to an error, a cognitive misassociation; Bordeu, Tissot, Cabanis, and Pinel had allowed for sensibility to dysregulate a reasonable citizen into a maniac. However, Immanuel Kant placed a distorting force inside reason itself. For Kant, "I think, therefore I am" had become "Who is the I that thinks and is thought?"

Kant's work unleashed a flurry of responses and generated a widening gyre of post-Kantian philosophers, poets, doctors, and scientists. Hailed as a genius, even a new Christ, Kant became the subject of a series of generative readings, misreadings, and improvisations. He spawned Kantians in German-speaking lands and then, thanks to proselytizers like Madame de Staël, followers in France and Britain. As the new century beckoned, Kant's prediction proved quite right: his challenges could not be ignored.

Among Germans, Kant rejuvenated metaphysics: Karl Leonhard Reinhold concluded that a rigorous study of the phenomena of consciousness should be the critical task for this branch of philosophy and inaugurated this effort at the University of Jena. During her visit to this university town, Madame de Staël discovered a collection of extraordinary thinkers had gathered there to interpret and reinterpret Kant. Critical to this effort was their reinterpretation of Kant's "transcendental *a prioris*" as mystifications. The thing-in-itself, Johann Gottlieb Fichte wrote, "is the fundamental principle of the dogmatist, is nothing and has no reality." It was not something transcendent but something subjective that altered our experience of reality. Focused on self-creation and the active powers of intuition and reflection as molding forces in inner life, Fichte, along with Friedrich Wilhelm von Schelling and Georg Wilhelm Friedrich Hegel would dominate German philosophy over the next decades.

While these idealists embraced the powers of human subjectivity to create its own realities, others followed the empirical Kant and turned their sights to scientific physiology and psychology. For example, in medicine, one of Kant's greatest advocates was Marcus

Herz. At fifteen, Herz had been sent by his parents to Königsberg to study commerce, but somewhere along the way he had taken a turn into metaphysics. He fell in with Kant and became one of his most dedicated students. In 1774, Herz went to Halle to study medicine, and after graduating, he moved to Berlin, where with his wife, Henriette de Lemos, he established one of the most fashionable salons for intellectuals.

Herz hoped to create a Kantian medicine. In 1777, he wrote an epistolary book for doctors that mixed practical advice with calls for epistemological restraint. However, Herz would discover, uncertainty did not suit practitioners and their frequently desperate patients. And so, Herz disobeyed his master and postulated that the brain was the home of a life force, a *Lebenskraft*, that regulated nervous flow and linked the body to the mind. In one fell swoop, he had betrayed Kant and he knew it. To his teacher, the doctor jauntily confessed: "I am much more a deserter who still wears your uniform and who, while associating with other (not hostile) powers, is still in your service. Or to express myself less Prussianly, I enjoy wandering around the border towns of both countries, philosophy and medicine, and it gives me joy when I can make arrangements for their common government." If such border crossings protected medical men from succumbing to dumb empiricism, Dr. Herz added, they would also protect philosophy from descending into useless rumination.

Kant was not immune to the charge that philosophy did nothing. He himself was eager to put his thought to work by, for example, establishing a new human science that he called "practical anthropology." In 1773, Kant had started to lecture on this subject, and in a jab at Herz, he retorted that his mental medicine would avoid the speculative excesses of the "philosophical *medici*."

In fact, Kant began writing about mental disease as early as 1764. By 1781, he had concluded that reason and unreason could only be discerned by evaluations of external behavior. Our minds and inner states were mostly filled with unconscious ideas that only indirectly entered consciousness. The capacity for misperceptions of the inner and outer world, delusions or illusions or bewitchment, were great, as were errors of inner perception such as religious enthusiasm and spiritualism. Practical anthropology should stick to readily observable phenomena.

However, Kant could not follow his own advice. Of the mental aberrations that he discerned, many required conjectures about the patient's psychic world. Kant divided illnesses into those of reason, judgment, and will, then subdivided each of these again and again. He both employed familiar German terms for madness—*Wahnsinn, Unsinnigkeit, Wahnwitz, and Aberwitz*—and concocted some weird ones like *Grillenkrankheit*, literally "cricket-disease." This sort of melancholic, Kant explained, had his peace of mind and sleep disturbed as if by a constant chirping of insects. Major illnesses included melancholia and mental derangement; idiocy was not a sickness of the *Seele*, but of the absence of one, a point that forced readers to recognize that the author was not referring to an immortal Christian soul, but rather a mind.

Like the ancient Greeks, Kant believed mental ills were philosophy's domain, and he argued that medicine had little to offer when it came to insanity. In forensic cases, physicians called upon to explain bizarre behavior had nothing to say since no physiology of such acts existed. Forensics, save in a few cases, depended on the state of mind of the defendant. Judges needed to know whether an individual had a sound understanding of his actions. Such an accounting could only come from Kantian anthropologists.

Surprisingly. Kant's claim for philosophy's role in forensic assessments was supported by some physicians, like the powerful Christoph Hufeland. Hufeland opposed incursions of doctors into mental matters, out of fear that the line between mind and body would collapse and lead to atheism. And so in 1804, a Hamburg theologian accused of murder and deemed psychotic by two physicians was nonetheless put to death thanks to the testimony of Kantian experts.

A philosopher and theologian testified that the man had not allowed moral law to govern his actions, though like all men, he possessed the free will to do so.

While the inner world of the mad was philosophical terrain, Kant believed the causes of madness were biological and hereditary. Pinel and others had confused causes with effects. The melancholic boy whose heart was broken was not made mad by failed love; he overly suffered because of an underlying instability. Psychic cures were fruitless, and mental illness was incurable.

Kant's notion of a deeper biological cause beneath the superficial flow of conscious phenomena would be greatly influential in German medicine. However, with this claim, Kant exposed himself to those who might exclaim, how did he know? Hadn't the great epistemologist broken his own rules and pressed past the boundaries of reason?

WHEN THE FRENCH REVOLUTION commenced, Immanuel Kant, the thinker who counseled intellectuals to behave, was ecstatic. Following the death of Frederick the Great, Prussia had returned to a repressive, authoritarian rule, which soured the Königsberg philosopher on enlightened leadership. Even as the Revolution became quite bloody, Kant remained a staunch defender of the Republican cause. He hurried to get mail from France and was whispered to be a Jacobin. Among friends, he made no secret of his conviction that Reason was on the march in France.

Many German-speaking intellectuals shared his enthusiasm. Among them were members of the generation born after 1750, those nourished on the promises of the Enlightenment. Jews—who watched as France emancipated their brethren in 1791—and women both sought increased freedom and equality. In salons that cropped up in urban centers, these ideals were fostered. For example, in the Herzes' salon, hosted by the Jewish doctor who oversaw the publication of the *Critique of Pure Reason* and his impressive wife, the illustrious and enlightened of Berlin congregated to share their progressive visions.

One of the Herzes' frequent guests was Karl Philipp Moritz, a central figure in Berlin thanks to his popular *Magazine for Empirical Psychology*. A Rousseauian figure who buzzed with worry and mistrust, Moritz was Dr. Herz's friend and patient. Moritz required much attention thanks to ailments both real and imagined. After the writer declared himself near death once too many times, Dr. Herz sternly encouraged his patient to get on with it and die *well*. Moritz was suddenly cured. Marcus Herz later claimed this intervention was a calculated psychic cure, not an act of utter exasperation, but perhaps it was both.

Moritz suffered from repeated bouts of intense, often groundless, suspicion. This proclivity to paranoia may have eventually led him to a central recognition: no one could claim to know another until he knew himself. Moritz dedicated his new magazine to an exposition of the labyrinth of the self. In addition to linguistic study, he solicited first-person accounts of mental life. Essays and memoirs were assembled under headings like *Seelenkrankheitskunde*—mental disease; *Seelennaturkunde*—natural history of the mind; and *Seelenheilkunde*—psychic healing. For Moritz's readers, this wholesale co-optation of the *Seele* as the natural mind was clearly not news.

Moritz's magazine amazed readers. Reports on hallucinations of little men jostled with tales of mad murderers who sought their own execution, a woman who lost part of her finger each time she got pregnant, and compulsive shouters who could not resist interrupting Lutheran services. While stories like these filled the section on mental diseases, the normal mind was explored in vignettes on premonitions, waking dreams, and lost childhood memories.

Herz backed Moritz's documentation of the mind's weird world, as he pursued a merger between Kantian philosophy and medicine. However, the result of his efforts was mostly negative. Nerves could not be equated with individual ideas, nor should we accept exaggerated claims for sensibility. Forget Mesmer's nervous fluids. Associational psychology employed spatial metaphors, which was wrong, since as Kant showed, the deep structure of the mind did not exist in space. For this Kantian doctor, these critiques made sense, but they led to a question. What could a Kantian psychic medicine actually know, and how might it relieve suffering?

While Herz was struggling with his Kantian medicine, an inquisitive young doctor came to live with him. Johann Christian Reil was from Rhaude in the northwest of German lands. The son of a Lutheran pastor, born on February 20, 1759, he was nurtured on Enlightenment ideals. At the age of twenty, he began his medical studies in Göttingen and then transferred to Halle, where he graduated in 1782. Armed with an introduction to Dr. Herz, Reil traveled to Berlin. For a year, he resided with that family, where he was surrounded by the doctor's circle of Kantians, as well as his wife Henriette's friends, young Romantic critics and aesthetes like the Schlegels. This conflict between the Kantians and the Romantics that took place in their salon would become a guiding tension for young Reil as he strove to rethink medicine and the role of the mind.

Johann Reil returned home to practice medicine but was soon summoned to Halle by an admiring old professor, who set him up as a faculty member, then promptly died. Promoted to the vacated professorship, Dr. Reil taught in Halle for the next twenty-two years. And like Herz, Reil at first sought to bring Kant to medicine. In 1795, he founded the *Archive for Physiology* to promote a new physiology based on Kantian principles. Reil contributed a long essay on the most central question in physiology: "On the Life Force" took stock of the critical difference that distinguished the living from the dead. Spurred on by Newton's theory of gravity and Haller's sensibility, ideas of a life force had grown central to late 18th-century biology and medicine. However, in German lands, Haller's forces had encouraged more overblown theories, such as a five-pronged model of inner forces that included a *Bildungstrieb* for character development. As these claims sprouted, they became ripe for a Kantian pruning.

Reil discounted a number of theories and proposed that through a process of complex self-organization—his favorite metaphor was the process of crystallization—chemicals developed new properties that somehow made for living matter. Still, he reminded his readers that the experience of a force was a matter of subjective perception. In illness, we feel forces working upon us, but the true source of such experiences lay in the disruption of a bodily organ. Doctors must become fluent at translating subjective complaints into their objective determinants. Thus, the good Kantian critiqued physiology. But soon his own beliefs would be turned upside down by the wild-eyed friends of Henriette Herz.

AS KANTIANS CONSIDERED the mystery of force, an unstoppable one swept through Prussia. After Napoleon declared the revolution complete in his homeland, he commenced a series of military actions to spread it throughout feudal Europe. In 1795, a bankrupt Prussia sued for peace with the Republic of France and for the next decade enjoyed relative peace with its bellicose neighbor. Two years later, the Holy Roman Empire sought peace and agreed to withdraw from Mainz, beginning a series of setbacks that included the 1801 Treaty of Lunéville, which ceded control of the left bank of the Rhine to France.

Napoleon provoked mixed reactions in central Europe. He horrified those whose privileges were threatened, and provoked jubilation among a cadre of intellectuals who saw French troops marching for the Rights of Man, for the moderns, for science and reason. To some, Napoleon's armies seemed to be the Republic of Letters' warriors. French troops were welcomed by writers, lawyers, merchants, and physicians. In 1797, the German poet Friedrich Hölderlin wrote a paean to the heroic spirit, one too grand to be contained even in the vessel of poetry, that great being who bursts forth with life. The poem was simply entitled "Buonaparte."

This exciting challenge to the feudal political and social order occurred alongside an aesthetic awakening. In the 1770s, the *Sturm und Drang* movement had emerged, thanks to German writers who focused on the soul within. Not a Christian soul, but one that loosely connoted one's innermost being. Unlike the *esprit* of French rationalists and sensationalists, the *Sturm und Drang* writers' *Geist* carried mystery and throbbed with dark meaning.

Some of the impetus for this literary revolt against classicism was obvious. During the 1770s, many German readers had been swept up by Rousseau. They too recoiled against the dehumanization and mechanization tied to rationality and science. If Pietists searched for intensely lived religious experience, that same passion was transferred to a search for earthly epiphanies, as epitomized by these new writers, especially Johann Wolfgang von Goethe.

Born in 1749 and schooled in the law, Goethe gave up revealed religion early and turned to writing. In 1770 in Strasbourg, he met the Prussian clergyman Johann Gottfried Herder, a literary critic, Francophobe, and student of German myth. A former student of Kant, Herder had turned from his teacher and proclaimed, "Come Rousseau, and be my guide!" Herder and Goethe became fast friends. Then in 1774, at the age of only twenty-five, Goethe published a novel influenced by Jean-Jacques, *The Sorrows of Young Werther*. A tale of anguished, unrequited love leading to self-murder, the work was so powerful that it resulted in a rash of suicides. It also became a runaway best-seller that made its author a celebrity.

Werther placed his own interior life at the center of his universe. In his soul, the place of his passions and his inner truths, lay the source of his happiness or misery. This was his obsession, for it was both a reflection of God and the source of sincere, honest humanity.

Werther scoffed at the classical models of sanity, like those that balanced reason and passion:

> Oh, you rationalist! Passions! Drunkenness! Madness! . . . all the extraordinary people who ever achieved anything great, anything that seemed impossible, were always certain to be vilified as drunks and lunatics.

Goethe's artistry pulled his readers into Werther's desperate, impossible love for Lotte, a passion that soon landed the hero in crazed despair. Stray impressions tortured him, his inner tranquility vanished, and Werther dove toward self-destruction. Attempts to save him were futile. His sickness, the hero noted, was incurable.

After 1781, that same obsessive inner focus would be reconfigured by the supposed followers of Kant, many of whom wandered far from their teacher's thought. For if Locke was wrongly said to have proposed a passive mind, Kant had the honor of being misread in many ways. He had hoped his style, which could resemble a logical vice, would compel assent from defeated skeptics, dogmatists, and other disputants. Instead, his obscurity made him immediately lose a grip on the reception of his own work. His first great acolyte misconstrued his teacher and then popularized *his* Kant. Through enthusiastic essays on the *Critique of Pure Reason* and packed lectures in Jena, Karl Leonhard Reinhold's understanding of Kant—or the Kant-Reinholdian philosophy, as it was known for a fleeting time—was one the master would have hardly recognized.

Reinhold proposed that the distinction between the noumena and phenomena was merely one of degree. The parade of conscious experiences was distinguished from the noumena of being merely by the fact that those mental contents were clear, rather than murky and unconscious. Thus, in one fell swoop, Reinhold transformed Kant's transcendental distinctions into mental ones, and metaphysics became psychology.

If the facts of consciousness were not just metaphysically structured by considerations of space and time, but also distorted by
unconscious mental forces, what did that mean for reason and science? Consciousness was based on mental representations, so if Reinhold was right, cognition became the process of understanding these
representations through—well, more representations. If one followed
this logic forward, objective knowledge became the representation of
another representation. Plain facts began to be sucked into a vortex
of symbols and signs. Leaving a transcendental essence behind, Reinhold's illustrious students eagerly sought to account for this language
of reflection and self-reflection in the mind.

The most famous of these Idealists, Johann Gottlieb Fichte, was
committed to Reinhold's Kant. He developed not transcendental idealism, but what others called subjective idealism, which focused on
the absolute self and its constitutive powers. For Fichte, in everyday
experience, the knower becomes invisible to herself. The "I" behind
the curtain orchestrated sensations into perceptions and thoughts.
This unconscious subject lurked behind consciousness without ever
coming onstage. Far from being passive clay, subjectivity was a creative powerhouse that shaped the outside world, the not-me. There
was no thing-in-itself, only an Absolute Self constantly striving and
making realities. For Fichte, an ardent republican and atheist, psychological, political, and moral freedom was at the core of human
subjectivity. If reality was the creation of the subject, it could be
changed by him. Fichte's packed lectures were given with the gusto
of a political rally, in which he urged his listeners to embrace his
radical vision of freedom.

Fichte was not much interested in the natural sciences or medicine, yet his model had serious implications for those disciplines.
For him, that bastion of modern knowledge, empiricism, was thin,
simple, and quite deluded: it pretended that stimuli from "out there"
were transferred into the mind without distortion. It ignored the
biases and transformations required for inner representation. Bacon,

Locke, Helvétius, Condillac, and Cabanis did not consider such matters. Thanks to Kant's critique, Fichte recognized that when we perceive the world, we do it with a mix of amnesia and creativity. We forget ourselves, our inner skewing, our misknowing. Reality only emerges after the subject disappears into herself. "Self-forgetting," Fichte wrote, "would be the character of reality."

Robert Boyle and his colleagues at the Royal Society constructed empirical science around the common sense that said seeing was believing. A trustworthy gentleman need only witness and judge for himself. The members of the Royal Society did not consider the possibility that different white gentlemen, not to mention women, slaves from Santo Domingo, or bitter *sans-culottes* might witness some of the same things differently. For Fichte, reality could not be so blithely assumed to be consensual. It was dependent on not just the universal *a prioris* of Kant or the cultural relativity of Montesquieu, but on individuality. Thus, empirically based attempts to create universal laws for man, including Cabanis's *science humaine*, Kant's anthropology, and Bonnet and Wolff's psychology were all fatally flawed.

In the 1790s, Fichte and a cadre of other post-Kantians proposed a model of the mind that answered French Lockeans. While Locke's faculty of reflection was dropped by Condillac, Fichte reinserted and magnified that creative capacity. The French sensationalists gave man no active, natural force by which he could choose, will, and decide, hardly a model of mind compatible with a citizen capable of exercising individual rights and participating in a democracy. In contrast, Fichte's mind was empowered with a freedom that was nearly unconstrained. We naturally create our world and our reality and should be free to do so.

The basis for enlightened societies was thus challenged. Empirical science and universal reason no longer served as a reliable compass. Reason, on close examination, had become the representing of representations. The groundwork for secular ethics seemed like quicksand, with an endless regress of symbols that crumbled under inspection. If consciousness was once a clear reflection of the world, for the followers of Fichte, it was now a hall of mirrors where reality could disappear.

Once the source of enlightenment, reason began to resemble, in the phrase of the English poet Samuel Coleridge, a serpent intent on devouring its own tail. Reason was now a risk, a problem. Hyper-rationality could lead to a loss of touch with the real, as one got lost in the signs of signs. Fichtean man did not worry about cognitive errors or the passions run amok. Consciousness itself was a fallen state, a misrepresentation of the world, and to think about these mis-representations meant to risk falling further into an abyss of illusion. Far from quelling superstition and acting as a strong bulwark against a torrent of emotions, consciousness became something one could have in unhealthy excess. For G. W. F. Hegel, consciousness itself was a state of alienation, like the ones he read about in Pinel's work, in which the self grew disconnected from its own authentic state.

While different in many ways, August Wilhelm Schlegel and his brother Friedrich, Caroline Böhmer Schlegel Schelling, Friedrich Schelling, Clemens Brentano, Ludwig Tieck, and the writer Nova-lis all urgently sought to further uncover what Kant's critique had exposed: the underbelly of reason, the diseases of reflection, and the truths offered by sublime eruptions of beauty, authenticity, and states that had once been called madness.

Madame de Staël was swept up in this same search for that barely glimpsed inner being. And she spread the word with a fervor. When her *Germany* was completed in 1810, the plates were destroyed by Bonaparte's police, but a copy was smuggled out to England, where the book was first published in 1813. The author extolled the *l'âme romantique* and the breakthroughs of German philosophy, writing, "The Germans are to the human mind what pioneers are to an army: they try new roads, they try unknown means: how can we avoid being curious to know what they say when they return from their excursion into infinity."

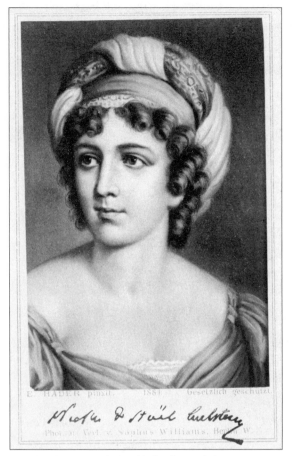

Figure 38. Germaine de Staël helped spread German critiques
of the Enlightenment throughout Europe.

For German romantics, the mind was not a machine, but an artist, creating and erasing realities. These thinkers revolted against the
Newtonian, the mechanical, and the hyperrational, and took a stand
for individual truth, poetry and art. The French Revolution, in their
view, had been a great act of subjective freedom. For Fichte and others, this uprising demonstrated the validity of their beliefs. Metaphysics must allow for a mind that was free to follow the ideals of justice,
equality, and fraternity. Subjectivity was not merely a problem for
objective science, but rather the source of liberty, ethics, and sanity.

From the small university town of Jena, near Weimar, these ideas flourished. For the Romantics, old models of sanity needed to be challenged. If to be mad was to break free of dry rationality, it was a necessity. Only unreason held the possibility of authenticity and freedom from unending alienation. It was the price to pay for the Age of Reason, and a way to break free—not of the Old World with its feudalism and superstition—but, as the English poet William Blake would later put it, the chains inherited "from Bacon, Newton, and Locke."

Rhapsodies for Psyche

T HE JENA IDEALISTS turned their scrutiny from the dream to the dreamer. With so much weight now placed on the self and its capacities, experiences were sought out that foregrounded the normally invisible director of subjective experience. Nightmares, fantasies, and ruptures of ordinary consciousness became more than curious: they became valuable opportunities to glimpse that deeper self. And nothing revealed the hidden recesses of the mind more than madness. Mental aberrations became a critical part of Romantic ideology, and Romanticism helped transform German thinking so as to give rise to a discipline called psychiatry.

A long-standing question for everyone from Thomas Willis and Descartes on was to explain how an array of disparate sensory and cognitive inputs led to a unified, relatively stable state of consciousness. For Kant and the post-Kantians, this unity was a sign of mental health; it was the central task of the self, the "I," to unify inner experience. Mental illness, conversely, manifested itself in fragmentation. For Kant, madness resulted from the mind's failure to synthesize representations. Hallucinations and delusions, in his view, pointed to some biological deficiency. However, as Karl Moritz's magazine showed, seemingly normal humans were filled with strange, frag-

mented happenings. Impossible beliefs, illusions, and waking fantasies seemed to be just another day in the life of the psyche. Were all
these the result of incurable mental illness?

In Jena, the answer would be a resounding no. There, everyday bits of madness were embraced. Their philosophical positions on
reality made it seem as if sanity was little more than a commonly held
dream, one that, as the Bedlam inmate Nathaniel Lee complained,
was based on majority rule. In addition, for them madness was not an
abstract concern, something that happened to others. Many in Jena
suffered from alterations in their own minds, such as melancholia,
hallucinations, suicidality, and psychosis.

Madness became a defining metaphor for this vanguard. Being a
bit mad made sense in a world where to be otherwise was to become
a passionless automaton. The ethos that once drove *philosophes*, their
dare-to-know thirst for knowledge, could result in a life of cold,
meaningless facts. Following Rousseau, the Jena Romantics called
for a new age, where the ideals of reason and moderation were seen as
life-killing. A dictatorship of reason drove one into despair. Enthusiasm, that folly that Enlightenment thinkers dreaded, was restored
to its original meaning. It was again a precious gift, a force, not necessarily for Christian revelation, but for a way past cold logic, a path
perhaps to the Absolute.

Surprisingly, the defining parable for these young and tempestu-
ous Jena Romantics came from a middle-aged dignitary in nearby
Weimar. Famous for his *Young Werther*, Goethe had been enno-
bled and now served in the ducal court of Carl August. From this
perch, he received luminaries who came to drink in his erudition.
He himself continued to thirst for knowledge and not only wrote
plays and poems, but also assiduously took up scientific studies on
metamorphosis in plants and color perception. However, the hunt for
knowledge never altered the fact that thoroughout his life, Goethe
remained a fool for love, repeatedly becoming deeply infatuated
with women and landing in emotional turmoil. "Great passions are

a hopeless sickness," one of his characters wearily declared in 1809, echoing Werther's complaint thirty years earlier.

In the 1770s, Goethe had set his imagination to work on an old tale about a doctor who made a deal with the Devil. Dr. Faust had had a number of other interpreters, including Christopher Marlowe, whose 1604 morality play showed how an arrogant rebel's lust for truth led to disbelief and damnation. Goethe put his *Faust* away for a long period of time, and then in 1790, published *Faust: A Fragment*. This short work was received ecstatically among the young radicals assembled in Jena.

The affinity between the great man of German letters and the younger Jena circle was not obvious. As an advisor to the Duke of Saxe-Weimar, whose territories included Jena, Goethe played a significant role in that town's cultural and intellectual life, but he stood on the other side of a wide political divide. In 1792, when the French army approached, Goethe marched with the duke against the republican forces and wrote verses against mob rule, while in Jena, the young mavericks agitated for a republic. Fichte's boom-ing speeches extolled humans to seize the day as free moral agents, unconstrained by either transcendental or material overlords. Car-oline Böhmer Schlegel, the woman at the center of the Jena com-munity, was also a diehard radical. An admirer of Mirabeau and Rousseau, Caroline was eager for the French Revolution to make its way into Prussia. When Goethe declared himself for the duke, she denounced him as a traitor.

She would pay heavily for her beliefs. In 1792, when she lived in Mainz, the French took over the city and "Jacobin marriages" allowed betrothed locals to sleep with French soldiers. Caroline was said to be the Jacobin wife of a French general. When the French were forced to retreat, a now pregnant Caroline was beaten by a mob and thrown into jail. Friedrich Schlegel reported to his brother that Caroline had grown "mad with grief," could only speak sin-gle words, and suffered from hallucinations and deranged thoughts.

While delighted when her little "citizen" was born, she was crushed when the infant died. Pilloried and tormented, Caroline's imprisonment was meant to teach her a lesson; as with other abused prisoners, the lesson was one of lifelong rage and indignation. She emerged from her ordeal hardened in her support for the revolution. And so, she made her way to Jena.

Old Goethe understood that these radicals did not share his views, but still he advised the duke to appoint the firebrand Fichte to his professorship in 1794. That same year, Goethe met another thinker, Friedrich Schiller, at a meeting of the Jena Natural Research Society. Schiller was enchanted by *Faust: A Fragment*, and urged the poet to complete his drama. For Goethe, Faust's rebellion, while Satanic in Marlowe's hands, was heroic and tragic, a futile attempt to escape the chokehold of reason. Schiller's friend, Wilhelm Schlegel, heralded Goethe's *Faust* as a story for the times. Faust was the new man whose Enlightenment ideals had debilitated him. The doctor's pact with the Devil was a desperate attempt to embrace Nature and life. The melancholic Friedrich Schlegel added to the applause; Goethe's Faust, he proclaimed, was the German Hamlet.

Buoyed by this praise, Goethe continued to work on this story, a labor that would last his lifetime. By 1808, the initial fragment had grown into *Faust: A Tragedy*, an epic in which this scholar falls into despair. What had his *saper aude* search yielded? Suicidal, sick from too much logic, he returned to Nostradamus and alchemy, hungry for the supernatural and revelation. His mind became a source of illusion and his soul was entrapped in a "cave of grief." Then, Mephistopheles descended. As Madame de Staël trenchantly observed, Goethe's Devil was no ghoul. Wry, ironic, cutting, Satan was a slick, cultivated seducer who employed sarcasm and the blade of reason to slice up human meaning. Philosophy, theology, and law were easy prey; they were mocked as sophistries. Medicine was a straight swindle. Amid the deceits of civilization, only sensual delight could cure the doctor. Feverishly, he and his new companion hunted for the burning fuse within being, and in the process, set in motion a cascade of catastrophes. *Faust: A Tragedy* became very successful and, in the process, it showcased a new Goethe, the duke's advisor in league with the rebels from Jena.

Madame de Staël also came under Jena's sway. In 1796, she had taken a classical view: the passions caused unhappiness and must be tamed by reason. One of her lovers, Benjamin Constant, however, had begun to see reason as the source of misery. He wrote about the man of indecision, torn up by his restrained emotions, half alive. Chateaubriand also concluded that the progeny of the Enlightenment had grown sick with anxiety and indecision. After befriending the Schlegels, Germaine de Staël soon agreed. Passionate suffering, she now decided, could be a source of rebirth. In the same way that plant life was regenerated through destruction, human feelings even when painful could lead to growth and happiness. That once dreaded disease, enthusiasm, was an antidote for modern ills. It gave meaning and force to lives otherwise filled with cool detachment, alienation, and ennui. A gift, an elevation, such inspiration made for love, joy, and life's grandeur. It was not madness, but that precious, epiphanic moment of "God in us. "

The German Romantics attracted followers from university students, salon society, republicans, writers, artists, and mystics, but they did not speak with one voice. They split with regard to both politics and religion. Some became reactionaries. For example, Novalis sought a return to the ancient order, and asked the Church to again take up the moral education—the *Bildung*—of the people. Friedrich Schlegel would also advocate for a return to King and Christianity. A host of others, like Schiller and the followers of Fichte, stuck to their beliefs.

Furthermore, no single response to Kant prevailed among this school. While the daring and difficult Fichte inspired many, he convinced few. Schiller mocked him for creating this new divinity, the "I." It was F. W. J. Schelling who labeled Fichte's thought "subjective

idealism," which was not intended as a compliment. Friedrich Schlegel wrote a friend and reported that, to his surprise, in Jena almost
no one took Fichte seriously. "Fichte," he continued, "is really like a
drunk who does not tire of climbing up on one side of a horse, tran-
scending it, and falling off on the other side."

Instead of Fichte's subjectivism, the Schlegels and others sought
to break free of reason's limits through aesthetics. The mind's inability to grasp anything other than its own representations created a
deadening distance from the world: conscious introspection led only
to more and more abstract representations. Art could break this cycle,
and become civilized man's cure, his new religion. Friedrich Hölderlin wrote:

> I am attempting to prove that what must be continually
> demanded of any system, the union of the subject and the object
> in an absolute I (or whatever name one gives it) is undoubtedly
> possible on the aesthetic level in intellectual intuition, but not
> on the theoretical level except by means of an infinite approx-
> imation. . . .

The Jena intellectuals also varied greatly in their approach to
science. The Schlegels believed science and poetry should be one,
but did not attempt to merge these seeming opposites. That marriage
was presided over by a new powerhouse in Jena, Friedrich Wilhelm
Joseph von Schelling. Born in 1775, Schelling was a child prodigy
who at the age of fifteen took up university theological studies at
a seminary in Tübingen. There, he befriended Friedrich Hölderlin
and G. W. F. Hegel, and with them, turned to the study of Kant,
Spinoza, and Fichte. When news of the French Revolution arrived,
this son of a Lutheran preacher grew so enthused that he translated
"The Marseillaise." He and his two friends formed a secret society.
They were eager to end orthodoxy and despotism, and ambitiously
plotted a three-pronged assault. Hölderlin would attack conventional

education, Hegel would take on the historical roots of Christianity, and Schelling would critique contemporary theology and the foundations of science.

After completing his studies at the seminary, Schelling became a tutor for a baron's family in Stuttgart. In 1796, he traveled to Leipzig, where his charges had begun the study of law. He aided the boys in their legal studies, and in his free time attended lectures on electricity, magnetism, chemistry, and medicine, a profession that he informed his parents was easy and could be learned swiftly. The young man also told his parents that these classes were critical for him, since he was constructing a new theory of life.

At the time, Schelling was a devotee of Fichte. However, soon, having climbed up onto Fichte's horse, he would tumble down the other side. Schelling concluded that Fichte's idealism, his subsuming of Nature into the transcendental subject, was one-sided. The mind of the subject should not obliterate the world, any more than the world could erase the mind. Nature and consciousness needed to be conceptualized in unity; idealist philosophy needed to be balanced by empirical, scientific study.

In 1797, Schelling's *Ideas for a Philosophy of Nature* appeared. It was intended to be a new foundation for both philosophy and natural science. In its outlines, *Naturphilosophie*—Nature philosophy, as it became known—had a biblical cast. In the beginning, man and Nature existed in an Absolute Unity. This was sundered by human reflection. "Henceforth," he wrote, man "separates what nature had forever united: object from intuition, concept from image, and finally, by becoming his own *object*, he separates himself from himself." The power of human reflection, which Locke relied on to guide mankind beyond sheer sensation, had become a blinding light. Having eaten from the Tree of Knowledge, men and women were forever cast into a shadowy world filled with only their own signs and symbols.

Schelling conceived of the natural world as polarities in dynamic opposition, a model that followed Fichte's dialectic of subject and object. In addition, his theory was critically aided by his observations of magnetism and electricity, where contrary forces from differing poles faced off. Nature consisted of a balance or disruption of such opposed forces. Physics, chemistry, biology, and psychic life could not be comprehended through isolated mechanical causes and effects, for they were all a set of dynamic relations of attractions and resistances. Polar forces in conflict compel the natural world and result in a purposiveness of the whole. All of Nature was a unity, a self-enclosed system, a circle that returned to itself. The outer world of objects and the inner world of the mind were similarly one. As Schelling wrote: "Nature should be visible Mind, Mind being invisible Nature."

At times arcane and quizzical, Schelling's 1797 inauguration of Nature philosophy nonetheless grew in popularity and won its

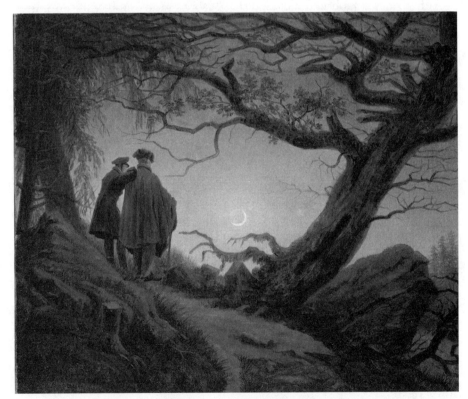

Figure 39. Caspar David Friedrich, *Two Men Contemplating the Moon*, 1819–1820, reflected Nature philosophy's pantheism.

twenty-three-year-old author a professorship in Jena. This success befuddled critics, who point to Schelling's flights of speculation and his grandiose theorizing. However, in his zeal to overcome the fragmentation that modernity engendered, this curly haired prodigy had accurately homed in on a profound set of problems. After Novalis met the youthful professor, he dug into his writings and emerged to confess to Caroline Schlegel: "The more deeply I penetrate into Schelling's world-soul, the more interesting do I find his mind—which seems to intimate the ultimate and to lack only the pure gift of rendering. . . ." With an intoxicating urgency, Schelling conveyed the need to reestablish contact between Nature and the mind, in a manner that harkened back to Renaissance animists and mystics and mirrored the despair of Faust. In 1798, Friedrich Schlegel joked about the youth's zeal, asking his brother's wife, Caroline: "But where will Schelling, the granite, find a granitesse?" To the great dismay of many, Caroline would soon volunteer for that job.

Schelling aimed to encompass subject and object, science and the soul, mechanistic matter and human freedom, all the great rifts that attended the birth of modernity. Nature philosophy took up that fragmentation not as a historical problem, but as a timeless one. And Schelling added another division derived from Fichte. Split off from an original holism, humans became divided from themselves. He wrote: "This mere reflection is a mental disorder in man, and when it takes control of the whole person, it kills the seed of his higher existence and the root of his spiritual life, which proceeds only from identity."

Schelling contrasted the ills of dry reflection with the aims of true philosophy. Philosophy began with the *premise* of the mind's freedom and demonstrated the moral agency of human beings, a commitment for Schelling that was both political and logical. As for the French sensationalists and the Lockeans, "They are caught up in the mechanism of their thought and presentations; *I* have broken through this mechanism." He went on:

Whoever is nothing more for himself than what things and circumstances have made of him; whoever, having no control over his own representations, is caught and swept away in the current of causes and effects, how should he know where he comes from, where he is going, and how he has become what he is? Does the wave that sweeps him away in the current know this?"

Schelling acknowledged the impact of that philosopher who, a century earlier, sought unity between Nature and the soul, Spinoza, the renegade pantheist. Spinoza and Leibniz, he believed, both refocused philosophy on the active forces within man, the subject that represented, rather than mere representations. After 1797, Schelling's Nature philosophy was laid out in a series of works over the next six years, and during that time his stature grew. In 1799, when Fichte was run out of Jena because of charges of atheism, Schelling moved to the center of the Romantics' circle, a place he held even more firmly after he won Caroline Schlegel's heart.

Some of the most receptive followers of Schelling's *Naturphilosophie* were physicians and scientists. Goethe was taken by this brilliant youth, since he too valued scientific methods and viewed nature nonmechanistically. Some doctors, caught up first with Kant, also perceived the necessity of comprehending Nature in its unity, and of developing a medicine that did not overly focus on appearances, but discerned what lay beyond the empirical senses.

The bond between German doctors and Schelling was no accident. After his 1795 classes in Leipzig, Schelling fancied himself a medical expert. In 1798, he chastised his parents for the silly notion of sending his brother to Tübingen for medical studies. No one there knew a thing about healing, he assured them. If the boy came to study with his older brother, he would become one of the greatest doctors in the German lands. In January of 1801, Schelling did not hesitate to treat the great Goethe for a cough: unfortunately, Peruvian bark and opium didn't do the trick. Apparently, his confidence had not been shaken, even by another notorious, failed medical treatment. A year earlier, when Caroline Schlegel left Wilhelm to join Schelling, she had brought her daughter with her. The sixteen-year-old fell ill and died. Rumormongers spread the word that Schelling insisted on treating the girl and therefore hastened her end.

Despite this disaster, Schelling continued with his medical studies. When the second edition of his *Ideas for a Philosophy of Nature* came out in 1803, the author was now advertised as a professor of philosophy and a medical doctor. A year earlier, Schelling had been awarded the title of doctor of medicine from the University of Bamberg. It was there that he had studied with Andreas Roeschlaub, the man who made that school a center for Brunonian medicine. The Scottish doctor John Brown had constructed a medical theory that was gloriously simple: all illnesses were based on disruptions of excitability. Diseases were due to overstimulation or understimulation. Treatment called for agents to counter these effects.

In 1803, after becoming a physician, Schelling delivered a lecture in which he insisted that medicine must become the universal science of Nature. To do so, it must be based on first principles, not scattered empirical facts. The Brunonian theory of excitability—which dovetailed nicely with his notion of bipolar forces in conflict—offered that possibility. In 1805, Schelling launched *Yearbook of Medicine as Science* with the Brunonian doctor and psychiatrist Adalbert Marcus. In the opening editorial of this journal, Schelling announced, "Medical science is the crown, the epitome of all natural science." The time was now, he urged, to forge a scientific medicine by bringing together philosophers, scientists, chemists, and clinicians.

Many German doctors were ready to hear out this celebrated doctor and philosopher, who wrote extensively not just on ontology and epistemology, but also physiology, chemistry, magnetism, electricity, and the interactions of body and mind. Schelling's Nature philosophy seeped into a medical world that was thirsty for a new philosophy. Marcus Herz, Johann Reil, and others initially hoped Kant would provide answers. The Brunonians also emerged with their philosophical brand of medicine. Schelling's Nature philosophy offered another alternative.

After his studies with Roeschlaub, Schelling had developed Brown's views of animal excitability into a broader theory that merged irritation and sensibility into what he called "Instinct." He critiqued Reil's "life force" and was especially appalled by those who casually made their way from physiology to psychology, from the body to the mind. From light and the stimulation of the optic nerve to internal experience, a crucial leap had to be made: "You can insert as many intermediate members as you like between the affection of your nerves, your brain, etc., and the representation of an external thing. Yet you deceive only yourselves; for according to your own representations the transition from body to soul cannot be continuous, but must be made in a leap, which you purport to wish to avoid." That impossible step was from quantities of matter to qualities of experience.

For all his criticism of rationality, Schelling did not (yet) advocate a return to Christian metaphysics. He was quite disturbed when some of his Jena brethren turned to Christian mysticism and later would find himself attacked by the church as well as advocates of the Enlightenment. Schelling believed that Nature philosophy offered a path between mechanism and religion, and that path opened up when one recognized that the innermost aspect of all Nature and all men, the essence of soul and body, was not an unknowable thing-in-itself, but rather *Geist*.

This word immediately grew opaque after Schelling offered it up as a grand solution. *Geist* literally meant "spirit," but by 1800 it could also connote "mind." What exactly was it for him? Schelling expended a good deal of energy explaining that and other weighty words, like "world-soul" and "absolute," which were central to his theories. He began with the notion that a nonmaterial *Geist* united idea and matter; it placed man within Nature and Nature within man. External irritations of nervous sensibility were ordered and integrated by this unifying power. Neither life nor consciousness could be explained by physical facts alone, but must take in the unifying forces that organized whole structures.

Geist was the spirit that animated life, the force often called psyche, anima, or soul. Dualisms that split mind and body were wrong; reductive materialism and mechanical notions of life were impossible. Nature and man were a purpose-driven unity, animated by *Geist*, driven not by a linear chain of causes and effects, but rather feedback loops within a dynamic system. To grasp the ultimate realities of the Absolute, beneath appearances, we must leap past the empirical world and, through self-reflection, merge subject and object together in true knowledge.

Schelling's model seemed to reclaim the animating soul from theologians. His world-soul was clearly not a Christian soul, but closer to Spinoza's pantheism. That inner essence was at the heart of Nature and throbbed in the recesses of consciousness too. It was the beating pulse of human life, and if it did not hold out the promise of celestial salvation, it did control health and vigor, meaning and happiness. Through self-reflection, shocks of sublime insight, art, and unreason, one might enter the vault of the unknown.

If Schelling's philosophy distinguished itself from other post-Kantian approaches by its employment of an animistic soul, it also adopted another orphan of modernity: teleology. The notion that natural processes had a fate, a final end, had been mostly banished by modern science. And that meant that any phenomena that one explained through the use of human intention was seen as forever on the wrong side of natural science. It was not scientific to explain an event by saying that it was motivated, that some force wanted it to happen.

Schelling was not the first to insist that teleology was necessary for the life sciences. Kant recognized the need for teleology when it came to the study of the phenomena of the mind: "Certain mental products from the special constitution of our Understandings, must be considered by us, in regard to their possibility as if produced designedly and as purposes." In Göttingen, the medical faculty boasted the influential Johann Friedrich Blumenbach, who in 1781 posited a formative drive in nature, a *Bildungstrieb*. From this vantage point, biological complexity did not derive solely from mechanics. Rather, inorganic matter led to an emergent vital force that led to complex living beings. Schelling adopted an inner formative drive: the world-soul was a constant striving force in Nature. It endlessly sought to organize itself and structured living matter in a dynamic evolution. Hence, a polyp regenerated, a young girl matured into a woman, and the mind created consciousness.

By 1806, Schelling had established Nature philosophy. He would abandon his own project and turn back to myth and mystical religion, especially after the sudden death of Caroline in 1809. Nonetheless, his child went on without him. For the next four decades, Nature philosophy remained a force among German scientific and medical thinkers, for it offered a viable theory of the active forces and transmutations in life forms, including the human mind. Modern conceptions of the mind now included this theory of striving forces. Nature philosophy represented a powerful counter to mechanistic thought. From this perspective, one discovered a dramatic world of purpose and agency, a world that Goethe's Faust pointed to when he wrote that in the beginning was not the Word, but rather the Deed.

SCHELLING'S NATURE PHILOSOPHY made inroads in the universities of Freiburg, Leipzig, Heidelberg, and Erlangen. In Halle, by the 1790s, a circle of enlightened elites discussed the Jena writers and welcomed visitors like Novalis and Tieck. When the university sought to recruit from this new breed of thinkers, they turned to Johann Christian Reil, whose days in Henriette Herz's salon had well familiarized him with this group. Thanks in part to him, by 1803 one of Schelling's most avid followers, Henrik Steffens, had moved to Halle.

Reil knew Schelling's work, for the philosopher had critiqued the doctor's essay on life force. Having already rejected Blumenbach's *Bildungstrieb*, it seemed likely that Dr. Reil would have tossed aside Schelling's even more speculative world-soul. However, by the time Steffens arrived, Dr. Reil's Kantian physiology was a mess. To consider matter only as an appearance might be fine for metaphysics, but would not suffice for medicine. As Marcus Herz admitted, the only way for doctors to proceed—given the restraints of Kantian epistemology—was to break the rules.

And so, Reil found himself attracted to Schelling's notion of organic life and the post-Kantian emphasis on the self-creating capacities of the mind. He began to turn his attention to subjectivity and its breakdowns, and returned to the extraordinary events that led to his Halle professorship. The mentor who called Reil to Halle, a Dr. Goldhagen, had suffered from striking delusions. As Reil later recalled, the old professor would wander through his home looking for a sick patient, only to discover that patient was himself. Freed from his Kantian reserve and armed with Schelling's model, Reil approached these weird phenomena anew.

An opportunity arose to develop his ideas. As the director of the medical clinic and city physician of Halle, Reil was asked by a poorhouse pastor, Heinrich Wagnitz, to write something that advocated for the humane treatment of the mentally ill. By then, Dr. Reil was a prominent academic who had been recruited by the medical school in Göttingen, an offer he turned down after extracting a ransom from his present employers. A committed liberal, Reil had already published a book dedicated to Bonaparte, whom he described as a friend of science.

Reil accepted Wagnitz's offer and prepared to add his voice to a growing chorus. By the 1780s, humanitarian outcries against infernal conditions for the mentally ill could be heard across Europe, including German lands. One outraged commentator had written that in "any of the institutions for the insane in Germany," one found fellow human beings who cried out in rags, freezing and dirty, chained and brutalized by their keepers. A movement to more fully medicalize the treatment of madness also had made progress. For example in 1785, new regulations had been laid down in Frankfurt that legally required medical oversight of the mentally ill. In 1788, Ludwigsburg opened a madhouse staffed by doctors, and in 1789, insane patients in Berlin were moved into the Charité Hospital where under Ernst Horn patients were categorized by illness and no longer subjected to bloodletting and old-time purgative medications. Instead, they were treated with mental means and their chains were replaced by modern forms of restraint. In Vienna, along with liberal reforms like the cessation of serfdom and laws that called for the toleration of Jews, the care of the insane was also a focus of reform. In 1783, it was discovered that certain Capuchin monks made a practice of placing exorcised parishioners who stubbornly remained mad in subterranean cells. A decree was issued that demanded all mentally ill cared for by religious orders be reported to the state to prevent such abuses.

In Halle, Heinrich Wagnitz himself had written a treatise cataloguing the abuses of prisons and arguing for the segregation of the mentally ill from those dumped in the poorhouse. He hoped Reil would add his prestige to this effort with a book that the pastor promised to see into print.

When Johann Reil was done, he had completed a book dedicated to Wagnitz, but it was a wide-ranging 500-page account that included merely 40 pages on humanitarian reform. Worse, at the heart of this volume was a shocking assumption that the pastor could never abide: the soul was a myth, Reil asserted. All the functions of the mind and the self were natural. Not surprisingly, the pastor declined to publish the book.

Rhapsodies on the Use of Psychological Therapies for the Mentally Disturbed appeared, nonetheless, in 1803. Never before had such a significant medical treatise been advertised as an ecstatic form of verse. Reil was intent on signaling that this was not a dry collection of facts. Something new was happening, his title announced, something poetic, antimechanical, and unconventional. Something allied with aesthetes and idealists in Jena.

In his hope to establish a German mental medicine, Reil had been preceded by a number of mid-century physicians who had clambered onto the moral therapy bandwagon, men like Christian Gottlieb Ludwig, Johann Christian Bolten, and Johann Friedrich Zuckert. And others had seen the opportunity to deploy post-Kantian theories of the mind to reconsider mental illness. After studying law and theology, in 1794 Dr. J. G. Langermann arrived in Jena, took philosophy classes with Fichte, did his medical training, and became friends with Goethe and Schiller. In 1797, he produced a dissertation on melancholia that echoed the concerns of his philosophy teacher. The free soul created its own misery through misguided strivings and desire. Passions were the cause of this deformity, and the self must be the locus of self-correction. Mind doctors must help the misguided tame their passions and regain their equanimity.

He never wrote on insanity again, but Langermann went on to become an influential administrator who advocated for reform in the treatment of the mentally ill. In 1804, he proposed a plan to modernize the asylum in Bayreuth and have it staffed not by preachers, but by doctors. This proposal became the basis for the first mental sanatorium for the poor in Germanic lands, a place in which cure came through mental pedagogy and physical therapy. Langermann's Fichtean psychiatry was mirrored by Horn at the Berlin Charité Hospital, where this doctor combined strict Prussian morality with notions of individual responsibility for madness. For him, French concerns about sensibilities were weak; his patients were coerced back to health through a range of demands, lectures, forced labor, strict discipline, and finally torments, such as his rotating machine.

While some doctors saw the opportunity for employing post-Kantian thought for a mind medicine, so too did the growing middle class, the *Bildungsbürgertum*. They had followed the *Sturm und Drang* focus on interiority, the Kantian revolution, and the rise of the Romantics with their focus on the dark side of reason. For them, there was an obvious overlap between philosophical doctrines that insisted the mind's grasp of reality verged on being a hallucination and the doctors of hallucination. Take for example, the case of the psychotic Christoph Friedrich Nicolai. After finding that his own case had been inaccurately reported by his doctor, Nicolai asked for equal time, and instead of being dismissed as a madman, he was invited to address the Berlin Royal Society. His illness, Nicolai contended, proved that Fichte's theories were wrong. He recounted how, in 1790, while suffering a nervous collapse, he began to see and converse with ghosts. By his reading of Fichte, these specters should have behaved *no differently* than his daily perceptions. But not at all!, Christoph declared. After laying out many careful distinctions, Nicolai concluded that these unreal visitations were distinctly different from everyday experience.

Johann Reil's work built on these prior efforts, but not just those. The Halle physician demonstrated familiarity with the work of mind doctors starting with the Ancients such as Hippocrates, Celsus, and Al-Rashid; the English mad doctors like Willis, Pargeter, and Tuke; the Italian Chiarugi; and the French physicians like Tissot, Cabanis, and Pinel. He had studied Kant and Fichte, and benefited from Karl Moritz's magazine. *Rhapsody* was littered with citations to mentalists whose discussions and examples he freely employed.

However, Reil was no parrot. He sought to unify these voices into one coherent model. No one, he believed, had done that well, especially not his rival, Pinel. Though the Frenchman's case histories were excellent, his conceptual framework was simplistic. Reil spent a good deal of energy castigating French arrogance in medicine.

Still, commentators would add up Reil's numerous citations of Pinel and write him off as an imitator. Some called him the German Pinel. That was misguided. Reil's assumptions not only differed from Pinel's, they emerged from a stinging critique of the two pillars that guided Pinel: sensationalism and vitalism. Following Kant, Reil focused not on external stressors so much as the essence of the individual, the dreamer behind the dream. Underlying psychic structures drove mental phenomena. Reil hoped to define the emerging field of psychical medicine as the science of these deep inner causes.

Despite his title, there was little poetry in Reil's book. Alongside some lyrical flights, Reil laid out a quite rational dissection of the mind and mental illness, as well as the possibilities for a new psychical medicine. The book did, however, open with gusto:

> It is a remarkable experience to step from the whirl of a large city into its madhouse. One finds here repeated the same scenes, though as in a vaudeville performance; yet, in this fool's system, there exists a kind of easy genius in the whole. The madhouse has its usurpers, tyrants, slaves, criminals, and defenseless martyrs, fools who laugh without cause, and fools who torture themselves without cause. Pride of ancestry, egoism, vanity, greed and all the other idols of human weakness guide the rudder in this maelstrom, just as in the ocean of the large world.

The Halle doctor suggested that inside the madhouse one might find men like Newton, Bacon, and Leibniz. Reason, even of the superior sort, was no guarantee of sanity.

While liberally using terms like *Geist* and *Seele*, Reil redefined them as naturalistic, if at times quite speculative, notions. If a limb and its nerves were amputated, he wrote, part of the *Seele* would be lost. More so, he turned to the Greek word for soul, *psyche,* and defined it as a material entity that possessed free will and depended on the body. Of course, this word had been central to Wolff's psychology, which used that root, and had been adopted for journals such as the *Psychological Magazine* founded in Jena by Karl Schmid in 1796. Armed with this term, Reil developed a psychology for doctors, a psychical medicine, made of psychic illnesses and cures.

Reil liked triads. People interacted with the world in three ways, he proclaimed. The first was mechanical, the second was chemical, and the last was mental. Three distinct sciences accounted for each: anatomy, physiology, and psychology. Three medical approaches organized the understanding of illness in each realm; surgery, medicine, and psychical medicine. Finally, each of these forms of medicine had distinct therapies: surgery, pharmacology, and psychic cures.

Thus, against Kant, Reil insisted that psychical matters were medical. Doctors, he admitted, were often too unphilosophical for psychological medicine, but philosophers were not medical enough. A new kind of medicine was needed, a psychical medicine and science.

Like Hobbes, Locke, and the Montpellier vitalists, Reil believed that the mind arose from the body. Living matter, like an embryo, grew by adding new parts: it developed more and more complex organizations with novel properties, including the mind and its cognitive processes. Lower forces were synthesized into higher ones that possessed new qualities and operated by new laws of operation, including free will and reason. Physicochemical forces gave birth to physiological forces, which then supported the emergence of mental capabilities.

So far, students of Pinel and Cabanis might have yawned, but their eyes surely widened as Reil continued. An inner drive, a *Bildungstrieb*, established antagonistic polarities that then drove development. Like the rest of the body, the mind was governed by a dynamic equilibrium of these forces. And they were not the classic faculties of reason, passion, and will, but another threesome.

Self-consciousness was the most critical function; it was the force of mental integration. From the multitude of experiences and the many selves one possessed, it created unity and allowed us to awake each morning with the same identity:

> The mind in self-consciousness rolls up the immeasurable thread of time into a ball, reproduces the long dead centuries, and gathers into the miniature of one of its representations mountain ranges, rivers, woods, and the stars. . . . The mind senses itself as if it were in each representation, it relates what is represented to itself, as the creator of the same, and it maintains thereby a special rule over the world outside itself insofar as it is representable.

Reflection served as a compass in "a sea of sensibility." The mind responded to sensations and focused on appropriate objects thanks to this capacity. Finally, mental attention allowed for selective processing and proportion, the scaling of mental objects and the focus on some, which required the abandonment of others. When these three mental forces flowed together, the result was harmonious mental health. A disruption of the equilibrium could result in madness, crazed obsession, or murderous enthusiasms.

Reil especially cast light on the risk of psychic fragmentation. While children demonstrated an immature form of self-consciousness, the mad had faults in this critical function. For them, inner and outer, fantasy and perception, could lose distinction. The result was patients like old Dr. Goldhagen, who searched for himself in his own home, or the patient who believed he was two individuals and ate accordingly.

When it came to naming mental illnesses, Reil did not stray

far from Pinel and his taxonomy of melancholia, mania, idiocy, and dementia. However, he expressed the concern that some of these categories might contain multitudes. Given that mental illness was the disruption of a dynamic that stretched back and forth between anatomy, physiology, and psychology, Reil urged doctors to understand the specific causes of illness, for the suspects were many.

Reil's psychical doctor should start by mapping his patient's inner landscape, understanding symptoms, and the often secret motivations beneath such phenomena. Such an outline of the sufferer's mental world would reveal what aroused their pleasure and pain. Only then could the doctor of the mind begin to reeducate the patient and return him to inner peace.

But how? Since the body and mind affected each other, treatment would occur on both fronts. The doctor might approach the mind by altering physiology or proceed through consciousness and the senses. Reil denounced cruelty in asylums, but he had no qualms when the violent acts were not blows against a person, but rather against insanity. Patients would be forced out of their illusory reveries through a sudden dousing with water, being dunked in baths, having food withheld, or even being thrown into a pool of eels. Pain and fear, Reil believed, would provoke "reflections upon reflections within himself and therefore about himself." Tortures of this sort stimulated whatever remnant of self-consciousness the patient possessed. While such pain could be reorienting, pleasure could be too. Melancholic patients should be coaxed back to life with sexual activities, warm heat, and baths.

Direct cognitive cures also abounded. Through writing, reading, and talking, delusions and fixed ideas could be confronted. Reil's mental therapeutics included a full-scale retraining with elaborate contraptions. He described exquisitely created boxes of objects, in which the distracted and delusional patient would pull one item out, be asked to name the object, list its qualities, and finally combine all of that into a written description. Impressed by Pinel's success with the delusional watchmaker, Reil also advocated for engaging the senses with jigsaw puzzles, painting, music, and poetry which thereby pushed sick fantasies to the side.

Every mental hospital should have a theater; patients should be encouraged to read their lines, add the appropriate affects, then memorize it all. Thus, they would literally begin to act human. When necessary, the playhouse could be used to combat delusions. Reil, who had no asylum at his disposal, repeated cases reported by Pinel and others, in which fixed delusions were dramatized in the hope of guiding the patient away from them. Attendants stuffed in a casket rose up to eat and proved that a fixed idea about the dead starving in their coffins was not so. These high jinks, empiricism turned to mad charade, were considered a powerful way of subduing paranoid thought. Even the mentally ill believed what was there before their own eyes.

Mental hospitals were required to provide bodily and mental treatment on pleasant grounds that did not resemble jails or poorhouses. They should be run by the state, so that the motive for profit did not rule. After *Rhapsody* was published, Reil hoped to build such an establishment in Halle, and he advocated for a new field of psychical medicine and science.

In 1805, he started the *Magazine for Psychic Healing*, coedited by a Halle philosophy professor, Anton Adalbert Kayssler. The journal seems to have been almost exclusively written by Kayssler, though that remains unclear, since in the first volume over 200 pages of work went unsigned. Articles developed strange geometries based on the polarities of life, described horrors to be found in Dr. Horn's Charité in Berlin, and detailed Reil's *Rhapsody*, which was taken as a foundational text.

After three issues, the journal expired in 1806 as Reil's efforts were overwhelmed by political events. Flush from his victory in Jena,

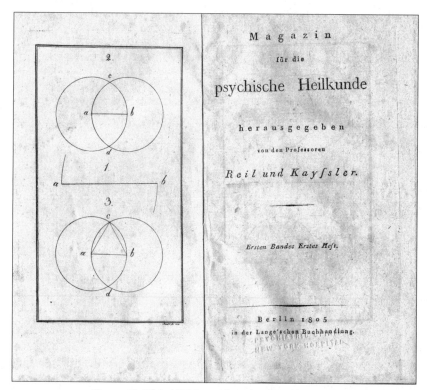

Figure 40. This 1805 journal was coedited by Reil,
who coined the term "psychiatry."

Napoleon met the Prussian army outside of Halle and routed them.
The French closed Halle University and quartered their troops in the
homes of the locals. As Prussia fell and French taxation began, early
advocates for the Rights of Man like Johann Reil stopped whistling
the Marseillaise.

With the university shuttered, the doctor stubbornly launched
another journal of psychical medicine. For this one, he recruited a
different Halle philosopher, Johann Christoph Hoffbauer. In 1807,
the new journal appeared. This time the editors had managed to
muster a few contributors, and before this effort also went the way
of most small magazines, Reil contributed a seminal article. In it, he
reiterated much that he had argued for in 1803: the three modes of
human life—the mechanical, the chemical, and the psychical—had

corresponding medical disciplines. Surgery and medicine were now joined by the third domain, which Reil christened *"psychiaterie."* This neologism, soon to be altered to "Psychiatrie," combined the Greek *psyche*, or "soul," with *iatros* for "physician." For Reil, he and his colleagues would become the modern doctors of what once was the soul.

The Promise of Phrenology

B Y 1805, Russia, Austria, and other continental powers that
opposed Napoleon rose up against the French. The result was
catastrophic for Bonaparte's opponents. The massive French army
marched forward and destroyed the opposition at Ulm in October,
Vienna in November, and then Austerlitz in December. By 1806,
Austria and Russia had been routed. The Prussians were next. They
broke their peace with the French, declared war and were humbled.

In the coming years, the reign of Napoleon Bonaparte would
result in the modernization of feudal economies, some liberal reforms,
and new political rights for some. However, the French occupation
would also stoke a fierce anti-French nationalism based in part on the
everyday recognition that the ideals of the Revolution now seemed
to justify theft, murder, blackmail, rape, and dispossession. As the
French armies moved in to conquered places like Halle, those who
once welcomed the armies of the universal rights of man grew bitter. German nationalism and identity emerged from the negation of
French values, and in opposition to Napoleon and his lustful cam-
paigns that marched under the banner of Universal Reason.

After the military collapse of 1806, Halle became a depressing
place. Even after the French allowed the university to reopen two
years later, few students returned. However, in Berlin, liberals had

instituted some reforms and, thanks to the energetic efforts of Wilhelm von Humboldt, a new university opened with great hopes. Humboldt sought to add *Geisteswissenschaft*—human science—to the traditional curricula of law, theology, and medicine. He recruited a stellar faculty that included Fichte and Hegel for philosophy. With regard to the medical school, Humboldt lured Johann Christian Reil away from Halle to join Christoph Hufeland.

Reil left Halle in excellent hands; his former student, Dr. Christian Friedrich Nasse, took over his professorship and began to deliver the first lectures in psychiatry in 1810; he would remain a strong advocate of Reil's "moderate" Nature philosophy, as one student would call it. When Reil and Hoffbauer's psychiatric journal failed in 1812, Nasse became the next editor of such an undertaking, the *Journal for Psychical Doctors*, which ran from 1818 to 1822. Reil's tripartite division helped organize medical reform in Halle. His influence extended to others who took up the study of self-consciousness and fragmentation, as well as those who penned rhapsodies on psychical topics. And so, as moral therapeutics were riding high in liberal England and Philippe Pinel's mental medicine sought to establish itself in Napoleonic France, Reil's psychiatry gathered adherents in German lands.

Still, by 1800, over a century of efforts to integrate mind into matter had resulted in a resounding maybe. Seemingly insoluble problems had been finessed and managed through the use of metaphors, plausible hypotheses, more or less tenable models, and promissory notes, often based on the fleeting prestige of new advances in medicine or science. From Willis's brain anatomy to Locke's thinking thing and Priestley's pneumology, from Haller's sensibility to the vitalistic models of Bordeu and Barthez, from Schelling to Reil, one thing was true. These were the offspring of Hobbes and Gassendi, not Descartes. They sought to plant the mind firmly in Nature, while not disavowing its capacities that may not be found elsewhere, active functions like consciousness and free will. To do so, they employed linchpin concepts that stretched from physics to ethics, culture, and creative human life. Through these efforts, reformers hoped to establish an array of fields: *science humaine*, a psychology or *anthropologie*, as well as a medical discipline variably called alienism, mental medicine, and psychiatry.

These efforts were critical for the advocates of modernity. If universal reason was to be their guide, a natural home for that faculty was required. And with such a faculty, some amount of teleology would need to apply to human desires and voluntary actions. Otherwise—against all common sense—science would be forced to insist that no human capacity for intentional action existed. Medical psychologies from Locke to Pinel and Reil, all allowed for a measure of free will within the workings of the body. And thanks to that, their psychologies could be extended and applied to ethics and politics. An active mind that possessed some free will was a necessary belief for those who wanted to consider individuals as autonomous agents.

However, while the links between the physical and the mental seemed necessary, they were difficult to empirically verify. Skeptical members of scientific societies were awaiting direct, "ocular" proof. And so, when thusly examined, the bridge between body, brain, and mind could not hold. While every breathing, thinking human lived each day convinced of their own intentionality and its connection to consciousness, advocates of the soul, Cartesians, and Newtonians were happy to point out that those commonsense conclusions had scientifically established nothing.

Since Thomas Willis, many hoped brain anatomy would establish the anatomical basis for a science of consciousness. However, for those with such hopes. brain research had been a terrible disappointment. By the middle of the 18th century, the very study of the brain had hit hard times. Some concluded that there was nothing left to be learned from this grey, wrinkled flesh.

Then surprisingly, around 1800, a Viennese doctor, who disdained vitalist and Romantic conceptions of the body, reenergized the search for spots where the mind and matter met. He launched a new science that brought together behavior and the brain. Using the language and logic of empirical science, he announced clearly testable, definitive solutions. He had found reason's bodily home, uncovered the biology of desire, and by adopting teleology, created the first science of character and personality. His work promised to underwrite a new pedagogy, a new model of crime and justice, and new views of mental illness. He presented discoveries that, if correct, would be the ultimate solution to 150 years of debate between advocates of the soul, the brain, and the mind.

WHILE NAPOLEON'S MASSIVE armies swept across the continent, a Quixotic little band of Austrians quietly made their own assault on the status quo. In 1805, they left Vienna for Berlin and assiduously avoided battlegrounds. However, they would not rest until they had toured over thirty cities. Their caravan made for a ghoulish image: armed with a trunkful of human and animal skulls, some plaster brains, and two ill-fated monkeys, they consisted of a personal servant, a young expert with a scalpel, and a short, pallid Viennese doctor said to possess a capacious head. After two years of commanding lectures and demonstrations, both the doctor and his assistant settled in Paris, where they continued to amass skulls and attack conventional notions of the brain, the mind, and the soul. In the spirit of the *lumières*, they deployed empiricism to banish illusion, even if those illusions seemed to be *égalite* and *liberté*.

Very early in his European tour, the doctor, Franz Josef Gall, brought his new truths to Halle. His long season of demonstration and debate had just begun, for he had so far made his case only in Berlin, Potsdam, Leipzig, and Dresden. He came armed with discoveries all the more stunning for being so obvious. Freed from ancient dogmas about immortal souls and their traditional faculties, contemptuous of Cartesian dualism, Gall linked anatomy, physiology, and psychology in a massive synthesis. After Halle, he swept through Jena, Weimar, and twenty other locales from Zurich to Amsterdam. Before crowned heads and professors, with clarity and careful logic, he demonstrated the exact location of the mind in the body. What that meant for the soul, he insisted, was not his problem.

Born in 1758 to a wealthy Catholic family, Franz Gall was raised in a Swabian village, part of the Grand Duchy of Baden. An easily excitable child, he suffered from insomnia, somnambulism, and childhood visions. In 1777, he traveled to Strasbourg to study medicine, then completed his studies in Vienna. Having received his medical degree in 1785, Gall married and set up a successful, private practice in the capital of the Holy Roman Empire. However, his ambitions were greater. In 1794, in a stunning act of hubris, Gall turned down an invitation to be among the personal physicians to Emperor Franz II. He saw this as an unnecessary intrusion on his freedom.

Gall had become obsessed with philosophical questions in medicine, so much so that often he needed to calm himself down at the end of his day by gardening. His first publication appeared in 1791 as *Medical-Philosophical Investigation into the Nature and Culture of the Diseased and Healthy State of Man.* It took aim at speculation in medicine, especially from the soul-based medicine of the Stahlians, and lauded standard authorities such as Haller and Tissot. More interestingly, the young Austrian doctor focused on the innate differences that result from variables like age and gender, and in the process revealed his debt to Johann Gottfried Herder.

Herder was controversial. In Königsberg, he studied with both Kant and Johann Georg Hamann, a central figure of the growing anti-Enlightenment movement. Hamann believed reason had desiccated the soul and employed Hume's skepticism to justify the possibility of miracles. Herder would be poised between these quite different positions. He shared Kant's belief in philosophy as a liberating force but did not share his teacher's enthusiasm for universal values. He believed in natural law but denied that that meant human nature was always and everywhere the same. He hated smug French claims of progress and worried about the destruction of local cultures and the domination of foreign peoples, all in the name of Reason. A believer in democracy, he despaired over the cozy alliance between the *lumières* and their supposedly enlightened but often despotic rulers.

All this made Herder, now a Lutheran pastor, turn his sword against the *philosophes*. He challenged their ideals of progress and perfectibility. Their abstract, grandiose notions, he argued, alienated the masses from their folk traditions and their personal histories. Between 1784 and 1791, Herder pressed forward these alternative views in *Ideas for a Philosophy of the History of Man*. In the process, he helped launch what has been called the "Counter-Enlightenment."

Individuals, nations, and cultures must be understood in their historical specificity. Herder rejected the notion that to be modern and rational meant that one must wipe away "superstitious" traditions, culture, and language. And Herder remained skeptical about the power of reason. As Hume had shown, causal knowledge was not objective, but highly contingent. Reason was just a tiny light in the thick, immense jungle. History moved in ways that overwhelmed the capacities of human understanding. "What am I supposed to say about the great book of God that extends over all the worlds and times, when I am barely a single letter in that book and when, looking around, I can scarcely see three more letters?"

What distinguished Herder from other Counter-Enlightenment thinkers was his reliance on natural arguments, not theological ones. Nature—and for Herder that included individuals, nations, and cultures—was an organism driven from within by an inner purposiveness. While this student of Kant never turned his back on the critical import of reason, he privileged this inner will. Like Blumenbach, he considered human development to be the unfurling of a drive that was modified by the environment. Herder's notion of historical development encouraged notions of Providence or fate, for much of what was to come had already been written. This stood in sharp contrast to the narratives of the self and mind created by Locke and his followers in France.

While the *philosophes* proclaimed all men equal, Herder used the philosophical language and logic of the Enlightenment to argue that humans were unequal. He called for the study of humanity and human cultures in their distinctive richness and unique complexity. Herder dreamed of a comparative anthropology for Africans, Asians, Americans, Islanders, denizens of the North Pole, and those from European countries. However, unlike Montesquieu, he did not ascribe national and ethnic differences to external factors such as diet and temperature, geography and climate, but rather looked to innate ones.

Human individuality, Herder concluded, was mostly not the result of accidental events, but rather the twists and turns of our inheritance. Humans were part of the divine, organic plan. They emerged from an active, self-organizing force. To comprehend the source of their complex organization, Herder turned to zoology. Comparative anatomy demonstrated that the orangutan was not far from man. One could even study the emergence of mental life, he concluded, by comparing us with those apes who stood at the brink of reason.

From these studies, Herder developed a hypothesis. Animals for whom smell was essential often possessed large, projecting noses. Upon dissection, these long snouts reflected extended olfactory nerves and an abundance of brain matter. Perhaps the outer form of humans, Herder suggested, might also reflect what was inside. Since innate forces blossomed into external forms, the brain and its relative capacities should be reflected in the contours of the head, not just for foxes and rabbits, but for Asians, Europeans, and Africans, men and women. The Greek male, for example, possessed a fine "crown," with a distinct and ample frontal area, a spacious temple for clear and beautiful thought. "I am persuaded," Herder wrote, "that on this . . . may be erected a valuable science."

⁓

PHYSIOGNOMY WAS NEITHER reputable nor new. As old as the ancient Greeks, this line of inquiry had been revived by Herder's friend, the Swiss priest Johann Lavater, who considered facial characteristics to reveal the contours of a man's soul. Lavater developed a popular following and general opprobrium from the scientific elite. However, casting the soul aside, Franz Joseph Gall took Herder's suggestion for a science of brains and heads and made it his life's work. The science, which Gall called organology, would eventually be remembered as phrenology.

The discovery of Gall's new science remains distorted by the self-promotional narratives that he and his followers created. While he cited Herder often, Gall never publically acknowledged that this author bluntly put forward one of the main theoretical paradigms that, for better or worse, made Gall's name. Against his diverse crit-

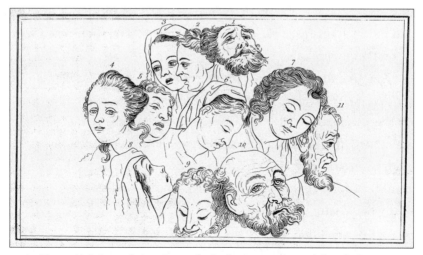

Figure 41. Johann Caspar Lavater's physiognomy proposed that character types could be discerned by facial features.

ics, he never tired of insisting that he was an empiricist who had come to his ideas by observation alone. Much later in life, Gall repeated a tale from childhood: he had been amazed by classmates with a facility for memorization; he not only envied their mammoth memories, but noticed that these lucky boys and girls *always* possessed bulging eyes. He also observed that his playmates and siblings had varied talents—from flowing penmanship to musical gifts—as well as distinct psychologies. Some were arrogant, others meek; there were the frank ones and others who were always secretive. Furthermore, he noticed those personal qualities did not alter. The girl who could easily recite Homer, the boy who sang perfectly on pitch, the bully who was cruel, all carried these traits into adulthood. Years later, a little liar could be counted on to keep telling fibs.

Like Herder, Gall had dissected enough beasts to recognize that different species' brains mirrored the shape of their skulls. The flat skull of a snake and the round skull of a fox held flat and round brains. What if the orators' eyes bulged because of excess brain beneath his orbits? What if liars had different cerebrums? Gall began to link brain structure with discrete mental functions through the use of his new measuring stick, the human skull. If the shape and size of the skull was a valid marker of brain difference, as it was for the snake, the dog, and the monkey, then these observable forms should correlate with mental differences.

The first step was to study hundreds of skulls and see if anything on this outer surface could be found that matched some extraordinary psychic characteristic. Over the next years, Gall sought out anomalies: the absurdly talented and monstrous, the famous, the mad, the ethnically and racially exotic, and the criminal. Vienna's Minister of Police gave him access to prisoners whose histories and skulls the doctor carefully pored over. Another supporter was Dr. Johann Peter Frank, who in 1795 was appointed professor of medicine, head of the Vienna General Hospital, and director of the lunatic asylum. Frank had embraced Brunonian medicine and would transform Viennese medicine into a center for thinking on excess and insufficient excitability within the mind and body. Gall adopted a similar model by which inherited qualities could be exaggerated or diminished in this manner.

Gall spent countless hours trying to categorize various behavior while fingering heads. He began to collect plaster casts of the cranium as well as real ones. His intense desire for strange and special skulls won him a ghoulish reputation. If the Exterminating Angel was under his control, he himself once joked, it would be a dangerous time to be a genius.

As for his method, Gall dismissed critics—he had no need for "the language of Kant" and did not fret about the distorting power of his own subjectivity. Gall confidently strode into the chamber filled with Nature's secrets, secrets that were hiding in plain view. He quickly proclaimed that all mental faculties were obviously housed in the brain, which was the structure that gave rise to the mind and its functions. There were no vital spirits in the brain's ventricles, no moral sentiments bubbling about in the heart, and no passions convulsing the gut. The mind, Gall believed, had become mystified due to its rivalry with the soul. It was simply a natural organ and could be studied in the same scientific manner as the rest of Nature. That study would quickly yield a crucial truth. Just as the nerves of the nose traveled back to a special spot on the brain, mental functions had discrete, independent locations on the cerebral surface. By 1793, even before Gall began to actually dissect brains, he had already come to these conclusions.

At the time, cerebral localization theories had been mostly dropped. After the promising 1672 studies by Thomas Willis, which claimed that memory resided in the cerebrum, research that sought to pin down other mental functions in specific brain locales continued for a while, then collapsed. Modest efforts by researchers like Haller, Vicq-d'Azir, Xavier Bichat, and Samuel Thomas von Soemmerring made some strides, but the complexity of this organ outstripped the capacity of even the most brilliant researchers. By the middle of the 18th century, Albrecht von Haller convinced many that the brain worked as a unity and was not divided into discrete functional parts. Johann Frank, Gall's eminent medical colleague in Vienna, advised him to desist from his studies: there was nothing left to learn from brain anatomy.

Still, Gall began to dissect, guided by the organic principles of Nature put forward by Herder, in which even reason and creativity flowered from the roots and trunk below. His dissections were aided by another premise of Herder's philosophy: as animals became more complex, they added structures and functions to their nervous systems and brains. This led Gall to buck conventional wisdom and approach the brain not from the top, but from below. He was therefore able to track the spinal cord into the midbrain and, through careful dissection, trace the cords and strands of tissue into the lower aspects of the brain.

The results were amazing: discoveries tumbled forth. Gall became the first anatomist to locate the origin of eight cranial nerves and track them up to their homes in the brain stem. He was the first to discover why injuries to the left side of the brain led to right-sided paralyses, and vice versa: the nervous cords twisted and flipped in the lower brain, the so-called pyramids. He was the first to note that different kinds of fibers made up the cerebellum. These discoveries and others would have been enough to immortalize Franz Joseph Gall.

Gall's neuroanatomical researches, however, would fade into the background as he began to make startling claims about the psychological properties of brain regions. Gall first reviewed the literature on the highest faculties. It was a mess. Authorities like Aristotle, Bacon, Descartes, Locke, Bonnet, and Kant differed about the faculties of the mind. While Descartes counted four faculties, Hobbes described two, Locke had a different duo, Bonnet discerned six, and by Gall's count, Kant had some twenty-five. Over time, he correctly noted, the list of mental functions had become indiscriminate, up to the whim of each author.

Gall sought to isolate psychological faculties that could be empirically and biologically confirmed. Prior authors, often uncomfortable or uninterested in the material basis of the mind, did not believe these functions to be organically rooted. Hence, their concepts remained high-minded abstractions, so general in Gall's view as to be meaningless when it came to the biology. The doctor believed it was up to him to establish new and clear categories based on organic structure.

Moving back and forth between his observation of behavior and his study of skulls, Gall set to work. In the end, he postulated that the brain was not one organ but twenty-seven little ones that existed on the surface of the grey matter. Gall accepted a critical analogy from Charles Bonnet; the brain was like a sense organ. It had its equivalent of eyes and ears and taste buds. Each brain organ carried a unique mental function, for a total of twenty-seven in all. Gall discarded the old, abstract faculties like reason, imagination, and will for specific, observable behaviors. For Dr. Gall and the next half-century of phrenologists, human character, behavior, and mental pathology were to be understood by variations of these twenty-seven capacities, such as hope, religious feeling, mathematical facility, consciousness, cunning, thievery, self-esteem, veneration, a sense of metaphysics, and wit. Each of these, he claimed, had been closely observed and each had been scientifically correlated to a spot on the skull.

Much of this can be seen as a desperate attempt to force empiricism to yield answers that the German idealists claimed it could never provide. But Gall also gathered credibility from his exacting study of natural history. Animals, he believed, far from being Descartes's *bête-machines*, had a robust psychology. Animals possessed cunning and experienced joy, pain, and sorrow. The difference between the brains of humans and those of higher mammals was no more than

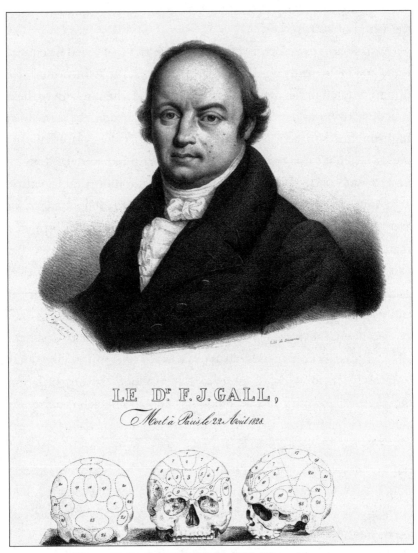

Figure 42. Dr. Franz Josef Gall and his 27 cranial regions.

eight faculties. All humans—no matter what gender, ethnicity, or race—possessed the same functions. However, innate differences in the size and strength of these regions accounted for individuality. In support of this view, Gall cited somewhat similar views that had been voiced by Bonnet, Herder, Cabanis, and Reil. Armed with this new map of the brain/mind/skull, Gall also declared that mental illness could now be diagnosed in a scientific manner. These confusing illnesses could be simply divided up by the particular faculties that were affected. Skull elevations and depressions revealed excessive or defective brain areas and, hence, impaired mental functioning such as megalomaniacal grandiosity or suicidal self-hatred.

While others had hypotheses about the unity of mind and brain, and while some before him had wondered about the relation between the skull, brain, and mind, no one before Dr. Gall had so confidently forged links between all three. By 1796, Dr. Gall began to deliver public courses that described his new *Schädellehre*, his doctrine of the skull. Curious educators, court officials, and theologians flocked to hear him. Two years later, in December of 1798, Dr. Gall wrote a public letter to a censorship official that laid out his basic premises and sought to pacify concerns about his teachings. While human difference was innate, that did not mean that healthy human beings had no capacity to resist an inclination, that man had no free will to make moral choices. However, for some who were ill, there was an irresistible impulse to steal or kill, and in those cases punishment did nothing. These brain defectives were beyond reform. It was crucial for society to recognize that.

Gall's work called for a new age. While Kantians complained about his crude way with causality, Gall brushed them aside, admitting he "never sufficiently appreciated the *a priori.*" His rise in Vienna seemed secure, when on December 24, 1801, Emperor Franz II suddenly decreed that Dr. Gall would no longer be permitted to lecture or publish, for he posed a risk to ethics and religion. The decree indulged in a bit of black humor; Gall's doctrine, it suggested, might cause some to turn to materialism and "lose their heads."

Gall's threat to religious doctrine was real. However, his censoring may have been but a pretext for the machinations of one Andreas Joseph Stifft, the personal physician of the emperor, who maneuvered against not only Gall but also his ally, Dr. Frank. In 1804, after being declared a Jacobin by Stifft, Frank departed Vienna for

Russia. On March 6, 1805, three years after the emperor's decree against him, Gall fled too. He packed up his plaster and wax brains, his collection of skulls, and his monkeys, and with a small entourage left Vienna forever.

GALL'S ARRIVAL IN a new city became a much anticipated event. In Halle, his lecture attracted not just physicians like Johann Christian Reil, but also musicians, artists, and writers, including the author of *Faust*. This wise elder who was by Herder's side when he wrote *Ideas on the Philosophy of the History of Man* seemed eager to see how those speculations had turned out. And Goethe was so intrigued with Gall's claims that he hosted the itinerant doctor in Weimar. Goethe shared Gall's conviction that neither nature nor the mind were machines, but rather organic forms. Despite serious reservations about Gall's twenty-seven mental functions, the great man of letters came away impressed.

Not all were won over. Gall's visit to Halle was recorded by Henrik Steffens. Nature philosophers like him thought Gall's neat division of the self was ludicrous. Through Steffens's eyes, so too was Gall's performance in Halle. He portrayed Gall as a sycophant who sought to win over his audience with fawning praise. He recorded how the Viennese lecturer pointed to the first row, directly at the greatest German writer alive, and asked the crowd to contemplate Goethe's large, evenly contoured cranium, clearly one of universal genius. As the crowd murmured, Gall then pointed to a well-known musician in the audience and proclaimed him to have the typical head shape of musical genius, distinguished by certain bulges above his ears. As Gall moved on to the next prospective genius, his praise was preempted by that man's mocking display of coquettish vanity, which brought down the house.

In some university towns and cities, Gall's craniology was seen as rather close to the hocus-pocus of physiognomy. However, his careful dissections of the brain were revelatory. He exposed structures never before seen. In Berlin, Gall won praise from Dr. Christoph Hufeland, who wrote a long account that defended Gall's brain anatomy while distancing himself from the Viennese doctor's "cranioscopy," his skull-based method of diagnosis. After witnessing Gall's dissections in Halle, Johann Christian Reil also began to passionately immerse himself in brain anatomy. For much of the rest of his career, the man who coined the term "psychiatry" tried to map brain matter. His new method for hardening the brain resulted in discoveries such as the *insula Reili*, the *sulcus circularis Reili*, and *vallecula Reili*. Around Europe, Gall would stimulate such excitement in others: he left behind a mix of serious interest, skepticism, and muffled laughter.

In 1807, Gall's tour left German lands. Though he had influenced university professors like Hufeland, Reil, and Blumenbach, his organology and cranioscopy diminished in Prussia and Austria after Gall immigrated to Paris that October. His work was criticized by post-Kantians for its lazy epistemology; it was anathema to Nature philosophers, for it broke up the unity of self-consciousness. And it was poison to republican Romantics because of Gall's claim that man's inner being was not free, but biologically determined. The influential physician and Romantic biologist Lorenz Oken firmly opposed Gall over the next decades, as did the rising star of the post-Kantians, G. W. F. Hegel, who devoted a number of pages in *The Phenomenology of Mind* to physiognomy and phrenology, and the ridiculousness of regarding bone as a manifestation of man's inner spirit and reality. Had the grandeur of Hamlet's reflections on poor Yorick's skull come to this? he demanded.

In Paris, however organology received serious consideration. In January of 1808, Gall first lectured to the general public. Not surprisingly, Gall's appearance was scrutinized and recorded. He was said to be of middling stature, with large though not coarse features. With a burly chest and strong muscles, a firm step, and a vivid expression, he was not someone who backed down easily. His head, naturally, was "strikingly developed."

In his first lecture in Paris, Gall argued that the most important part of natural history was a bit of unfinished business; a *science humaine*. If known, this would aid individuals in their search for happiness and would guide governments and institutions, so that they fell into harmony with man's natural inclinations. Such a science must bind physiology, psychology, and ethics. More so, if successful, it would reveal the mysteries of discrepant talents and disabilities and offer a deeper understanding of science and art, vice and virtue, crime and insanity, idiotism and the genius of a Bacon or Voltaire.

Science humaine, of course, was Cabanis's term and the ideologues' domain. Paying little attention to their efforts, the Austrian announced his conclusions, which were backed up by "thirty years" of research. As with his earlier attempts at flattery, Gall again went too far in his efforts to win over the audience. The fifty-year-old could not have been working on organology for thirty years; a more truthful number would have been eighteen. However, the neuroscientist was a salesman who meant to impress and persuade. And so, his excessive flourishes continued. He had brought organology, he told these Parisians, to the "center of civilization," the home of the *lumières* and their great sovereign, Napoleon, a vast genius. Later, phrenologists worried that this last bit of obsequiousness had been ill conceived. Napoleon's cranium, like the rest of him, was diminutive. And after making some inquiries, the emperor would take a deep dislike to Gall's notions.

Winning over a popular audience was one thing. Gall knew that oozing praise would not be enough to win over the French experts. Many of these thinkers were devoted sensationalists, such as Maine de Biran, who thought human difference stemmed wholly from varied experience. They scorned organology. Gall would be ready, and ask these skeptics to account for the six-year-old Mozart. Surely, innate differences existed in our brains and minds; in fact, there were twenty-seven differences.

Gall grabbed the attention of the French scientific elite. On March 14, 1808, he presented his findings to a commission of the Institute of France, which included the hospital reformer Tenon, the brain anatomist Antoine Portal, the famous alienist Philippe Pinel, and the naturalist Georges Cuvier. With this group of experts, Gall's hopes for official recognition in France would crash.

The committee observed Gall as he performed his dissections and demonstrations. The chairman, Cuvier, was a well-connected, notorious debunker; he had already taken aim at Germanic Romantic chemistry and had won the nickname "legislator of science" by strictly defining what was and wasn't science. When the Institute's report was published, only his name appeared on it, but it would later become clear that others like Pinel were delighted with the outcome.

Gall had presented his novel and persuasive method of dissecting the brain from the bottom up, as well as his twenty-seven different brain organs, each with their discrete mental functions. The commission disapproved, and their language was harsh: Gall's connections between structure and function were never established. Thus, the doctor's discoveries were nothing but grandiose pretensions. As for his "discovery" that the brain was the organ of the mind, that was hardly news. However, what all serious explorers had discovered, from Democritus to Haller, was a grave, insurmountable problem: "The function of the brain supposes the mutual and still incomprehensible influence of divisible matter and the indivisible Me." This ignorant Viennese had been blind to such troubles. In addition, his claim of being an empirical observer was a farce: organology was his naked conjectures wrapped in the robes of science.

Gall and the master dissector in his entourage, Johann Spurzheim, reacted with a 274-page rebuttal. The brain was the sole source of mental activities, they insisted, pushing back ancient claims made by Aristotle and echoed by some French doctors, like Cabanis, who believed the epigastrium played a role in the passions. And if the examination of the brain led to no overt observations of mental functions, so what? When one dissected the visual nerves, did one expect to see blue skies and green trees?

Scorned, Gall nonetheless refused to be run out of another city. And so, despite this opprobrium from official science, he stubbornly settled in Paris for the rest of his days. He would come to believe that Napoleon himself had condemned his science, but still, his theories spread and his practice thrived. Ambassadors and royalty sought out his services. His theories of cerebral localization and the fixity of human difference penetrated into medicine and anthropology. While Pinel refused to consult on any case that involved Gall, other prominent alienists were not unwilling to share cases with the Viennese doctor.

In 1810, Gall and Spurzheim began publishing their lavishly illustrated account of *The Anatomy and Physiology of the Nervous System in General and the Brain in Particular,* a multivolume work that was only completed nine years later. Their prestige was such that they were asked to contribute the entry on the brain for a French encyclopedia. Gall failed to win over official French science, but he had not been vanquished. He flattered the ambitions of all those who would wish for a stable and empirical mind and brain science. For it would seem that he had united matter and brain anatomy with human agency, will, and action.

In France as in Vienna, Gall's organology would be accused of materialism by religious authorities, who believed it eliminated the soul. Chistoph Hufeland had tried to defuse these attacks when he suggested Gall believed the soul infused the brain and worked through its organization. Gall himself was cagey and mostly sought to distance himself from such questions. At times, he talked about the eternal soul, while at others his soul was mortal. An understandably confused

English commentator wrote that Dr. Gall asserted "the Brain is the organ of the soul, mind, or whatever we please to call it. . . ."

In France, unlike Austria, theological concerns could not kill organology. However, Gall's claims were challenged on scientific grounds. His extravagant claims for brain, mind, and skull forced serious naturalists like Cuvier to study brain anatomy, which one skeptic suggested was the only good Gall accomplished. A surge of interest in brain anatomy followed organology. One of Cuvier's students, Pierre Flourens, developed the important method of ablation experiments, in which aspects of the living brain were destroyed, in the hopes of understanding what function then became altered. His motive was to expose Gall as a fraud, and in the process, he noticed that the cerebellum controlled coordinated movement. While Gall and Spurzheim rejected Flourens's "mutilation experiments," other French doctors began to turn up at the morgue to check Gall's claims for themselves. In the process, they reopened a question that Pinel had shut off when he declared that the brains of the mad were no different from those with other illnesses.

For Gall, proof of his tenets came in part from the study of disease. Since the inception of the mind, great theoreticians had carefully constructed paradigmatic diseases, pathologies that revealed the truth of their own normative generalizations. Followers of Galen pointed to the sluggish, darkened melancholic; Lockean doctors focused on the wacky delusions of enthusiasts; Pinel described driven maniacs, and Reil explored the cracking of the self into madness. For Gall, organology's truths were confirmed by the extreme genius of a child prodigy as well as specific "partial" insanities, in which one highly specific behavior, but not others, became disturbed.

And so Gall butted heads with the celebrated Philippe Pinel. Pinel himself had seriously studied animal skulls and brains, and even considered that human skulls might reflect underlying mental illness, only to explicitly reject that notion. Since skulls hardened at a young age, he concluded, they could not bear the traces of ills that developed mostly after adolescence. Pinel did notice that in one form of mental alienation, idiotism, skull malformations were present. However, after numerous autopsies, Pinel came to the conclusion that mental illness was due to functional changes that occurred without any alteration in brain structure.

Gall allowed for the influence of shocks and environmental influences, but he argued these things were incidental: mental differences were inherited and rooted in brain anatomy. As the Scottish philosophers and doctors once stood for the forces of Nature in opposition to Locke's emphasis on Nurture, Gall challenged the environmental perspective that made Pinel's diagnoses and treatments famous. While Gall tended to be discreet in his opposition, his younger colleague Spurzheim was not. "Moral treatment," he declared, was "synonymous with ignorant and stupid."

In the first years of the 19th century, neither Gall nor Spurzheim possessed anything like the authority of Philippe Pinel. Gall's writings on mental ills were themselves much indebted to the Frenchman's case histories, such as the irresistible tale of the watchmaker who sought perpetual motion. However, the Austrian pressed the view that Pinel's mania was a mixed bag. This category was really a heterogeneous bunch of specific brain disruptions. A man lost his capacity to remember names after a shock; another whose ambition was crushed became convinced he was a general; an upright, reliable woman became a thief for no reason. In all these cases, much of the mind remained intact. Even the wild boy of Averyon preserved a healthy sense of order, the Viennese doctor noted. And so, where Pinel spoke of mania, Gall sought to delineate kinds of mania.

The critique had some appeal, since Pinel was overly fond of handing out this diagnosis. Still, it must have been shocking for the founder of French mental medicine to find his most prestigious follower, J. E. D. Esquirol, and his students, moving toward his rival. Esquirol would remain torn between Pinel and Gall. He would please the latter by successfully replacing mania with numerous monomanias, a diagnosis indebted to Gall that eventually dominated mid-century French asylums.

WHILE GALL'S AUDACIOUS merger of brain, mind, skull, and behavior seemed to be a godsend for those mentalists who yearned for a way to root the mind in the body, it also posed a serious challenge by its emphasis on inheritance. From the start, mentalism held profound political and legal implications. Locke's tabula rasa gave philosophical and scientific standing to Thomas Jefferson's proclamation that "all men are created equal." Sensationalism, ideology, and *traitement moral* all supported this egalitarianism as well as underwriting optimistic efforts at social reform and ameliorative progressive endeavors. In this tradition, human difference was accounted for by experience. Intelligence and stupidity, poverty and wealth, criminality and moral soundness, sanity and madness, were in good part due to the environment that then populated the mind with its myriad of influences. Impoverished circumstances led to impoverished minds. At the same time, through this lens, rights based on supposedly inherited superiority or inferiority were simply masks for the maintenance of feudal privilege. Reparative influences could alter a man: the mind was malleable.

However, following the Counter-Enlightenment ideology of Herder, Gall insisted that humans differed primarily because of their endowment. A being's destiny was mostly dictated by the brain, which had been sculpted by a Hand much greater than reason. A panoply of forces, call it history, went into the making of a body, a self, a family, a village, a city, or a way of life. Through their frail powers, reformers could grasp only so much, and could not presume to improve anything. For Gall, inheritance held a great deal of human fate, as it did for a rabbit or a fox. While some of his followers would try and amend this pessimistic conclusion, it could not be avoided. The individuals with the largest cranial region for intellect would always be the smartest, no matter where they were born. And those whose biological foundation was deficient, would remain that way, even if they were graced by the best of upbringings. And so, Gall's theory posed a direct challenge to faith in the power of enlightenment itself. If the *lumières* wanted to be free of illusions, Gall seemed to announce, here was one: human beings were born wildly different and fully determined, while everywhere they were proclaimed to be equal and free.

Gall made a show of benevolent tolerance; all members of society, no matter how misbegotten, should be accepted. However, democracy was unnatural. Revolution by the masses was a form of insanity. A healthy society took into account different human proclivities: for example, he reported that Negroes had a passionate love for their children, but little capacity for cunning and poor musical capacities. Such endowments could be modified a bit by education, but no amount of practice would make for a Negro Mozart.

Though surrounded by post-Kantian critiques of false objectivity, Gall seemed unperturbed. As with his claims about Negro musicians, he simply banked on widely held social assumption to strengthen his case. In this way, organology never surprised: it did not show that science proved the Greeks were lousy at abstract thought. Without self-consciousness, it used its own methods to reach conclusions that were already widely known. Goethe's head was that of the universal genius. In this way, conventional notions of difference between genders, classes, and races were legitimized, then fed back to the people as science.

The risk that such biases would loop back to the populace as proven certainties never became more apparent than when Dr. Gall discussed a favorite topic: criminals. At the beginning of his tour of German cities, Gall had visited the Berlin and Spandau penitentiaries, where he palpated hundreds of heads. His view was not uncharitable: he believed these individuals suffered from an illness, which compromised their ability to make moral choices. Hence, they should be pitied, not hated. However, there should be no illusions regarding their rehabilitation. Again and again, in these physical examinations, Gall discovered what he knew in advance: thieves all seemed to have elevations in Section 16, the "Organ of Theft." Swindlers inevitably possessed a massive endowment in Section 15, the "Organ of Trickery," a faculty also enhanced in actors and large cats. Apparently, these criminals, like large felines, could not but deceive, for that is what their brains made them do. Against those who denounced Gall for sweeping away free will and moral responsibility, he would allow that education could result in self-control, though it never created or destroyed these constitutional variants. And an inherited faculty did not *totally* determine one's future actions. A patient with a hypertrophic faculty of trickery might become a forger, but if schooled by actors, he could become one himself.

Dr. Christoph Hufeland deeply appreciated Gall. He considered him one of the most remarkable men of the age, one thankfully not possessed by the fashion of Germanic transcendental nonsense. But he anticipated grave social danger if organology was adopted. Gall's desire to apply his science to education, justice, and ethics was unwarranted and perilous. It would lead to a dystopia filled with legions of miserable children whose possibilities had been unjustly neglected and constrained. Based on their skull examinations, "criminals" would be proactively removed from society before they committed a crime. And the dire prediction that all reform was futile would mean "justice more severe not less, to prevent future crimes."

While a number of doctors and men of science were taken in by Gall's logic and language, philosophers, coming after Hume and Kant, saw this as a vulgar parody of empiricism, a crude effort to claim objectivity through experiences that were shot through with subjectivity. They could see how correlations became causal inferences that then hardened into truths, which were then confirmed by the original correlations. When Gall cheerfully admitted that he never quite understood Kant, they could reply that it showed.

And yet, all these defects did not stop phrenology from becoming the single most influential theory of the mind over the next four decades. After so many partial and tentative efforts, theories couched in uncertainty, analogy, and speculation, this siren song linked that elusive entity, the mind, to the brain in the most concrete manner imaginable. It proclaimed itself to be the final chapter in the struggle to establish the mind–brain as a unified natural object. Increasingly the great hopes of over a century of effort to supplant the soul with an embodied mind seemed to be perched on the capacious head of Franz Josef Gall.

The Mind Eclipsed

L ONG BEFORE HIS disastrous Russian campaign, his exile in Elba, and Waterloo, Bonaparte had suffered a crippling defeat. Much of the Frenchman's power lay not just in his vast armies and military brilliance, but also the ideology he wielded. As long as Bonaparte marched under an internationalist, liberationist banner, as long as he fought for reason and freedom against serfdom and the injustice of the old order, he possessed a mighty tool to raise and rally troops, as well as win over oppressed plebeians and reformers inside enemy states. Between 1810 and 1814, the Corsican and his forces squandered that advantage. Despite some reforms, the emperor gradually lost the allegiance of those who once so eagerly placed their liberal hopes in him.

Instead, Bonaparte and his troops became a fearsome tornado. As crops were confiscated and art masterworks were carted off to Paris, around Europe, the supposed champion of *égalité* became a hated figure. The man that Hegel considered the *Weltseele*, this great rational Spirit of Europe, this lover of science and Goethe and Jean-Jacques, became a machine of death. And since he cloaked himself in the rhetoric of the Enlightenment, Bonaparte called into question the very nature of that movement.

By 1812, numerous intellectuals who had welcomed Bonaparte

now fomented popular resentment. In Berlin, Johann Fichte implored his listeners to rise up, and Johann Christian Reil, the fifty-four-year-old medical professor, became so incensed by the injustice of the French that he volunteered for service. Placed in charge of Prussian field hospitals, Reil contracted typhus as it swept through the ranks and died on November 22, 1813. Far away, across the Channel, one-time supporters of Napoleon like the Romantic poets William Wordsworth, Samuel Coleridge, and Robert Southey could not help but concede that their hero had become a festooned thug.

After the Russian debacle, the 1814–1815 Congress of Vienna brought together diplomats to resolve issues that arose during Napoleon's attempt to take over Europe. Negotiations led to agreements between the great powers: Austria, Prussia, Britain, France, and Russia. France brought back the Bourbons and the deceased king's brother, Louis XVIII. Germanic principalities were transformed into a confederation of thirty-four sovereign princes and four free cities, dominated by two large states, Austria and Prussia, run by divine-right monarchies. In Russia, Tsar Alexander, once a devotee of enlightened absolutism, discovered that he preferred plain old-fashioned absolutism.

The great states had taken care to construct a new balance of power that would discourage any future tyrant from seeking total domination. However, as the diplomats returned home, they encountered other fears. In the wake of the French Revolution, monarchs across Europe feared the enemy within. And these concerns were not unfounded: over the next three decades, battle cries would be heard not from foreign states, but from frustrated liberals and angry revolutionaries within their borders. For while new governments sought to turn back the clock, large sectors of the population had not abandoned the promises of freedom, equality, and democracy.

To contain the threat of an uprising, the monarchies of Europe employed large secret police forces and networks of spies; they returned to censorship and cracked down on universities and mass gatherings. Anything that might smell Jacobin, republican, atheistic, or revolutionary was a potential sign of revolt. And so efforts were begun to roll back scientific and medical claims that did violence to the Christian soul.

LOUIS XVIII, the morbidly obese Bourbon king, called for amnesty and a constitutional monarchy in an attempt to win over the throngs who once howled for his brother's head. Prison reform, the abolition of slavery (which Napoleon had restored in 1802), and attempts to alleviate the plight of the mentally ill commenced. Such moderation, however, was short-lived. In 1820, the murder of the king's right-wing nephew provoked a purge in the government and the universities. That year, the École Normale was shut down. Liberals in the philosophy faculties lost their posts. On November 21, 1822, three days after anticlerical demonstrations by medical students, the government dissolved the entire medical faculty. The Chair for Mental Maladies was eliminated and that old revolutionary, Philippe Pinel, was shown the door. When the newly appointed professors convened, they shared a clear purpose. They would cause no problems for the monarchist government or the souls of its Catholic people. The head of the University of Paris declared that religion no longer had to fear false knowledge coming from medicine and physiology. The course on mental pathology, which dared to discuss the interactions of the mind and body, was canceled.

This counterrevolutionary push increased in 1824, when the reactionary Charles X took the throne and reasserted divine right. By then, theological philosophers like Joseph-Marie de Maistre had risen to prominence. Alongside him was the devout Paul Royer-Collard, professor of philosophy at the Sorbonne and archopponent of the ideologues, who were withering under the watchful eyes of the Catholic Church. By 1820, one former proponent, Maine de

Biran, had returned the Holy Spirit back into his model of inner life. But that betrayal would be outweighed by another. In 1824, sixteen years after his death, a secret document appeared that was said to be Pierre-Jean-Georges Cabanis's deathbed conversion.

In fact, the lengthy essay was not such a dramatic departure from Cabanis's earlier writings, but the editors clearly hoped this document would rehabilitate this thinker for more religious times. The short text was larded with 96 pages of editorial commentary that anxiously sought to explain away unacceptable comments. For example, when Cabanis asserted that ancient philosophers dreamed up religions, the editors jumped in with long dismissals of this error. However, one assertion was not contested. Dr. Cabanis seemed to adopt the view that the vital principle could be degraded but never destroyed. It was a line of thought not far from other vitalists like Sauvages and Barthez, but was presented as an end-of-life epiphany of the everlasting life of the soul. While heated debates ensued, it now seemed possible to claim that the fiercely anticlerical founder of ideology had recanted. It was just another nail in the coffin of the human sciences.

Meanwhile, a new philosophical position emerged that was well suited for the times. It was the brainchild of Victor Cousin, a philosopher who had first studied with Royer-Collard and Pierre Laromiguière. Cousin lost his job at the École Normale during the purge of 1820. However, after eight years of wandering, when he studied Schelling and befriended Hegel, Cousin was called back to Paris and restored to his university position. From there, he offered a new philosophical psychology that would be opposed to Locke, phrenology, and human science. Cousin's "eclecticism" merged sensationalism with Catholic faith. It called for the close internal observation of the workings of consciousness, all of which ultimately would be rooted in the soul. His disciple, Jean-Philibert Damiron, started his psychology class at the École Normale by making it clear that the self was merely the face of the soul.

This mix of psychology and religion, Cousin believed, resolved the conflicts of his people and his time. Mental models that denied the soul had led to rampant atheism, lack of personal responsibility, and the French Revolution. Eclecticism would not call for a return to clerical dogma, but would call for a naturalistic investigation of a new unit, the *"moi"*—the me. This unified self was available for empirical study, critical for morality, and did not challenge one's faith. Cousin's "me" was also filled with ambiguity; it could at times be sensational, Cartesian, or Christian. Nonetheless, this confused doctrine shot to prominence.

In 1830, the overthrow of Charles X and the rise of the more liberal July Monarchy ushered in a time of more open debate. Just as the new citizen-king, Louis-Philippe, was neither republican not absolute monarch, France now hovered between its more extreme pasts. In this setting, Cousin's neither-here-nor-there psychology flourished. In 1832, he was appointed director of the École Normale, then was elevated in 1840 to Minister of Public Education. His détente between empiricism and Christianity proved popular and was widely disseminated in schoolbooks.

However, after 1830, such accommodations with the Church could be openly opposed, and they were, not just by an old guard of ideologues, but also by a new generation of even more radical materialists, most importantly Auguste Comte. Born in Montpellier, Comte had come to Paris and lived on the margins of society. In 1830, Comte began to publish a series of works that laid out his positive philosophy, or positivism.

Comte believed that knowledge moved from the theological to the metaphysical to the scientific or positive. For Comte, introspection, central to Cousin's method but also a necessary part of any psychological inquiry that included inner experience, was merely a way to get lost. It could never be the basis for true knowledge. Comte placed his hopes for scientific knowledge about the inner world in phrenology, the teaching of which had been outlawed in 1820, but with the rise of the July Monarchy had been reestablished with the Paris Phrenological Society.

Victor Cousin staunchly opposed Comte and phrenology and, in the subsequent contest of ideas, he held one distinct advantage. As Comte noted, Cousin's psychotheology was not falsifiable and could not, in its essential assumptions, be challenged with evidence. The phrenologists were not so lucky. In 1822, the pious scientist Pierre Flourens presented ablation studies on birds, rabbits, and dogs, and they seemed to show that Gall and the theory of cerebral localization was false. Most brain regions, when destroyed, did not affect discrete functions. Flourens' results were themselves riddled with errors, but his widely proclaimed scientific victory over Gall revealed the receptivity of a community that preferred to follow men who allowed for the soul. Without the soul, both Cousin and Flourens were convinced that the social order would be imperiled.

And so, after 1830 in France, the foundations of mentalism became increasingly tenuous. The mind-body interaction allowed for in vitalism and human science waned. The hoped-for final solution, phrenology, was increasingly doubted. "Psychology" was a term that increasingly returned to spiritualists; it was opposed to physiology, which was studied in a manner that held no possibility of an emergent mental entity.

French practitioners of mental medicine were caught in the crossfire. Given these definitions of psychology and physiology, there would be no mental medicine, for there would be no mind. In this charged atmosphere, French alienists could not easily evade the fact that their field had been founded by a revolutionary who placed no faith in the soul. Clerical pressure was at times acute. An old adage began to circulate: it had it that for every three doctors, one would find four atheists. Since revolutionary times, it was widely assumed that most French doctors were secretly materialists. Now competition with the Church had again become direct: after 1815, religious institutions for the insane made a comeback, run by the Brothers of Charity along with the Grey Sisters.

Some alienists began to advocate for a return to dualism. Their leader was Paul Royer-Collard's brother, Antoine-Athanase, who in 1805 was appointed to direct the Charenton, a position he held until his death in 1825. During the years before the Restoration, this zealous Jansenist opposed Pinel and Esquirol, and stood against the secular tide. When the Bourbons regained power, he was well placed to push for a return to the old Cartesian lines. When Royer-Collard lectured on "mental medicine," there was no mind, only brain physiology and the soul.

However despite these broader pressures, Royer-Collard and his followers remained outmatched by Pinel's prized student, Jean-Étienne-Dominique Esquirol. Born in Toulouse in 1772, Esquirol's early life had been upended by the Revolution. His father was initially in favor of the uprising, but the Terror made him switch sides. In 1799, Esquirol's brother took up arms with Royalist forces, was captured, imprisoned, and executed. With his family now in ruins, Esquirol having already studied medicine in Toulouse, then Montpellier, headed to Paris.

In 1802, he began work in Pinel's private *maison de santé* located on 8 Rue Buffon. On December 28, 1805, Esquirol received his medical degree with a thesis on the passions as causes of illness. Childless, he threw himself into his work, conducting research, dedicating himself to his patients and fostering students, who eventually grew into an impressive network. With the rise of Charles X and his reactionary government, Esquirol benefited from another fact. Pinel was now considered a radical, but Esquirol, whose brother had died for the Royalist cause, was deemed safe. After Pinel was forcibly retired, Esquirol was handed his mentor's job as *inspecteur général des facultés de médecine*.

Esquirol began to refine Pinel's work. Fascinated but also skepti-

cal of phrenology, Esquirol hoped for a more precise diagnostic system for mental maladies. Over the next decades, he chopped Pinel's
mania into three distinct entities: a pure form, another close to melancholia, and a third called monomania. This last illness was Esquirol's invention, but it bore some resemblance to the phrenologists'
partial insanities. However, rather than being due to an overly or
poorly developed brain region, these highly specific forms of insanity
were the result of "fixed ideas" hypercharged by an expansive passion.
Monomanias had no other sign of delirium and otherwise resembled sanity, which meant they made terrible trouble for societies.

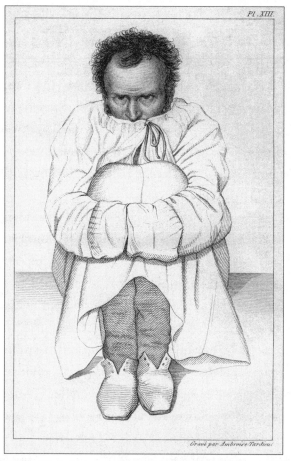

Figure 43. A depiction of paranoia from J. E. D. Esquirol's
Mental Maladies, 1838.

The Crusaders suffered from monomania, Don Quixote was a classic monomaniac, and Martin Luther had a monomania of ambition.

After Royer-Collard died in 1825, Esquirol expanded his power and took charge of the Charenton. Almost overnight, the most common madness in France—nearly 45 percent—became some form of monomania. Esquirol seeded his loyal students throughout the provinces of France. And while his position could at times seem equivocal, he never abandoned mental causes and cures. In fact, they were central to his argument for the most important mental health legislation France had ever considered.

Like Pinel, Esquirol had long advocated for the construction of public institutions to care for the mentally alienated. With the rise of the July Monarchy in 1830, reforms like asylum care were again possible. At the time, there were only eight specialized establishments in France that took care of the mentally ill. In his testimonial in favor of the seminal Law of 1838, Esquirol argued that those struggling with mental illness were often monomaniacs, who suffered from limited, periodic disruptions. Why deprive them of liberty? Many were curable, but healing required isolation to alter bad habits. Asylums were required to pull the mad out of the social network that had contributed to their pathology. Passage of the Law of 1838 made these hopes materialize. Overnight, every *département* in France was ordered to construct a specialized public establishment to receive and treat the mentally ill.

As French mental medicine won its greatest victory, it began to break apart. By 1840, a series of events led doctors to turn against mentalism. The Paris School of Medicine emphasized the search for a lesion in illness, and that model had a great success for the alienists. Many of the mentally ill developed paralyses that did not respond to moral methods, and one of Esquirol's students, Étienne-Jean Georget proposed that some might suffer from brain abnormalities. However, in 1822, a young Royalist doctor, Dr. Antoine-Laurent-Jessé Bayle, working under Royer-Collard, published an astounding new finding. The brains of the mentally ill, he announced, were marked by sickly, hardened outer membranes. In 1826, Bayle expanded his claims: essentially all mental diseases were due to these spiderweb changes of the brain's outer membranes. Madness, he declared, was a meningeal disease.

Esquirol's allies launched a counterattack, and after Royer-Collard died, Bayle had little support. This distant descendent of Pierre Bayle drifted away from medicine. Only later was his discovery recognized as a great one: he had found the residue of neurosyphilis.

Still, Bayle's disease model raised questions about mental theories of alienation. Others, with different kinds of evidence, would soon follow with more challenges. One of Esquirol's students, the doctor Jacques-Joseph Moreau de Tours was sent by his teacher to the Middle East on a therapeutic trip with a patient. In 1840, he returned to France with an astonishing substance called hashish. He joined the Club des Hashischins alongside writers like Charles Baudelaire and became an opponent of one of the last of the fervent mental therapists, the increasingly isolated François Leuret. For Moreau de Tours, hashish chemically induced hallucinations, Esquirol's sine qua non for insanity. Clearly then, insanity was due to this drug, which, he proposed, altered blood circulation. Following Moreau, others would look to ether, opium, alcohol, and cocaine as artificial means to expose the physiological basis for normal mental life and the ruptures of alienation.

With little support from positivist philosophy or natural science, fractured from within, French mental medicine began to lose its mind. The once mutually reinforcing connections of mental medicine with secular liberalism and its ideals of autonomous freedom, equality and toleration, as well as the supporting theories of ideology, sensationalism, and vitalism, unraveled. With phrenology on the decline, French doctors anxiously searched for a way to root their work in the body, and after 1850, they would increasingly turn to a model that opposed any of the sunny environmentalism of Locke's mind. A student of Gall, Bénédict-Augustin Morel, believed original sin found its biological confirmation in brain disease, which was the result of a previous generation's vice. Degenerative heredity accounted for mental illness as a brain disease that was unalterable. It ran in families and ethnicities and was quickly attributed to minorities like Jews.

In 1823, Citizen Pinel died poor and outcast. However, his public image as a humanitarian would be later enshrined. In 1849, a heroic painting was commissioned and hung in the National Academy of Medicine; it depicted the benevolent doctor as he unshackled the mad and tamed them with reason. Though this event never occurred, Dr. Pinel, now an icon of the Revolution, became part of French lore, even as his theories of the mind and his vision of mental health and illness collapsed.

AFTER BONAPARTE HAD been defeated, Germanic reaction was intense against perceived Jacobins, atheists, and rebels. In Habsburg Austria and Höhenzollern Prussia, large, repressive bureaucracies employed police and informants to monitor and control those in the populace who might foment dissent. Archconservatives like the late Justus Möser, who warned that the rule of reason would result in the catastrophic destruction of traditional beliefs and values, seemed vindicated. For the next thirty years, the nobility retrenched and made only minor concessions to liberals and the bourgeoisie.

In this charged atmosphere, as in France, support for claims about the mind began to erode. In philosophy, German idealism, always a mix of naturalism and metaphysical speculation, turned to the latter. Schelling, the founder of Nature philosophy, broke away from his former positions and dove deep into a philosophy dominated by world-souls and the role of the divine spirit, positions he held until his death in 1854.

The later work of Schelling did not win many over. Instead, German universities became filled with the followers of his childhood friend, Georg Wilhelm Friedrich Hegel. In 1806, Hegel published his fascinating, if at times impenetrable, work on the phenomenology of *Geist*—the English translation of which alternated between mind and spirit, and for good reason. For Hegel, sensory perception presupposed a mind that discerned the laws of nature. Therefore, knowledge of the outer world was always predicated on self-knowledge, a turn inward that characterized German idealism and offered the possibility for a naturalistic psychology. However, Hegel then went on to conclude that only *Geist* was real, and that it was infinite, immortal, and free. He created a metaphysics around world-spirit, a willful force that led to progressive change in history like the French Revolution. Hegel's lectures at the University of Berlin, where he taught from 1818 until his death in 1831, spawned a generation of followers, who applied his thought to logic, metaphysics, theology, history, art, law, and politics.

However, after 1831, divisions in Prussian society intruded into these rarefied discussions. Hegel did not believe in individual revolutionary action; the spirit moved in an inevitable manner to the Whole and the True. Older academic followers of Hegel believed that he had determined that what was real was rational, hence right; thus, they could happily support the status quo, including the Lutheran Church and the monarchy. However, a group of students, the Young Hegelians, began to use their teacher in a new way. They believed their teacher claimed the present was an imperfect, alienated state. Orthodoxies must be critiqued and opposed to create the tension required for a new step forward. In the service of such advancement of the world-spirit, these radicals rejected Christianity and, soon, the state. Alarmed, the King of Prussia cracked down on these firebrands, men like Ludwig Feuerbach, Arnold Ruge, and, famously, Karl Marx.

With the return to monarchy and the rise of Hegelianism, the fertile, if at times complex, marriage between German post-Kantian philosophy and the psychology of the mind came undone. Some continued on the older path, such as Johann Friedrich Herbart, who filled Kant's chair in Königsberg and in 1824 proposed to integrate Locke with Romantic notions of inner conflict. But most followed the paths of the Hegelian *Geist*, whether it led them to the Absolute Spirit of God or dialectical materialism and revolution.

And so, when the last and greatest of the post-Kantian idealists, Arthur Schopenhauer, published his extraordinary magnum opus, *The World as Will and Idea* in 1819, it was born out of time. Having studied medicine with Blumenbach, Schopenhauer put forth a biologically rooted philosophy of perception, inner drive, and mind that was no longer in fashion. His epiphany—that Kant's thing-in-itself was an inner, natural drive called the will—would have to wait, as would his psychological model of subjectivity based on an unconscious need. When this brilliant summation of post-Kantian thought appeared, to Schopenhauer's dismay, it was ignored. In Berlin, when he boldly came to challenge the Hegelians, five students signed up for his class, while Hegel's auditorium overflowed. His work would be forgotten until the end of the 19th century, when it was rediscovered.

In biology, the models that linked mind and body, such as vitalism, and Nature philosophy, held on at first; however, by the 1830s, as philosophy split into connoisseurs of spirit and materialist revolutionaries, natural science changed too. In 1839, the biologist Theodor Schwann attacked the Nature philosophers as nonsensical and asserted that the life force in Nature and the mind was not due to sensibility, but rather to God. Other dualists followed and argued for both a pure science of the body and a return to the Bible for the soul.

However, a new, more radical critique emerged and would prove decisive. This *coup de grâce* for German theories of an embodied mind came not from Pietists, but was delivered by a graduate student rebellion against the scientist Johannes Müller. Müller was one of the greatest biologists of his time, a man who like J. C. Reil was a vitalist as well as a materialist. Between 1833 and 1840, he produced a mammoth authoritative compendium, *Handbook of Human Physiology*, which included 82 pages on mental processes. There he discussed associations, sensations, ideas, as well as illusions and hallucinations. His own landmark research into the nature of visual illusions seemed to verify a basic tenet of German idealism. Müller showed that manual pressure, electrical stimulation, and light stimulation on the optic nerve all produced the exact same effect: light and color. Hence, it followed that external stimuli were not directly recorded in the brain, but were in part created there. The mind, he concluded, made its own reality.

As Johannes Müller established the subjectivity of perception, his students revolted. Disgusted by Hegelian speculation, they also became skeptical of their teacher, and became eager to turn physiology back to mechanistic models. To do so, they rejected the methods that allowed for life forces and mental causes: in opposition to this, they adopted a strict reductionism. All complex life phenomena including mental ones, they declared, must be explained at the level of physics and chemistry. Those were the only determining forces. And unlike Theodor Schwann, these doctors and men of science did not also resort to religion. They believed that a fully materialist and reductionist model of life would require no inner force, no active matter, no mind, and shockingly, no soul or God-force. The brain and the body's matter would alone suffice.

Müller's students would go on to greatness. By 1842, Emil du Bois-Reymond had recruited Ernst Brücke to his cause: Hermann von Helmholtz and Carl Ludwig soon joined in their lab conspiracy. In 1847, they declared in unison that they would pursue the processes of life with physics and chemistry only. While some prominent French physiologists like Louis Pasteur and Claude Bernard maintained a commitment to vitalism, that would not be true in German labs. The Biophysics Movement of 1847 would spread out from Berlin to dominate German biological science for the next half-century. It was not until three decades later, after their research program ran aground, that Hermann von Helmholtz would acknowledge the failure of their approach with regard to the mind and return to a mixed model of physiological forces and ideas.

This hard shift toward materialistic reductionism caught up with Reil's psychiatry, which had only just begun to be institutionalized. In 1805, at Bayreuth, the first state mental asylum hired a doctor and a teacher to be supervised by the judiciary, thanks to the efforts of J. G. Langermann. In 1806, the Association of German Alienists was founded. During 1810, in Heidelberg, a Nature philosopher and doctor, Alexander Haindorf, was the first to teach psychiatry at a university. In 1811, the first university chair for psychical medicine was established at the University of Leipzig; the recipient was the most important of Reil's followers, and the man who would do the most damage to his legacy.

As the first professor of psychiatry in German lands Johann Christian Heinroth was poised to spread Reil's model, much as Esquirol had done for Pinel in France. However, Heinroth injected the Holy Spirit into his idea of the mind. He proposed that there were three levels of consciousness. World consciousness was the experience of pleasure and pain, which all animals possessed. Self-consciousness was a state that organized inner human longings. And the highest and God-given level of consciousness, the conscience, regulated mankind by frequently opposing the desires of the other two forms of consciousness. Through this inner voice, the elect transcended the self's narrow confines and became dedicated to Him.

Reil had no supernatural forces in his theory of the mind, and this difference between the two became stark when Heinroth discussed mental illness. Mental suffering and madness were failures to abide by the demands of conscience. Since the conscience came from Heaven, it was pure and blameless. Those who chose to defy the Lord would suffer, because the wages of sin was madness. To treat such failures of conscience, Heinroth called for "psychical doctors."

The Leipzig professor used the term psychical doctor interchangeably with psychiatrist, and his hierarchy of consciousness along with his theory of inner conflict leading to illness manifested his debt to Nature philosophy and the Romantics. However, Dr. Heinroth's theory of the conscience represented a rearguard action in which the insane were again guilty sinners whose transgressions made them mad. Critics assailed him, but Heinroth remained unmoved. The psychical doctor must establish a close alliance with the patient, he advised, so as to penetrate his guilty states, provoke a confession of sin, and then proceed with reeducation. This doctor's conviction was that biblical ethics alone would preserve one's sanity and that the mad had been bad. No one who was innocent could be found in an asylum.

The prolific Heinroth wrote extensively and applied himself to anthropology, criminology, and the history of his new field. His account of psychiatry paid homage to Chiarugi, the great Pinel, Langermann, and Reil. He also took pains to distinguish himself from Reil and saved his highest praise for the soon-to-be disgraced Ernst Horn. A psychical therapist, Horn nonetheless had adopted the same brutal means once meant to tame the madman's body. He preferred an alternative to the straitjacket called the "sack," into which an unruly patient was stuffed, a method that soon resulted in a patient's death and Horn's resignation. Heinroth similarly considered medications and restraints to be indirect psychical methods to control his mad sinners. He was not averse to an array of tortures such as confining belts and chairs, Cox's swinging chair, a device that stopped screaming by cramming a wooden pear into the mouth, and a casket called "the box." Far from the moral treatment of the Tukes or Pinel, Heinroth and Horn offered a treatment tailored to sinners who would be forced to repent.

With Reil dead, Heinroth helped precipitate a schism in the fledgling field of German psychiatry. He was joined by others who stressed the psychic and at times spiritual foundations of mental illness. Known as the *Psychikers*, these doctors broke apart the mixed models of body and mind. For example, in 1817, Albert Matthias Vering published *Psychological Medicine,* two hefty volumes in which he examined everything from the impact of a mother's fantasies on her fetus's growth to psychic cures of tetanus, paralysis, epilepsy, and hysteria. An 1824 textbook called *Contributions to a Purely Psychological Exposition of the Science of Mental Disorders* said it all in the title. A prominent exponent of this "its all in your mind" model was the influential Karl Ideler, who became chief of mental diseases at the Berlin Charité Hospital, a position he held from 1828 to 1860. Introspective, religious, and moody, Ideler saw morality as absolute and believed that secret contradictions in the mind led to mania, melancholia, and criminal violence. He preached reform to patients, and when that didn't work, resorted to the rotating chair, the box, and other devices that Dr. Horn, his disgraced predecessor, left behind.

The *Psychikers* were met by an opposing group of alienists known as the *Somatikers.* J. B. Friedreich, a professor at Würzburg, recoiled at the use of sin, guilt, or mental conflict in madness. His extensive studies, he believed, proved the somatic nature of all mental illness, a fact anyone could discern by the distinct odor each form of madness exuded! Like numerous other exclusively mechanistic thinkers before and after him, Friedrich was a dualist who thought it sacrilegious to speak of the soul in science. Dr. Heinroth, he believed, had returned medicine to premodern theories of guilt and possession. This was nonsense. Penitentiaries had little mental illness, and kind, virtuous people could go crazy.

From 1820 to 1848, the *Psychikers* and *Somatikers* traded polemics. For example, Karl Ideler accused the mechanists of eliminating human freedom, thereby absolving murderers of their guilt. Somaticists urged their colleagues to leave the inner world and moral questions to pastors. In this debate, Reil's few followers were caught in the middle. Some, like Christian Friedrich Nasse, held on, but others gave up their teacher's complex integration. From Bonn, where he ran an asylum, Maximilian Jacobi became a *Somatiker* and Heinroth's most prominent opponent. In his view, mental medicine required no mind. It should focus exclusively on the diseased brain.

After 1848, German psychiatry was dominated by brain doctors who joined forces with the biophysicists, who now dominated natural science. Doctors, it was declared, would no longer need to be concerned with false ideas, sensibilities, problems of consciousness, will, or inner conflict. The real culprit in mental illness was the brain's dysfunction. In 1845, Dr. Wilhelm Griesinger famously declared that all mental illnesses were localized brain diseases. While even a cursory reading of this doctor's writings shows how much he acknowledged psychic causes for illness, this adage took on a life of its own and was taken to support a brain-only model of psychiatry. In German lands, a science of the embodied mind was now considered a misstep, a conceptual error, and in the final affront to the radical naturalizing impulse of some of its originators, a puff of mysticism.

THE YEARS PRIOR to the French Revolution had been fairly tranquil ones in Great Britain. Thanks to decades of toleration and freedom of conscience, old dissenting sects lost their zealotry and become integrated into this constitutional monarchy. Censorship was on the wane, as rational religion as well as liberal proposals for social reform became commonplace.

The first tremors from the crumbling old order in Europe did not shake Britannia. However, by 1791, English Jacobins emerged to call for the dissolution of the monarchy, even an end to private property. Unrest now shook the homeland, which faced near-famine conditions, the threat of French invasion, and the prospect of an internal revolt. Those suspected of revolutionary sympathies were sought out by furious anti-Jacobins, such as the mob that burnt down Joseph Priestley's home. Four decades of counterrevolution commenced in England and Scotland.

Vitalism, post-Kantian idealism, Nature philosophy, and Romantic thought had all filtered across the Channel, inspiring British romantic scientists, doctors, and poets. Thought, Samuel Taylor Coleridge wrote, reflecting these sympathies, was a blossom of the human plant. Kantian critiques of British empiricism and the Jena school's emphasis on freedom stimulated radicals. They too concluded that the human mind was free, active, willful, creative, and distorting. It was neither soul nor machine.

The writers, William Wordsworth, Samuel Coleridge, and Mary Shelly were but a few who were waist-deep in this torrent of ideas, alongside natural scientists, none of whom was more influential then the physician Erasmus Darwin. A polymath whose work on biology, human evolution, the mind, and disease would be eclipsed by the monumental achievements of his grandson, Charles, Erasmus Darwin was a celebrity during his lifetime. After years as a busy physician, in 1768, after breaking his patella in a carriage accident, the housebound doctor began to pursue the nature of the mind with a private paper that conceived of it as part of the "animal System." When this alarmed Reverend Richard Gifford, Darwin, a Deist himself, assured the reverend that he would not publish anything that might endanger public morals.

Reputed to be the most learned man in England, Dr. Darwin began to construct a massive taxonomy for all living things. In 1794, his *Zoonomia* appeared, a 1,300-page account of the natural world dedicated to those who studied the operations of the mind and practiced medicine. Alongside his theory that the earth originated from a volcanic eruption on the sun, Darwin put forward an evolutionary model of animals and a theory of mental life based on conscious and unconscious streams of association. His efforts were initially applauded and influenced many. However, as the political atmosphere changed in Great Britain after the French Revolution, Darwin was cast in a new light. By 1798, this once-lauded genius was censured in reactionary periodicals like *The Anti-Jacobin*. Unbowed, he wrote his 1803 poem, *The Temple of Nature.* In iambic pentameter, Darwin described the emergence of life and the mind, and managed such feats as rhyming the nerve's silver train with its station in the brain. For his troubles, the doctor was accused of being an atheist, a Jacobin, and a miserable poet.

Even in stable, liberal England, angry arguments over vitalism broke out. In 1814, a famed London surgeon, John Abernethy, delivered a lecture in which the vital force in mankind was not sensibility, complex organic structures with emergent functions, or the natural forces of electricity and magnetism, but simply God. The rest was nonsense from godless Frenchmen and Germans. Abernethy was shocked to find his views quickly rebutted by his own protégé, Dr. William Lawrence. Having studied with Blumenbach in Göttingen, this physician to the Shellys openly leaned on French ideologues, theories of sensibility, and German doctrines of complex biological organizations with emergent functions. Abernethy's life force was nothing more than a primitive superstition, Lawrence declared. He called for a naturalistic psychology that would henceforth emancipate mankind from all religions.

So began the contest. Abernethy attacked Lawrence and his allies as Jacobin provocateurs. Lawrence shot back that only the Americans were still free to think, now that the mighty had turned Europe into "one great state prison." Students excitedly took sides, and Lawrence's patient, Mary Shelley, was inspired to write her 1818 novel *Frankenstein, or The New Prometheus.*

After the fall of Napoleon, liberal Great Britain became more repressive. In 1815, an archconservative Parliament raised taxes, which caused riots in London. The authorities restricted public assembly and even suspended habeas corpus. In 1819, radicalized workers tried

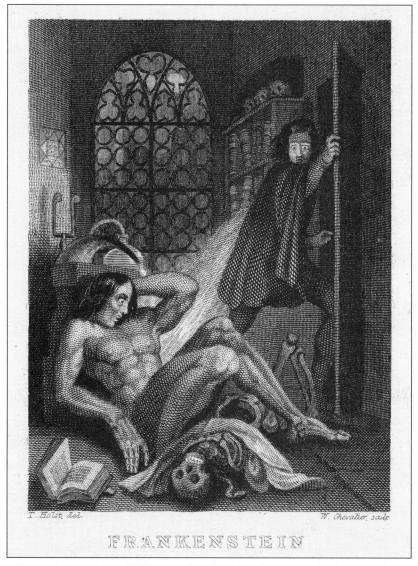

Figure 44. From Mary Wollstonecraft Shelley's *Frankenstein, or the New Prometheus.*
The scientist witnesses the stirrings of his monster.

to assassinate the entire Tory cabinet. In this tense atmosphere, in
1822, Lawrence had his copyright protections rescinded when his
writings were deemed to impugn the Scriptures.

The turmoil reached down into medical practice. The publica-

tion of Samuel Tuke's *Description of the Retreat at York* in 1813 brought
a damning critique of medical orthodoxy and painted a bright picture
of gentler, more effective treatment via nonmedical moral treatment.
In 1815, a Select Committee was ordered by the House of Commons
to consider abuses in the madhouses and the need for regulation.
Testimony revealed gruesome methods used by medical men. For
example, in 1806, Dr. Joseph Mason Cox, an insanity specialist, was
inspired by Erasmus Darwin to build a rotary machine, in which
strapped-in patients were swung in a circle until syncope and near
death. The Edinburgh-trained Philadelphia doctor and signatory of
the Declaration of Independence Dr. Benjamin Rush believed problems in blood circulation led to madness, so he thought it sensible to
employ his machine, the Tranquillizer. Perhaps these actions could
be medically justified, but what was the Committee to make of the
fact that some doctors sang the praises of one contraption, while
others thought it medieval torture?

Meanwhile, the rise of moral treatment among Quaker nonmedical practitioners had posed a direct challenge to the medical
monopoly on care for the mentally ill. And these treatments would
seem to be appropriate for a large number of sufferers, who, thanks
to Locke, Battie, Willis, and the British mad doctors, were deemed
to have a psychic cause for their illness. In 1810, Bethlem Hospital
admitted over half of its patients with causes that were deemed to be
mental. Sufferers were offered entry after misfortunes in love, grief,
jealousy, fright, and too much study.

However, while these were recognized psychic causes, most
British doctors had not been won over to mentalist cures. In Great
Britain, the most prominent research program concerned with the
mind had stopped trying to root psychic events in the brain. Associational psychology, fostered by James Mill, rejected the vibrating
mind-body connections of David Hartley. In his 1829 *Analysis of the
Phenomena of the Human Mind,* Mill quoted Locke's refusal to specu-
late on the physical roots of ideas. While some like Thomas Brown,

a Scottish doctor, tried to merge associationalism with nervous physiology, the dream of integrating these would recede.

A smattering of scientific theories of the mind popped up outside
of associational psychology. Edinburgh's Dr. Thomas Laycock called
for mental physiology, and the prominent London doctor John Con-
noly offered up his medical psychology. In 1835 the physician to the
King of Scotland, John Abercrombie, asked the British Association
for the Advancement of Science to include mental philosophy as a
branch of physiology, insisting it was critical for medicine. And in
America, Rufus Wyman and Amariah Brigham insisted mental philosophy was critical for medicine and the health of Americans.

However, despite these scattered efforts, none of these individuals had a novel approach or method, much less a powerful synthesis
that could solve the medical men's woes. Thus, they stood in peril of
being thoroughly discredited as unscientific ignoramuses and brutish, ineffective practitioners. Encouraged by Samuel Tuke and his
asylum's high rate of cure, the state began to plan the construction of
asylums. Scandal-ridden and internally divided, the mad doctors sat
on the outside looking in.

Their savior appeared on the horizon with a collection of skulls
and caged monkeys. Franz Joseph Gall visited England but once;
however, his colleague Spurzheim made two tours in a largely successful effort to gain a foothold for Gall in England and Scotland. In
his wake, a heterodox movement emerged led by devoted followers
like George and Andrew Combe. In 1815, one devotee, Thomas
Forster, coined a new term for organology that would stick: he called
this would-be science of the mind "phrenology."

Phrenology came at an opportune time for British doctors. They
were compelled by the clear and unequivocal statement that the brain
was the organ of the mind, and that functions of the mind when
pathologic must have structural disruptions in cerebral anatomy.
While some worried about the absence of the soul, one could sneak
the heavenly spirit into Gall's brain and make it the first cause.

Phrenology also allowed doctors to firmly oppose treatments offered by their religious or lay competitors. It linked the mind and mental ills to the brain and the skull, surely the purview of doctors. Insanity was a disease of the brain, an inherited abnormality that manifested itself in an illness of the mind. Disrupted mental functions emerged from different brain organs. Furthermore, followers of Gall could tout this as not just a theory of mental illness, but a new human science of behavior. It was almost too good to be true.

Then it got better. In Britain, phrenologists took a dramatic turn away from Gall's more gloomy conceptions of human possibility. For him, innate forces almost completely determined a woman or man's fate. When Christoph Hufeland first considered Gall's work in 1805, he recognized this fatalism and concluded that Gall had nothing to offer medical therapeutics. Instead, he seemed to have discovered how each of us was doomed. However, in Great Britain, liberal followers seized upon some of Gall's equivocal statements and sunnily emphasized phrenology's ameliorative possibilities. Exercise could build up weak faculties. Strengthening countervailing faculties could cure those who had a pathological excess. Battie and Tuke's therapies could now be woven into this medical science. Its effects could be framed as the result of specific exercises on specific brain regions.

Phrenology also complemented traditional authority since it naturalized social hierarchies. The elite deserved their privileged position, it could be argued, because they had inherited better brains. As the government clamped down on radical dissent from a growing class of workers, this conservative implication of Gall's thought was moderated by an array of bourgeois reformers who advocated, not for the end of property or monarchy, but more modestly, for better conditions for prisoners, paupers, aborigines, children, and lunatics. For these concerned citizens, phrenology became a congenial framework that guided their efforts. Against radical Levelers and Jacobins, phrenology supported the social status quo, while it left room for self-betterment. One philanthropist complimented Gall and Spurzheim for "having originated the simplest, and by far the most practical, theory of the human mind."

At the same time, there was a great deal to doubt in phrenology. Gall's "cranioscopy" was the least attractive part of his theory, but it served as a critical link from his otherwise debatable observations about the mind to the brain. Skull topography was proof that there were twenty-seven, not twenty-six or twenty-eight, faculties. Without those bony bumps and divits, phrenology dissolved into pure conjecture.

While British medical men adopted phrenology. Gall engendered a good deal of hilarity in the popular press. Magazines like the *Plain Speaker* ran scathing accounts of this new craze. Thomas Carlyle reported attending an 1817 lecture by a cranioscopist, a man much "addicted to building hypotheses," who nonetheless spurred Carlyle to study phrenology. All its precise measurements of the skull proved

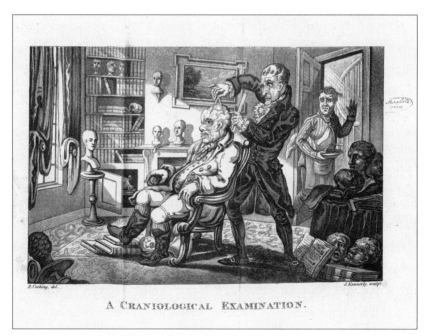

A CRANIOLOGICAL EXAMINATION.

Figure 45. From *Craniology Burlesqued in Three Serio-Comic Lectures*, by "A Friend of Common Sense," 1818.

nothing, he concluded. A man's soul was better reflected by the shape of his abdomen. However, phrenology, he predicted, if presented dogmatically, would win over many. A few years later when a phrenological journal verified his forecast, Carlyle wrote: "Error and stupidity are infinite in their varieties, eternal in duration."

Phrenologists fought back. Some of the fiercest debate took place in Edinburgh, where Spurzheim traveled to do battle. The philosophical descendants of David Hume rejected Gall's naïve causal claims, and brain anatomists dismissed his brain organs as quackery. Astonishingly, in the debate, neither of these groups of naysayers prevailed. In 1815, Spurzheim conducted a dazzling demonstration of brain dissection that was filled with so many new findings of lower structures that it became obvious he knew far more anatomy than his doubters. From there, he assumed the authority of science to dismiss their other claims. Phrenology had provided a straightforward answer to the problems of the mind and body. Q.E.D.

A few years later, in 1820, the Edinburgh Phrenological Society was established. In 1823, the London Phrenological Association was also founded, and that same year the Royal Society took up debate on the subject. Well-known alienists and distinguished asylum superintendents like W. A. F. Browne, John Conolly, and Richard Poole emerged as contributors to the *Phrenological Review*. For them, phrenology elevated moral treatment into a new psychobiology and psychopathology. It explained why one man was cunning, why a child could not read, and why a nymphomaniac could not stop herself. When in 1837, W. A. F. Browne, former president of the Royal Medical Society of Edinburgh, wrote his influential *What Asylums Were, Are, and Ought to Be*, he situated his efforts among progressive attempts to ameliorate the lives of the downtrodden and dedicated the book to the phrenologist Andrew Combe. Browne called for a new and "perfect Asylum, a Utopia" in which benevolence ruled alongside treatment of the human mind based on Gall's new science.

At the same time that phrenology was on the rise, mental medicine began to be institutionalized throughout Britain and the United States. In 1823, in London and Edinburgh, the first sparsely attended lecture courses in psychiatry were offered by Dr. Alexander Morison. Morison pressed Edinburgh for a professorship of mental diseases and helped reopen St. Luke's Hospital to young physicians who wanted clinical instruction. In 1841, an official British organization for mental medicine, the Association of the Medical Officers of Asylums and Hospitals for the Insane, was formed. Ten of the twenty-three medical superintendents of the public asylums in England and Scotland were phrenological doctors.

However, after 1840, a new generation of scientists and doctors increasingly considered phrenology an embarrassment. The Combe brothers did not help when they expanded the original number of faculties to thirty-six, which raised the question of why not forty-six? Was the answer based on scientific truth or dogma? Gall's original edifice shook again when George Combe attempted to integrate phrenology with Christianity and precipitated a schism among his loose alliance of pastors, jurists, and doctors. Meanwhile, autopsies continued to find nothing that supported the skull doctors.

By the 1840s, it became clear that the British alienists' grand wager on Gall was lost. A substantial number of doctors in the land of John Locke had committed themselves to a massive but ill-founded integration of thinking and the thing that did it. Draped in the garb of science, phrenologists had stretched past all evidence in the hopes of a final theory that tied empirically observable signs with specific mental functions in brain locales. In the end, they were left to inhabit a mansion made of air. As the prestige of phrenology plummeted, so too did that of mental therapies. During the second half of the 19th century, asylums began to be overcrowded dumping grounds, hardly a place of the individualized care of a Willis or a Tuke. Simultaneously, patients were now conceptualized not as vulnerable to the sensations and ideas that came from their environment, but rather as impermeable brain-disordered people who had little hope for recovery. English-speaking doctors on both sides of the Atlantic retreated from discredited mental treatments to practice their limited craft on diseased constitutions, nerves, and brains. The mind and its problems would be left behind.

Epilogue

IMAGINE A TIME in the future when your mind might travel. Perhaps it would fly from your flesh, a flickering theater of inner experience. Being immaterial and immutable, it might come to rest in a land of eternal consciousness. Call it Heaven. Early modern Christians like Marin Mersenne, René Descartes, and Robert Boyle preserved this hope in an increasingly desacralized world.

According to a different tradition, however, your mind could not travel so lightly. To make this trip, a host of Enlightenment thinkers insisted, the psyche would need to bring along the brain, hauling the grey and white organ that somehow held your faculties of cognition and memory. After 1750, some physiologists argued that your interior world would still not be whole, unless accompanied by its spindly tree of nerves. Others would go further and claim that a mind could not go anywhere without the entirety of the body. And off to the side, as this debate continued, laughter might be heard from those who considered all this a joke, since the mind was no more than a myth and a fallacy.

By 1815, all of these positions had been established. When a second wave of mentalism swept through the Western world during the 20th century, these positions would resurface and some of the same dramas would be restaged. Recurrent, unresolved battles over the mind, the soul, and the brain meant modernity would be characterized by these competing conceptions of human nature, each of which held powerful political, scientific, medical, and philosophical ramifications.

For religious traditionalists, Romantics, and Counter-Enlightenment thinkers, a naturalized mind remained a poor substitute for the life of the spirit. By embracing mechanical views of science for everything except inner life, post-Cartesian Christians believed they accommodated modernity with its skepticism and materialism, while also saving their souls. Truths about the soul were supported by Descartes's logical exercises and those of subsequent dualist philosophers, but more broadly were based on faith in Judeo-Christian authority. These commitments gave believers inspiration and resilience in the face of suffering, but as 17th-century thinkers could not fail to note, such nonrational, absolute beliefs also led to bloody strife. Too often, the result was soul doctrines that called for righteousness, virtue, and love, while their communities went to war led by zealots acting in God's name.

A modern circle of mentalists arose in reaction to this instability in Western Christendom. Following Hobbes, Gassendi, and others, John Locke established a competing tradition that centered on a natural mind endowed with capacities for rational reflection, ethical action, and free will. While the mind was the basis for consciousness, conscience, creativity, desire, and personhood, it was also limited and fallible, generating illusion, error, prejudice, and different forms of what could now be called mental illness. Nonetheless, political and social structures, it would be argued, should be constructed around autonomous individuals endowed with minds that afforded them the right to rationally choose their own beliefs and pursue happiness, as long as they were sane and did not endanger others or the state.

Mentalism thus helped give birth to secularism and liberalism. Theories of reason underwrote attacks on supernatural beliefs tied to theories of divine right and religious orthodoxy. A mind constructed from its earthly influences also gave support to doctrines of toleration. Since different ethical values and faiths sprang up from varied mental experiences, theoretically the Jesuit, the Quaker, and the Hindu should be all accepted. Insofar as the mind was structured by experience, mentalist theories were ameliorative and buoyed belief in human progress and social reform. And so, in these ways, the doctrines of naturalistic psychology, mental medicine, hedonistic ethics, environmental determinism, toleration, individual rights, and cultural relativism all stood together against the feudal order and the politics associated with the Christian soul.

However, despite the power of this theory of mind to unite so many strands of Enlightenment belief, mentalists faced grave problems of their own. The Terror and the turn to dictatorship in France seemed to prove that reason alone was not enough to secure public safety and morals; rather, it seemed to be a plaything that could be twisted by mad passions. Locke's emphasis on the contingency of human knowledge and the formative power of accidental experience did not reassure: it would be strongly challenged by those who looked to inherent capacities for more stable human attributes, thus setting in motion debates that continue to this day over what in human beings is acquired and what is innate. In addition, the initial assumption that conscious ideas were the mind's sole currency would engender rebuttals from Spinoza's theory of emotion, Scottish schools of sympathy, French accounts of sensibility, Puységur's unconscious ideas, and German theories of desire and will. In the future, advocates of the mind would bounce back and forth between these positions.

Alongside these internal disagreements, mentalists constantly struggled to secure the mind's status as a natural object. To do so, doctors, physiologists, and anatomists confronted the riddle of how passive matter might make for active consciousness. In the 18th century, influential schools of medicine adopted frameworks in which the body possessed not a divine *anima*, but a natural spark. Materialistic forms of vitalism and Romantic biologists claimed that mental activity was an emergent bodily property. From these generative, though highly problematic models, a psychobiological subject was constructed at the crossroads of nervous biology, selfhood, and culture. Like Rousseau's little Émile, this sensible being developed over time, was reactive to inner and outer forces, and could be susceptible to a range of disruptions from indigestion to mania to matter previously considered immoral but now considered unhealthy.

However, as Kant's critique exposed, attempts to close the gap between mind and body rested heavily on analogies and wishful thinking. Knowing the mind of another was no straightforward task. Introspection and analysis too often ended up serving preordained conclusions, as demonstrated by Christian rationales for religious toleration that managed to exclude Jews or male doctrines that confirmed their gender's superiority. The epistemological problems of creating an objective science of subjectivity could easily land one in a hall of mirrors. German-language doctors and writers embraced this vision of the mind as a willful and desirous force that figured the self and the world. Mental life, some post-Kantians concluded, was due to a powerful self's striving, and its ills came from fragmentation, inner conflicts, and the psyche's need to be blind to itself.

By 1815, these different conceptions of the mind had laid down roots in England, Scotland, France, Switzerland, the United States, and German-speaking lands. If no single theory conquered all, that was not just due to local allegiances and nationalism, but also to the fact that each model was clearly incomplete. No one explained the entirety of the intellect, passions, and will, the mind as constitutive and imitative, capacities that might be innate or learned, and the role of the conscious and the unconscious. No one could solve the riddle of how a book could write and read itself. The closest thing to an overarching synthesis was that disastrous failure, phrenology.

For years to come, Gall's project would act as a cautionary tale. His careful anatomical dissections granted him respect and authority to make broad claims that cohered with scientific principles but were otherwise empty. His map of skull bumps was no Holy Grail, but it did inadvertently expose a vexing problem. Unlike any other empirical object in Nature, the mind's presence is immediately apparent to itself, but opaque to all external observers. Mentalists therefore have been required to seek out indirect empirical validation of consciousness and its attributes. At times, these efforts could become desperate, stretch beyond evidence or legitimate theory building, and head down Gall's road to the town of make-believe.

For some, there was a different lesson to be learned from the failure of phrenology. After 1848, an intellectual community of radical reductionists coalesced who dismissed the soul and the mind altogether. Heirs to Mesmer and La Mettrie, these doctors and scientists proposed that the brain and its physical quantities alone accounted for reason, ethics, and psychic life ills. Minds, spirits, and souls were all superstitions. Man was a nervous machine, whose seeming self-regulating and creative properties were delusions. Focused on physics and chemistry, these researchers conceived of ideas and thoughts as effects, never causes. Reason and knowledge did nothing.

During the second half of the 19th century, these views, generated most prominently by French positivists and German biophysicists, carried beyond universities and labs into public discourse. However, while these scientists could point to new knowledge regarding basic processes of the nervous system and evidence that heredity was the cause of some mental traits and illnesses, they could do little more than stand quietly befuddled before the everyday workings of the mind. Their brain was a machine, and a machine did not grow, learn, or develop; it did not decide to change its hairstyle or learn a new language. If mentalists could not demonstrate exactly how ideas caused some bodily actions, brain anatomists could not prove otherwise.

Nonetheless, surrounded by speculations about skull bumps, world-souls, and vital forces, these scientists rose in prominence by positioning themselves as guardians of the Enlightenment. They offered to rid mankind of the superstition that reason and intention were anything more than a cascade of chemical and physical forces. Theirs then was a quite different kind of enlightenment, one that cast off many of the *philosophes'* beliefs. However, as with Mesmer, these radicals demanded a good deal of blind faith; they asked others to ignore everyday observations that defied not evidence, but rather closely held, scientific principles. Reductionism meant that, in the end, ideas had to be powerless. The extrusion of any intention, any *telos,* from Nature meant that any science of inner life—before it got off the ground—must be denied the possibility of motivated action. And yet, all day, people seemed to act based on their thoughts. Furthermore, while a comet did not streak across the sky to get to its destination, it seemed quite possible that men and women sometimes did walk, jog, or sprint to get to theirs.

Dismissive of *science humaine, Geisteswissenschaft,* and the humanities, this vanguard spread the hope that natural science could someday answer questions posed not just by anatomy and physiology, but also by ethics, politics, psychology, and history. As these scientists garnered power, however, their soaring ambition threw their own contradictions into relief. In Vienna, Berlin, and Paris, creative, rational scientists stepped forward to argue that the mind was incapable of reason and creativity. The more willfully they argued for their points, the more they seemed to nullify them.

During the *fin-de-siècle,* it became obvious that the brain-only reductionists, with their physiologies for ethics and poetry, had gone too far. In 1872, a founder of the German biophysics movement, Emil du Bois-Reymond signaled a retreat when he admitted that science could never account for free will and aspects of the mind, which he labeled World-Mysteries. Thus, after a determined struggle to rid mechanistic science of mysticism, du Bois-Reymond ceded the mind back to the mystics. Cornered by his own narrow method, he was forced to hand inner life back to faith. Marin Mersenne would have smiled.

Still, the desire to solve the mind-brain problem by eliminating mental attributes would not die. It periodically resurfaced, often encouraged by advances in genetics, neuroscience, and technology, or the demands of antiliberal political forces that favored doctrines of heredity that could be employed in support of gender, class, and race hierarchies. The willingness of some brain scientists to extrapolate beyond their actual findings to offer up such claims would prove perpetually problematic, dangerous even, because of these explosive ideological usages. If the mind was an empty fiction, then claims for individual liberties were meaningless, for humans in fact possessed no freedom to make such choices. For 20th-century leaders who would choose to translate these dictums into social policy, a brave new world lay ahead. Brute exercises of power could easily be legitimized against broken machines, beings that were both desacralized and dehumanized. The abuses of racial science, degeneration theory, eugenics, and finally euthanasia programs lay in the future, seeds that would bear monstrous fruit.

Near the advent of the 20th century, as the reductionist research program began to founder and mentalism reemerged, leaders in an array of new "psy" fields would seek to avoid the embarrassments of the past. As hospitals, schools, governments, armies, and courts throughout the West turned to experts on the mind, distinct professional disciplines emerged that cautiously delimited their own endeavors. The German founder of academic psychology, Wilhelm Wundt, advised researchers to focus on mental contents alone without attempting any link to bodily states. Across Europe and the United States, psychology labs would follow his lead. The founder of psychoanalysis, Sigmund Freud, after his own failed experiments with mind-brain integration, considered the quest a kind of madness, and urged his followers to adopt psychic determinism, in which the contribution from the brain on psychic states was considered unknowable. On the other side of the mind-brain divide, neurology was influenced by the British physician John Hughlings Jackson, who urged his colleagues to examine neural causes alone, without seeking to unravel interactions with mental ones. While numerous mavericks would not be impeded, these boundaries served to stabilize these growing fields by leaving the mind-body problem to others.

In this hurrying to solid ground, one group was stranded. Though they would often try, these experts could not easily avoid the mix of mechanics and psychic acts, for it had been their raison d'être. Moral medicine, alienism, mental medicine, and psychiatry were created on this troubled ground. Buffeted between their commitments to biology and inner experience, this field would periodically zigzag toward mind or brain, nature or nurture. However, unlike psychology and neurology, the heirs of Battie, Pinel, and Reil would never fully rid themselves of the dilemmas of an embodied mind. Thus, their field would remain distasteful to physicists and poets, churchgoers and secular humanists alike. Stuck in a no-man's-land, these physicians became custodians of modern problems that no science wanted.

We live in this divided world. Despite the unifying efforts of Enlightenment thinkers, modernity has been structured around fracture lines, like the mind-body problem, the Nature-Nurture problem, free will versus determinism, and secularism or faith. Riven by these seemingly unresolvable dichotomies, separate thought collectives have emerged to pursue favored answers. Inside each of these communities, there are distinct models of knowledge, coherent political values, and the support of legitimizing beliefs, institutions, and figures of authority. However, outside each domain, all face immense complexity and challenges for which they cannot account.

In 1959, C. P. Snow struck a nerve with his tale of the Western intellectuals segregated into distinct cultures, one scientific and the other humanistic. The dividing line between these two worlds was the nature of inner life. Without a scientific model of an intentional mind, what could measurements of electrical brain activity contribute to the understanding of Rembrandt's self-portraits, a lover's jealousy, or an adolescent's struggle for meaning? And what could the study of Shakespeare do to uncover the biology of language or the causes of schizophrenia? Humanists continue to defend values like liberty and individuality, while scientists look past all that to search for the rules of nature, rules that do not include exceptions for human free will. Thus, these disparate communities remain uninteresting to the other, for unlike the days of Diderot and Goethe, there is no accepted path from quantities to qualities, mechanics to creativity, facts to values, and brains to psyches.

A vast, attempted synthesis had failed and left behind modern men and women who now must navigate between competing notions of their own being. Western believers and the spiritual heirs of Romanticism, never vanquished by modern secularism, continue to look to their souls for hope, meaning, and salvation. When the room spins or spots darken our vision, however, whether religious or not, we become exquisitely aware of the complex, whirring mechanisms within our astonishing physiology and anatomy. Mostly though, we pass through our waking hours secure in the distinctly modern belief that we possess the power to think, choose, sympathize, create, love, learn, wish, and remember thanks to a domain once known as the rational soul, but now called the mind. Within its invisible labyrinth, we exist, creators and inhabitants of our inner worlds, modern hybrids of soul and machine.

Notes

PROLOGUE

xi **it surely does not exist:** Leading advocates for a stance that eliminates the mind include Patricia Churchland, *Neurophilosophy: Toward a Unified Science of the Mind/Brain* (Cambridge: MIT Press, 1989), and Daniel Dennett, *Consciousness Explained* (New York: Little Brown, 1991). Until fairly recently, this position was widely assumed among neuroscientists, as noted in an excellent assessment of these debates, John Searle's *The Mystery of Consciousness* (New York: New York Review Books, 1997), p. 193. Flipping this argument on its head, the philosopher Thomas Nagel has argued that neo-Darwinist accounts must be wrong because they cannot account for consciousness; see his *Mind and Cosmos: Why the Materialist Neo-Darwinian Conception of Nature Is Almost Certainly False* (Oxford: Oxford University Press, 2012).

xii **how the modern mind emerged**: Contemporary histories of the mind have been accounts of the history of the philosophy of mind, with some forays into evolutionary biology. For the former, see Richard Rorty's chapter "The Invention of the Mind" in his *Philosophy and the Mirror of Nature* (Princeton: Princeton University Press, 1981). For the latter, see Nicholas Humphrey's *A History of the Mind: Evolution and the Birth of Consciousness* (New York: Copernicus, 1999).

xii **ruling conceptions of Western belief:** Plato (ca. 395–380 B.C.), *The Last Days of Socrates*, trans. H. Tredennick (London: Penguin Books, 2003). On the origins of the Greek soul, see Bruno Snell, *The Discovery of the Mind: The Greek Origins of European Thought,* trans. T. G. Rosenmeyer (Cambridge: Harvard University Press, 1953). Arthur Lovejoy declared the dualism of the body and soul to be one of the dominant beliefs of Western thought, *The Great Chain of Being: A Study of the History of an Idea* (New York: Harper & Brothers, 1960), p. 198.

xii **consolation in the face of death:** Roger Smith, *The Norton History of the Human Sciences* (New York: W. W. Norton, 1997), p. 49.

xiv **psychology, mental medicine, and psychiatry:** Numerous historians have pointed out that as reformers and radicals looked to heal their society based on natural law, they turned to physicians. See, for example, Roy Porter, "The Eighteenth Century," in L. Conrad et al, *The Western Medical Tradition: 800 B.C. to A.D. 1800* (Cambridge: Cambridge University Press, 1995), p. 382. Also, Porter's "Medical Science and Human Science in the Enlightenment," in Christopher Fox, Roy Porter, and Robert Wokler, eds., *Inventing Human Science: Eighteenth-Century Domains* (Berkeley: University of California Press, 1995). pp. 53–87.

xv **one interconnected European story:** Historical debates over the Enlightenment are too vast to adequately review here. The critique of an excessive emphasis on one (mostly French) Enlightenment rather than different national enlightenments was made by, among others, Roy Porter, *Enlightenment: Britain and the Creation of the Modern World* (London and New York: Allen Lane/Penguin Press, 2000). The distinction between a Reform and Radical Enlightenment has been argued at length by Jonathan I. Israel, *Radical Enlightenment: Philosophy and the Making of Modernity, 1650–1750* (Oxford: Oxford University Press, 2001).

xv **pernicious aspects of this era:** The traditional interpretation focused on its progressive and French nature. See Ernst Cassirer, *The Philosophy of the Enlightenment*, trans. F. Koelln and J. P. Pettegrove (Princeton: Princeton University Press, 1951), and Peter Gay, *The Enlightenment: An Interpretation*, 2 vols. (New York: Knopf, 1969). The progressive nature of this period was challenged most influentially by Max Horkheimer and Theodor W. Adorno in their (1944) *Dialectic of Enlightenment*, trans. J. Cumming (New York: Continuum, 1994).

xvi **irrationality and mental instability:** See Michel Foucault, *Histoire de la folie à l'âge classique* (Paris: Gallimard, 1972). In English, see the unabridged translation, *History of Madness*, trans. Jean Khalfa and J. Murphey (London: Routledge, 2006). Also see the work of, among other Foucauldians, Nikolas Rose, *Inventing Ourselves: Psychology, Power, and Personhood* (Cambridge: Cambridge University Press, 1996). A number of Foucault's major claims, such as his notion that the leper was replaced by the madman and his belief in a Great Confinement, have not held up to scrutiny.

xvi **made and what was found:** Thanks to Michael Macrone for this etymological insight. On the history of the concepts of discovery and invention, see James D. Fleming, ed., *The Invention of Discovery, 1500–1700* (Burlington, Vt.: Ashgate, 2011). The notion of invention should not be equated with the unreal.

xvi **body, soul, and mind:** On this "trinity," see George Rousseau, "'Braino-mania': Brain, Mind and Soul in the Long Eighteenth Century," *British Journal for Eighteenth-Century Studies*, 30 (2007): 164.

PART I: THE LOST SOULS OF MODERNITY

1 **"Dare to know."—Horace:** St. Mark 8:36, *The New Testament,* in *The Holy Bible, King James Version* (Cleveland: World Publishing Co., n.d.), p. 40.; Horace, *The Odes, Satyrs, and Epistles of Horace,* trans. M. Creech (London: J. Tonson, 1730), p. 275.

1. A SOIREE WITH MR. SPIRIT AND MR. FLESH

3 **a Mr. Thomas Hobbes:** Thomas Hobbes, *The Correspondence,* ed. Noel Malcolm, vol. 2 (Oxford: Oxford University Press, 1994), pp. 818–819. The British still used the Julian calendar, so the date of Charles's return by the Gregorian calendar used in Europe was June 8.

3 **perhaps win his favor:** John Aubrey, *Aubrey's Brief Lives* (Ann Arbor: University of Michigan Press, 1957), pp. 147–159.

4 **forge the modern world:** On Hobbes, see G. A. J. Rogers and Alan Ryan, eds., *Perspectives on Thomas Hobbes* (Oxford: Clarendon Press, 1988); Samuel I. Mintz, *The Hunting of Leviathan; Seventeenth-Century Reactions to the Materialism and Moral Philosophy of Thomas Hobbes* (Cambridge: Cambridge University Press, 1962); and Steven Shapin and Simon Schaffer, *Leviathan and the Air-Pump: Hobbes, Boyle, and the Experimental Life* (Princeton: Princeton University Press, 1985).

4 **lingered over Western Christendom:** See Hugh Trevor-Roper, *The Crisis of the Seventeenth Century* (Indianapolis: Liberty Fund, 1967).

5 **chain of material bodies:** An excellent work on the many usages of soul words in Greek, Latin, Hebrew, and English is Paul S. Macdonald's *History of the Concept of Mind* (Burlington, Vt.: Ashgate, 2003). His book essentially ends where this one commences. Also see the classic text by Nietzsche's friend, Erwin Rohde, *Psyche: The Cult of Souls and Belief in Immortality Among the Greeks* (New York: Harcourt, Brace & Co., 1925); E. R. Dodds, *The Greeks and the Irrational* (Berkeley: University of California Press, 1951); and Bennett Simon, *Mind and Madness in Ancient Greece: The Classical Roots of Modern Psychiatry* (Ithaca: Cornell University Press, 1978).

5 **deemed eternal would perish:** These claims were made, respectively, by Democritus, Diogenes, Hippo, and Critias. See Aristotle, *De anima,* in *The Basic Works of Aristotle,* ed. Richard McKeon (New York: Random House, 1941), pp. 538–541. Also see Simon, *Mind and Madness in Ancient Greece,* pp. 158–228.

6 **intellect, was eternal and divine:** Aristotle, *De anima,* in *The Basic Works of Aristotle,* pp. 535–603. The Greek word *nous* can be translated as "intellect," "understanding," or "mind."

6 **gave life to man:** Genesis 2:7, *The King James Bible*.

6 **that of Ptolemy and Galen:** Against the brain-centered views of Plato, Hippocrates, and Galen, Aristotle believed that motion and sensation occurred most centrally in the heart, but he gave no corporeal place for the higher intellectual functions of the soul. See Charles Gross, "Aristotle on the Brain," *Neuroscientist* 1, no. 4 (1995): 245–250. Aquinas wrote his commentary on Aristotle's *De anima* in 1268. See Thomas Aquinas, *Selected Writings*, ed. Ralph McInerny (New York: Penguin Books, 1998), pp. 410–428.

6 **to be memory and reason:** Differences emerged, for example, among those who claimed the faculty of the imagination was housed in a sensitive soul and was therefore possessed by all animals, and those who placed the will in the rational soul, restricting that capacity to humans. See Dominick Perler, ed., *The Faculties: A History* (Oxford: Oxford University Press, 2015).

7 **a taste of godly power:** See the classic study of Arthur Lovejoy, *The Great Chain of Being: A Study of The History of An Idea* (New York: Harper & Brothers, 1960).

8 **no more than a mass delusion:** See Paul Hazard, *La Crise de la conscience européenne, 1680–1715* (Paris: A. Fayard, 1961). A translation of Hazard's book is also available as *The Crisis of the European Mind, 1680–1715*, trans. James Lewis May (New York Review Books: New York, 2013), p. 52. In French, *conscience* firstly was synonymous with the English "conscience"; only during the period in question did this word come to also connote consciousness. Therefore, the choice of the word "mind" in the translation of Hazard's title is at best confusing.

8 **no argument was too small:** The terms "scholastic" and "scholasticism" are arguably not so monolithic after being modified by 16th-century injections of Renaissance humanism; see Charles Schmitt, *Aristotle and the Renaissance* (Cambridge: Cambridge University Press, 1983), and Peter Dear, *Mersenne and the Learning of the Schools* (Ithaca: Cornell University Press, 1988). Still, most thinkers attacked the "schoolmen" and "scholastic Aristotelians" without making such refined distinctions.

9 **magic, alchemy, and secret potions:** On the decline of Galenism, see Owsei Temkin, *Galenism: Rise and Decline of a Medical Philosophy* (Ithaca: Cornell University Press, 1973), and Harold John Cook, *The Decline of the Old Medical Regime in Stuart London* (Ithaca: Cornell University Press, 1986).

10 **erudite, inquisitive monk Marin Mersenne:** On the underappreciated Mersenne, see Robert Lenoble, *Mersenne ou la naissance du mècanisme* (Paris: J. Vrin, 1943); Dear, *Mersenne and the Learning of the Schools*.

11 **heretical doctrines of Renaissance naturalists:** On Father Mersenne and the threat of skepticism and its extreme variant, Pyrrhonian skepticism, see Richard H. Popkin, *The History of Skepticism from Erasmus to Spinoza*

(Berkeley: University of California Press, 1979); also Dear, *Mersenne and the Learning of the Schools*, p. 25.

11 **while others simply became mad:** Christopher Marlowe, *Doctor Faustus and Other Plays*, eds. D. Bevington and E. Rasmussen (Oxford: Oxford University Press, 1998). This volume includes the 1604 and 1616 texts.

13 **a mechanistic understanding of Nature:** On differing definitions and conceptions of the mechanical, see Daniel Garber and Sophie Rous, eds., *The Mechanization of Natural Philosophy* (Dordrecht: Springer, 2013), and for alteration between mechanistic and nonmechanistic forms of scientific materialism, see, for example, Robert Schofield, *Mechanics and Materialism: British Natural Philosophy in the Age of Reason* (Princeton: Princeton University Press, 1970).

13 *The New Thought of Galilei:* In 1634, Mersenne translated Galileo's work into French in *Les mechaniques de Galilée*, and then again four years later with *Les nouvelle pensées de Galilée*. See Lenoble, *Mersenne ou la naissance du mècanisme*, pp. 336–357.

13 **philosophy of nature was mechanical:** Lenoble, *Mersenne*, p. 364.

14 **Father Mersenne turned him away:** Ibid., p. 42.

14 **greatly influential, if often unacknowledged:** On this underappreciated figure, see Antonia LoLordo, *Pierre Gassendi and the Birth of Early Modern Philosophy* (New York: Cambridge University Press, 2007); Lisa T. Sarasohn, *Gassendi's Ethics: Freedom in a Mechanistic Universe* (Ithaca: Cornell University Press, 1996); L. W. B. Brockliss, "Descartes, Gassendi, and the Reception of the Mechanical Philosophy in the French Collèges de Plein Exercice, 1640–1730," *Perspectives on Science: Historical, Philosophical, Social* 3 (1993); and Howard Jones, *Pierre Gassendi, 1592–1655: An Intellectual Biography* (Nieuwkoop, Neth.: Graaf, 1981).

16 **rewrite metaphysics and moral philosophy:** Pierre Gassendi, *The Selected Works*, ed. and trans. Craig Brush, 2nd ed. (New York: Johnson Reprint, 1972), pp. 24–25.

16 **"tragedy," no doubt his own:** Letter of Pierre Gassendi to Wilhelm Schickard, Aug. 27, 1630; see Jones, *Pierre Gassendi, 1592–1655*, p. 20. Also, Ira Owen Wade, *The Intellectual Origins of the French Enlightenment* (Princeton: Princeton University Press, 1971), p. 208.

16 **"Sapere aude." Dare to know:** Horace, *The Epistles of Horace, Book 1*, ed. E. S. Shuckburgh (Cambridge University Press, 1888), p. 7.

17 **natural world, ethics, and Christianity:** On Gassendi's promulgation of Horace's famous quote, see Wade, *The Intellectual Origins of the French Enlightenment*, p. 211. This call to intellectual courage is often tied to its use by Kant over a century later. On Gassendi's turn to Epicurus, see Jones, *Pierre Gassendi, 1592–1655*, p.25.

17 **"soul die with the body":** Dante Alighieri, *The Inferno of Dante Alighieri* (London: J. M. Dent & Co., 1903), p. 101.

17 **lechers, heathens, and anarchists:** On the rediscovery of Lucretius, see Stephen Greenblatt's *The Swerve: How the Renaissance Began* (New York: Random House, 2012).

18 **care hovered over all:** The world was not just atoms and immaterial void; there was also some incorporeal substance that made the soul. In addition, atoms were not infinite; only God could be that. For the debates regarding atoms and activity, see LoLordo, *Pierre Gassendi and the Birth of Early Modern Philosophy*, pp. 138–144.

18 **belief in atomism and materialism:** See Quentin Skinner, "Thomas Hobbes and His Disciples in France and England," *Comparative Studies in Society and History* 8, no. 2 (1966): 153–167. Also see Sarasohn, *Gassendi's Ethics*, p. 365.

19 **simple building blocks—matter and motion:** Thomas Hobbes, *The Elements of Law, Natural and Politic*, ed. Ferdinand Toennies (Cambridge: Cambridge University Press, 1928).

19 **the inner being of man:** Ibid., pp. 7, 21.

20 **physics, psychology, and ethics:** Richard Tuck, "Hobbes and Descartes," in *Perspectives on Thomas Hobbes*, ed. G. A. J. Rogers and Alan Ryan (Oxford and New York: Oxford University Press, 1988), p. 20.

20 **brilliant, and reclusive René Descartes:** From the large literature on Descartes, I have especially profited from Stephen Gaukroger, *Descartes: An Intellectual Biography* (Oxford and New York: Clarendon Press / Oxford University Press, 1995). Also see the excellent dissertation by Noga Arikha, *Adam's Spectacles: Nature, Mind, and Body in the Age of Mechanism* (Ph.D. diss., Warburg Institute, University of London, 2001).

22 **the royal gardens of Saint-Germain-en-Laye:** René Descartes, *Treatise of Man*, trans. Thomas Steele Hall (Cambridge: Harvard University Press, 1972), p. 21.

23 **"all other sorts of projects":** René Descartes (1637), *Discourse on Method and the Meditations*, trans. F. E. Sutcliffe (New York: Penguin Books, 1986), p. 91. Also see René Descartes (1637), *Discours de la méthode* (Paris: Bordas, 1965), pp. 162–163.

24 **his own "stay of execution":** Steven Shapin, "Descartes the Doctor: Rationalism and Its Therapies," *British Journal for the History of Science* 33, no. 02 (2000): 140–141. On Descartes and medicine, also see Richard B. Carter, *Descartes' Medical Philosophy: The Organic Solution to the Mind-Body Problem* (Baltimore: Johns Hopkins University Press, 1983), and Gary Hatfield, "Descartes' Physiology and Its Relation to His Psychology," in *The Cambridge Companion to Descartes*, ed. John Cottingham (Cambridge and New York: Cambridge University Press, 1992), pp. 335–370.

25 **Thomas Hobbes, and others:** René Descartes, *Méditations métaphysiques— Meditationes de prima philosophia—Méditations de philosophie première*, trans. Louis Charles d'Albert de Luynes and Michelle Beyssade (Paris: Librai-

rie Générale Française, 1990). In this, the original Latin and two French translations are published side by side. This important work first appeared in Latin in 1641, then in a 1647 French translation supervised by Descartes.

25 **passed for truth was absurd:** Descartes, *Discours de la Méthode*, pp. 27–44.

26 **I think, therefore I am:** This famous phrase, "I think therefore I am," was rendered in Latin as "*Cogito, ergo sum*," and in French as "*Je pense, donc je suis*." See Descartes, *Discours de la méthode*, p.100, and his *Discourse on Method*, p. 53.

27 **therefore a "thing that thinks":** Descartes, *Méditations métaphysiques*, p. 52. "*Ego sum, ego existo*," or "*Je suis, j'existe*." On p. 58, find the Latin "*res cogitans*," or "*une chose qui pense*." Despite seeming to make thought an entity, the thing that thinks for Descartes is immaterial substance.

27 **which must be the soul:** Descartes, *Méditations métaphysiques*, p. 58. The Latin used is *anima*, the French, *l'âme*. The French translation of Descartes's Latin text was done in 1647 by the Duc de Luynes, and the result so pleased Descartes that he reviewed, corrected, and endorsed this as the authorized translation. Scholars have since noted that it is not a fully faithful translation of the Latin.

28 **sixth and seventh possible meanings:** Randle Cotgrave, *A Dictionarie of the French and English Tongues* (London: Adam Islip, 1611). No page numbers. *Âme* is rendered as soul, spirit, or ghost. *Esprit* is defined as spirit, soul, heart, breath, beat, mind, or thought.

28 *anima* **becomes** *âme*, **or soul:** Descartes, *Méditations métaphysiques*, pp. 48, 58.

28 **words for mind and soul:** The varied usage of *esprit* and *âme* mark French translations of this important work. For example, in the title of the Second Meditation, the Latin *mentis* is rendered "*l'esprit*" in the 1647 translation, but in the Sixth Meditation, the same word is rendered "*âme*." This was altered to "*esprit*" in a recent French translation to try to make for a uniformity that did not exist in the original French text. Ibid., p. 202.

28 **"truly distinct from my body":** The French read: "Il est certain que ce moi, c'est à dire mon *âme*, par laquelle je suis ce que je suis, est entierement et véritablement distincte de mon corps. . . ." Ibid., p. 222.

28 **what made us human:** Scholars disagree about whether Descartes tried to distinguish the mind from the soul, an argument that hinges on the definition of the soul. I agree with those who suggest that he sought to equate the Latin *mens* with the rational soul. See Paul S. Macdonald, *History of the Concept of Mind*, pp. 281–283.

30 **Thomas Hobbes and Pierre Gassendi:** John Aubrey, Marin Mersenne, and William Cavendish's brother Charles all attest to this meeting, but Mersenne wrote of it taking place in 1647 and Cavendish had it in 1648. I follow Hobbes scholars like J. C. A. Gaskin and Noel Malcolm, who accept the close analysis of Helen Hervey in her "Hobbes and Descartes in

the Light of Some Unpublished Letters of the Correspondence Between Sir Charles Cavendish and Dr. John Bell," *Osiris* 10 (1952): 67–90. She asserts that this meeting took place in 1648. Descartes's biographer, Stephen Gaukroger allows that this meeting probably took place a year earlier, in May of 1647; *Descartes*, p. 407. Scholars also disagree as to whether Mersenne attended the meeting, or if it resulted in a significant improvement in the relationships between the three thinkers.

30 **corporeal God were absurd:** For Descartes's views on Hobbes, see, for example, his letters in Thomas Hobbes, *The Correspondence*, vol. 1, pp. 54–61, 118, and vol. 2, p. 826.

30 **they were ludicrous oxymorons:** For Hobbes's views on Descartes, see for example, Thomas Hobbes, *The Correspondence,* vol. 1, pp. 62–79, and Aubrey, *Aubrey's Brief Lives* pp. 94–95, 158.

30 **a clandestine conspiracy against him:** Gassendi, *The Selected Works*, pp. 153–154.

31 **process paid a heavy price:** See Thomas Hobbes, *The Correspondence*, vol. 2, pp. 70–79, 118–120, and the editor's notes on pp. 834–836. Also see Aubrey, *Aubrey's Brief Lives*, p. 95.

31 **he fell into a personal crisis:** Sarasohn, *Gassendi's Ethics.* During the 17th century, atheism was rarely the denial of the existence of God, but rather the rejection of a personal, providential God who interceded in human affairs. It was this that Gassendi feared, and it was for this reason, as we will see, that Deists were declared atheists.

31 **more than motion and matter:** On others who revived Epicurus, including Italian humanists and Erasmus, see Jones, *Pierre Gassendi, 1592–1655*, pp. 205–225.

31 **his admiring portrait of Epicurus:** Petro Gassendo, *De vita et moribus Epicuri libri octo* (Lyon: Guillaume Barbier, 1647).

32 **Gassendi's terrible inner struggles emerged:** Petro Gassendo, *Animadversiones in decimum librum Diogenis Laerti, qui est de vita, moribus, placitisque Epicuri* (Lyon: Guillaume Barbier, 1649).

32 **string of increasingly empty words:** René Descartes, *Objections to the Meditations and Descartes's Reply,* on www.earlymoderntexts.com/pdf/descartes1642_2.pdf, pp. 83–135. This Fifth Objection by Gassendi is often not printed with the book, since Descartes cut it out of later editions, assuring readers that they would not find any substantial claims there. See for example, René Descartes, *Meditations, Objections, and Replies,* trans. Roger Ariew and Donald Cress (Indianapolis: Hackett Publishing, 2006), p. 154.

33 **"(you want to go by!)?":** Descartes, *Meditations, Objections, and Replies,* pp. 86–96. I have followed this translation from the French; in Latin, the name calling was between "Mentis" and "Carnem." This reaffirms the notion that Descartes's readers, or Gassendi at least, considered his use of the Latin for "mind" as no more than an equivalent for a rational, immaterial soul.

34 **the immortal, rational soul:** Ibid., pp. 92, 89.

34 **"not answering either of them.":** Ibid., p. 146.

37 **warring sects in Western Christendom:** Hazard, *The Crisis of the European Mind*, p. 270.

39 **those raised on scholastic certitude:** Barbara J. Shapiro, *Probability and Certainty in Seventeenth-Century England: A Study of the Relationships Between Natural Science, Religion, History, Law, and Literature* (Princeton: Princeton University Press, 1983).

39 **the first diehard Cartesians:** Russell Shorto, *Descartes' Bones: A Skeletal History of the Conflict Between Faith and Reason* (New York: Doubleday, 2008), p. 21.

39 **made this compromise popular:** Ibid., p.71; Thomas M. Lennon, *The Battle of the Gods and Giants: The Legacies of Descartes and Gassendi, 1655–1715* (Princeton: Princeton University Press, 1993), pp. 1–26.

40 **France and became Cartesian:** Ibid., pp. 26–34.

41 **matter alone could think:** Ibid., pp. 26–34.

2. SCIENCE AND THE THING THAT THINKS

43 **"to stop further enquiry":** Francis Bacon (1620) "*Novum Organum Scientiarum*," in *The Works of Francis Bacon* (London: Jones, 1815), p. xvii.

43 **inferences might yield general principles:** Ibid., pp. 7–25. On the rise of Baconian thought in England, see Charles Webster, *The Great Instauration: Science, Medicine, and Reform, 1626–1660* (London: Duckworth, 1975). On Bacon's cure for his society, see Sorana Corneanu, *Regimens of the Mind: Boyle, Locke, and the Early Modern Cultura Animi Tradition* (Chicago: University of Chicago Press, 2011), pp. 14–45.

44 **physics, magnets, astronomy, and geometry:** John Willis cited in Marie Boas, *Robert Boyle and Seventeenth-Century Chemistry* (Cambridge: Cambridge University Press, 1958), pp. 5–6. Some held aspirations that went to the functions of the state, for they believed universal knowledge would lead to universal brotherhood. The groups in Oxford and London comprised the "Invisible College," as Boyle termed it in a letter to Samuel Hartlib of May 8, 1647; see ibid., pp. 7, 13.

44 **rigid, and sternly pious:** For Boyle's biography, see Michael Hunter, *Boyle: Between God and Science* (New Haven: Yale University Press, 1990). Also see Steven Shapin, *A Social History of Truth: Civility and Science in Seventeenth Century England* (Chicago: University of Chicago, 1994). pp. 130–192. Boyle's personality is vividly described in Aubrey, *Aubrey's Brief Lives*, pp. 36–37.

45 **one doctor as a hypochondriac:** Richard Alfred Hunter and Ida Macalpine, *Three Hundred Years of Psychiatry, 1535–1860: A History Presented in Selected English Texts* (Hartsdale, N.Y.: Carlisle Pub., 1982), pp. 246–247.

45 branch of Hippocrates' art—alchemy: Boas, *Robert Boyle and Seventeenth-Century Chemistry*, p. 19.

46 elaboration of Gassendi in English: Walter Charleton, *Physiologia Epicuro-Gassendo-Charltoniana* (London: T. Newcomb for T. Heath, 1654). Also see Robert Kargon, "Walter Charleton, Robert Boyle, and the Acceptance of Epicurean Atomism in England," *Isis* 55, no. 2 (1964): 184–192.

46 "without fayle to be burnt": Kargon, "Walter Charleton, Robert Boyle, and the Acceptance of Epicurean Atomism in England," pp. 187–188.

46 He made man: Robert Boyle (1681), "Discourse of Things Above Reason," in *Selected Philosophical Papers of Robert Boyle*, ed. M. A. Stewart (Indianapolis: Hackett, 1991), pp. 209–244. Also, Boyle (1663), "An Essay Containing a Requisite Digression Concerning Those That Would Exclude the Deity from Intermeddling with Matter," in ibid., pp. 155–175.

47 real, deadly, and powerful: Robert Boyle (1675), "Some Physico-Theological Considerations About the Possibility of Resurrection, in ibid., p. 207. J. J. MacIntosh, "Locke and Boyle on Miracles and God's Existence," in *Robert Boyle Reconsidered*, ed. Michael Cyril William Hunter (Cambridge and New York: Cambridge University Press, 1994), p. 206.

47 came from faith alone: Robert Boyle (1674), "The Excellence of Theology Compar'D with Natural Philosophy," in *The Works of Robert Boyle*, vol. 8, ed. Michael Cyril William Hunter and Edward Bradford Davis (London and Brookfield, Vt.: Pickering & Chatto, 1999), pp. 22–34.

47 he answered, a hundred nos: See Robert Boyle (1681), "A Discourse of Things Above Reason," in *The Works of Robert Boyle,* vol. 9, p. 369. The quotation is from Robert Boyle (1690–1691) *The Christian Virtuoso*, in ibid., vol. 11 p. 297.

48 could see for themselves: Robert Boyle (1661), *The Sceptical Chymist*, in *The Philosophical Works of the Honorable Robert Boyle*, vol. 3, ed. Peter Shaw, M.D. (London: W. and J. Inys & J. Osborn and T. Longman, 1775), p. 332. On Hobbes and Boyle, see the groundbreaking work of Shapin and Schaffer, *Leviathan and the Air-Pump : Hobbes, Boyle, and the Experimental Life*.

49 they were doing God's work: On the adoption of English gentle mores into the Royal Society, and the manner in which codes of civility undergirded reliable scientific testimony and allowed for dissent among reasonable gentlemen, see Steven Shapin, *A Social History of Truth*.

49 "zealots" who preached experimentation only: Quentin Skinner, "Thomas Hobbes and His Disciples in France and England," *Comparative Studies in Society and History* 8 (1966): 166.

50 "the affairs of the state": Huygens as cited in Roger Hahn, *The Anatomy of a Scientific Institution: The Paris Academy of Sciences, 1666–1803* (Berkeley: University of California Press, 1971), p. 12.

51 *the Royal Society* in **England:** See Tony Volpe, *Science et théologie dans les débats savants de la seconde moitié du XVII siècle: La genèse dans les Philosophical Transactions et le Journal des savants (1665–1710)* (Turnhout, Belg.: Brepols Pub., 2008).

51 **their side of the line:** James E. McClellan, *Science Reorganized: Scientific Societies in the Eighteenth Century* (New York: Columbia University Press, 1985), pp. 68–70.

51 **political life to the king:** Thomas Sprat, *The History of the Royal-Society of London for Improving of Natural Knowledge* (London: T. R, 1667), pp. 53–54.

53 **a board and carted away:** On Willis, see J. T. Hughes, *Thomas Willis, 1621–1675: His Life and Works* (London: Royal Society of Medicine, 1991), and Hansruedi Isler, *Thomas Willis, 1621–1675; Doctor and Scientist* (New York, London: Hafner, 1968). Also see the excellent introductions by Kenneth Dewhurst in Thomas Willis, *Willis's Oxford Casebook (1650–52),* ed. Kenneth Dewhurst (Oxford: Sandford Publications, 1981), and *Thomas Willis's Oxford Lectures,* ed. Kenneth Dewhurst (Oxford: Sandford Publications, 1980).

53 **existed so near to it:** On Willis and the brain, see William F. Bynum, "The Anatomical Method, Natural Theology, and the Functions of the Brain," *Isis* 64, no. 4 (1973): 444–468; Robert G. Frank, "Thomas Willis and His Circle: Brain and Mind in Seventeenth-Century Medicine," in *The Languages of Psyche: Mind and Body in Enlightenment Thought: Clark Library Lectures, 1985–1986,* ed. George S. Rousseau (Berkeley: University of California Press, 1990); and Robert L. Martensen, *The Brain Takes Shape: An Early History* (Oxford: Oxford University Press, 2004).

54 **hoped for wine, not vinegar:** Thomas Willis (1659), *Of Fermentation,* in *Dr. Willis's Practice of Physick Being the Whole Works of That Renowned and Famous Physician,* trans. Samuel Pordage (London: T. Dring, C. Harper, and J. Leigh, 1684), Part 1, pp. 13–14.

55 **focused on nervous life:** Frank, "Thomas Willis and His Circle," p. 122. It has been suggested that Willis's interest was primarily philosophical and based on a desire to rethink the soul; James O'Connor "Thomas Willis and the Background of *Cerebri Anatome,*" *Journal of the Royal Society of Medicine* 96, no. 3 (2003): 139–143.

55 **"and of every kind. . . .":** Thomas Willis (1664), *The Anatomy of the Brain* (Tuckahoe, N.Y.: USV Pharmaceutical Corp., 1971), p. 3. The original work is *Cerebri anatome: cui accessit nervorum descriptio* (London: Loundini, 1664).

55 **had been erroneously described:** Willis, *Thomas Willis's Oxford Lectures,* p. 149.

55 **"holy Alter of Your Grace":** Willis, *The Anatomy of the Brain,* p. 1.

56 **and the lower souls:** Isler, *Thomas Willis, 1621–1675,* p. 86.

57 **"mover of the animal Machine":** Willis, *The Anatomy of the Brain,* p. 58.

Two influential figures we will later encounter, Franz Gall and Julien Offray de La Mettrie, both carefully studied Willis.

57 **his ambition to go further:** Ibid., pp. 111, 119. In his original Latin text, Thomas Willis used the Greek word *psyche* which his English translator, S. Pordage, rendered as "soul"; see pp. 4,111. The soul was that which understands all but itself.

57 **or a "psychologie":** Thomas Willis, "Two Discourses Concerning the Soul of Brutes," in Willis, *Dr. Willis's Practice of Physick Being the Whole Works of That Renowned and Famous Physician*, Part XI, p. 7. On debates over the origin of psychology as a term and a project, see Fernando Vidal, *The Sciences of the Soul: The Early Modern Origins of Psychology*, trans. Saskia Brown (Chicago: University of Chicago Press, 2011).

58 **the brain ever created:** Anonymous review of *Cerebri Anatome* in *Le Journal des sçavans*, January 12, 1665, pp. 16–19.

58 **"but for sinning against it":** Nicolas Steno, *Discours de Monsieur Stenon sur l'anatomie du cerveau* (Paris, Robert De Ninville, 1669), pp. 2,3, 13. A student of Sylvius, Steno was the Latin for Niels Stensen. On Steno, see Stefano Miniati, *Nicholas Steno's Challenge for Truth* (Milan: Franco Angeli, 2009), and Gustav Scherz, ed., *Steno and Brain Research in the Seventeenth Century* (Oxford: Pergamon Press, 1968).

58 **straying beyond what was knowable:** Steno, *Discours de Monsieur Stenon sur l'anatomie du cerveau*, p. 11. Also see K. Dewhurst, "Willis and Steno," in *Steno and Brain Research in the Seventeenth Century*, pp. 43–48.

59 **"Lord Have Mercy on Us":** Samuel Pepys, *Passages from the Diary of Samuel Pepys*, ed. Richard Le Gallienne (New York: Modern Library, 1921), p.162. By Keith Thomas's calculations, the plague had spared London for only a dozen years in the 150 years before the Great Plague of 1665; Thomas, *Religion and the Decline of Magic*, p. 7.

59 **members fled to the countryside:** Thomas Birch, ed., *The History of the Royal Society of London*, vol. 2 (London: A Millar, 1756), pp. 57, 60. The dates of these transcripts were June 20 and June 28, 1665.

59 **"such great numbers forsake us":** Walter George Bell, *The Great Plague in London in 1665* (London: Lane, 1924), p. 63. Also Ernest Gilman, *Plague Writing in Early Modern England* (Chicago: University of Chicago Press, 2009).

61 **best-paid doctors in London:** On Willis's high fees and his amassing of a fortune, see Kenneth Dewhurst, "Some Letters of Dr. Thomas Willis (1621–1675)," *Medical History* 16 (1972): 63–76.

61 **"use of upon rotten sheep":** Birch, *The History of the Royal Society*, vol. 3 (1756), p. 227; also see pp. 179, 210, 225.

61 **sizzling juices, not something supernatural:** Thomas Willis (1667), "An Essay of the Pathology of the Brain and Nervous Stock," in Thomas Willis,

Dr. Willis's Practice of Physick Being the Whole Works of That Renowned and Famous Physician, Part VIII, pp. i–ii.

62 **women and hypochondria in men:** Ibid., pp. 6–7, 71.

63 **"as the first Mover":** Thomas Willis (1672), "Two Discourses Concerning the Soul of Brutes," in ibid., Part XI, pp. iv–v. This is the translation of *De Anima Brutorum* (London: Typis E. F. Impensis Ric. Davis, Oxon., 1672).

3. WITCHES, MELANCHOLICS, AND FANATICS

65 **the hand of God:** Hazard, *The Crisis of the European Mind*, pp. 155–161. On Divine Providence, see Thomas, *Religion and the Decline of Magic*, pp. 78–112.

66 **one from the other:** For an excellent summary of recent scholarship on medicine during the scientific revolution, see Harold John Cook, "The History of Medicine and the Scientific Revolution," *Isis* 102, no. 1 (2011): 102–108.

66 **tales of sorcery were fabrications:** Henricus Institoris and Jakob Sprenger (1486), *Malleus Maleficarum*, trans. Christopher S. Mackay, 2 vols. (Cambridge and New York: Cambridge University Press, 2006). The literature on witchcraft is immense. For a comprehensive survey, see Richard Golden, ed., *The Encyclopedia of Witchcraft: The Western Tradition*, 4 vols. (Santa Barbara: ABC-Clio, 2006). For witches and associated beliefs in England, see Thomas, *Religion and the Decline of Magic*. For an excellent overview of recent scholarship, see H. C. Erik Midelfort, "Witchcraft," in his *Witchcraft, Madness, Society, and Religion in Early Modern Germany* (Burlington Vt.: Ashgate, 2013), pp. 355–395.

67 **were diseased in their imaginations:** Johann Weyer (1583), *De Praestigiis Daemonum*, trans. John Shea (Binghamton, N.Y.: Medieval and Renaissance Texts and Studies, 1991). By the time Robert Burton wrote, it was commonly believed that humans could be made crazy by the Devil, or could seem to be possessed due to illnesses such as religious melancholy or, more rarely, hysteria. See Michael MacDonald et al., *Witchcraft and Hysteria in Elizabethan London: Edward Jorden and the Mary Glover Case* (London and New York: Tavistock/Routledge, 1991). Also see Stuart Clark, "Demons and Disease: The Disenchantment of the Sick (1500–1700)," in *Illness and Healing Alternatives in Western Europe*, ed. Marijke Gijswijt-Hofstra, Hilary Marland, and Hans de Waardt (London and New York: Routledge, 1997).

67 **the needs of the body:** Noga Arikha, *Passions and Tempers: A History of the Humours* (New York, N.Y.: Ecco, 2007), p.79.

67 **bleeding cups to prayer:** Judith Bonzol, "The Medical Diagnosis of Demonic Possession in an Early Modern English Community," *Parergon* 26, no. 1 (2009): 118.

67 **would be difficult to locate:** John Cotta, *The Infallible, True, and Assured Witch* (London: I.L., 1625), pp. 6, 95–101. On Cotta, see Frederick Valletta, *Witchcraft, Magic, and Superstition in England, 1640–70* (Burlington, Vt.: Ashgate, 2000), pp. xiii–xiv, 29. Other forms of proof included the presence of imps, such as cats or even butterflies, scratching tests, and testimony.

68 **war between Catholics and Protestants:** The theory that witchcraft persecutions occurred where confessional rivalries were strongest was put forth by H. R. Trevor-Roper, *Religion, Reformation, and Social Change and Other Essays* (London: Macmillan, 1967). Also see D. P. Walker, *Unclean Spirits: Possession and Exorcism in France and England in the Late Sixteenth and Early Seventeenth Centuries* (Philadelphia: University of Pennsylvania Press, 1981).

68 **through intense prayer and fasting:** Matthew 17:14–21, *The King James Bible*. In this passage, Jesus exorcizes a boy with seizures.

68 **"much counterfeited, little from disease":** Walker, *Unclean Spirits*, p. 33. Clark, "Demons and Disease: The Disenchantment of the Sick (1500–1700)," p. 48.

68 **seated beside the Pope:** A century later, this diagnosis was seized upon by the Huguenot skeptic Pierre Bayle, who memorialized this fraud in his famous dictionary; see ibid., p. 39.

69 **"or the Pope himself":** Hobbes, *The Correspondence*, vol. 1, pp. 46–47.

69 **"zeal and bitterness is displayed":** Ibid., p. 48.

69 **personally branded Scot a heretic:** Reginald Scot (1597), *The Discoverie of Witchcraft* (New York: Dover Publications, 1972), p. xxiii. Scot thought witches were either fakers, deluded, falsely accused, or true witches who harmed not with magic, but with poisons.

70 **caustically asked, "Can diseases hear?":** Thomas Hobbes (1651), *Leviathan* (Oxford and New York: Oxford University Press, 1998), pp. 37, 426–427.

70 **No witches, no miracles:** Mintz, *The Hunting of Leviathan*, p. 108.

70 **"nature, but of names":** Hobbes, *Leviathan*, p. 429.

72 **"unheard of prodigious monsters":** John Wagstaffe, *The Question of Witchcraft Debated* (London: E. Millington, 1671), pp. 2, 87, 127–130, 135. On other late 17th- and early 18th-century skeptics like John Webster, Samuel Harsnet, and Francis Hutcheson, see Thomas, *Religion and the Decline of Magic*, pp. 571–578.

72 **key to avoiding this disease:** Stanley W. Jackson, *Melancholia and Depression: From Hippocratic Times to Modern Times* (New Haven: Yale University Press, 1986).

73 **aid the tormented:** John T. McNeill, *A History of the Cure of Souls* (New York: Harper, 1951), pp. 17–41. Also see Sorana Corneanu, *Regimens of the Mind: Boyle, Locke, and the Early Modern Cultura Animi Tradition* (Chicago: University of Chicago, 2011).

73 **"what is sickness but vice?":** Boethius, *The Consolation of Philosophy*,

trans. S. J. Tester (Cambridge: Harvard University Press, 1973), pp. 364–365. The Latin *animorum* is rendered as "mind," but is more commonly and appropriately given as "soul." Despite his being sanctified as a martyr for the faith, the neo-Platonic Boethius's Christianity has been questioned by some, who see it as lapsed during his imprisonment. However in the *Divine Comedy*, Dante placed him in Paradise, not far from Thomas Aquinas.

73 **by the Word of God:** McNeill, *A History of the Cure of Souls*, pp. 171–172.

73 **weighted upon an afflicted conscience:** T. Bright, *A Treatise of Melancholy* (London: John Windet, 1586).

75 **"carried away by this by-stream":** Robert Burton (1621), *The Anatomy of Melancholy: What It Is, with All the Kinds, Causes, Symptoms, Prognostickes & Severall Cures of It* (New York: Vintage Books, 1977), p. 35.

75 **"who is not brain-sick?":** Ibid., pp. 38–39.

76 **"both make an absolute cure":** Ibid., p. 37.

76 **hence a true soul-doctor:** Ibid.

76 **distemper of the brain:** Ibid., pp. 126–127.

76 **only if that failed them:** Ibid., p. 97.

77 **did not doubt its power:** Ibid., p. 183.

77 **hung himself in Christ Church:** This was reported by Aubrey, *Aubrey's Brief Lives*, p. 52.

77 **half of these as mad:** The number was 264 of 513 cases. See MacDonald, *Mystical Bedlam : Madness, Anxiety, and Healing in Seventeenth-Century England* (Cambridge: Cambridge University Press, 1981), pp. 199, 243–245.

78 **bowed down in reverence:** Aubrey, *Aubrey's Brief Lives*, pp. 217–218.

78 **natural or theological in origin:** See Roy Porter, "The Eighteenth Century," in Conrad et al., eds., *The Western Medical Tradition, 800 B.C. to A.D. 1800*, p. 440. Also see Keith Thomas, *Religion and the Decline of Magic* (New York: Charles Scribners' Sons, 1971), p. 5, and Robert Lee (2009) "Early Death and Long Life in History: Establishing the Scale of Premature Death in Europe and its Cultural, Economic, and Social Significance," *Historical Social Research* 34, no. 4: 23–60. Before 1750, the average life expectancy of an English subject was 36; in France, it was 27.

78 **work suddenly stopped being read:** His magnum opus would remain almost unknown over the next century. Lord Byron and Charles Lamb fostered its revival in the early 19th century.

78 **might ignite a rebellion:** The groundbreaking work showing that religious enthusiasm in the late 17th century led to increasingly secular explanations of madness was done by Michael MacDonald. See his "Insanity and the Realities of History in Early Modern England," *Psychological Medicine* 11, no. 1 (1981): 11–25.

79 **madness called religious enthusiasm:** Michael Heyd, *Be Sober and Reasonable: The Critique of Enthusiasm in the Seventeenth and Early Eighteenth Centuries* (Leiden and New York: E. J. Brill, 1995).

79 **against the dictates of Heaven:** Ronald A. Knox, *Enthusiasm: A Chapter in the History of Religion: With Special Reference to the XVII and XVIII Centuries* (Oxford: Clarendon Press, 1950), p. 123.

79 **but rather the Redeemer:** Burton, *The Anatomy of Melancholy*, pp. iii, 311–312.

80 **"like a roaring lion":** Ibid., pp. 313, 321, 325.

80 **Age of Miracles had returned:** On the rise of radical groups during this time, see Christopher Hill, *The World Turned Upside Down: Radical Ideas During the English Revolution* (New York: Viking Press, 1972). On whether the Ranters were more invented than real, see J. C. Davis, *Fear, Myth, and History: The Ranters and the Historians* (Cambridge: Cambridge University Press, 1986).

80 **blasphemous language, hence their name:** Most of those accused of being Ranters rejected the charge. See Hill, *The World Turned Upside Down*, pp. 153–185.

82 **touched by the Holy Spirit:** Knox, *Enthusiasm*, pp.141–146.

82 **iron plunged through his tongue:** On Nayler, see Leo Damrosch, *The Sorrows of the Quaker Jesus: James Nayler and the Puritan Crackdown on the Free Spirit* (Cambridge: Harvard University Press, 1996). Also Hill, *The World Turned Upside Down*, pp. 186–207; Knox, *Enthusiasm*, pp. 161–166.

82 **threat to the regime:** Hill, *The World Turned Upside Down*, p. 200.

84 **"the same pranks in England":** Ibid., p. 174.

84 **"infect a whole Province":** Meric Casaubon (1655), *A Treatise Concerning Enthusiasme* (Gainesville, Fla.: Scholars' Facsimiles & Reprints, 1970), p. 173.

84 **divine grace and grave disease:** Susie I. Tucker, *Enthusiasm; A Study in Semantic Change* (Cambridge: Cambridge University Press, 1972), pp. 1–25.

84 **dreamt with their eyes open:** Henry More, *Enthusiasmus triumphatus*, excerpted in Hunter and Macalpine, *Three Hundred Years of Psychiatry, 1535–1860*, pp. 152–153. On More, see John Henry, "A Cambridge Platonist's Materialism: Henry More and the Concept of Soul," *Journal of the Warburg and Courtauld Institutes* 49 (1986): 172–195.

84 **"is a divine Impulse":** Thomas Green's 1755 work *A Dissertation Upon Enthusiasm* is cited in Tucker, *Enthusiasm*, p. 95.

84 **promulgated bloodshed, regicide, and war:** By the time Samuel Johnson compiled his dictionary, "Enthusiasm" had become "an excessive elevation of mind" and a definition of fury. See his entries for "Ecstasy" and "Fury" in *Dictionary of the English Language* (Dublin: W. G. Jones, 1768).

4. A CRISIS OF CONSCIENCE

87 **troubled the feudal order:** Hazard's claim for a European "crisis" between 1680 and 1715 has been challenged by those who thought he gave too

little importance to Renaissance developments, but nonetheless Anthony Grafton considered this book to be one of the "most revealing works of intellectual history ever written." See Grafton's "Introduction" in Hazard, *The Crisis of the European Mind, 1680–1715*, p. viii.

87 **work as a moral compass:** See Taylor, *Sources of the Self*, p. 159. Also see A. Anthony Levi, *French Moralists: The Theory of the Passions, 1585 to 1649* (Oxford: Clarendon Press, 1964).

89 **"tossed sometimes headlong into despair":** Charles H. Firth, *Oliver Cromwell and the Rule of the Puritans* (New York: G. P. Putnam's Sons, 1908), p. 70.

89 **inner motion spoke of "emotions":** Spinoza would term these "affects," while the French called them "sentiments." See Benedictus de Spinoza (1677), *Ethics*, trans. E. M. Curley (New York: Penguin Books, 1996), pp. 68–70.

89 **"nerves, and arteries, and veins. . . .":** Andrew Marvel, "A Dialogue Between the Soul and the Body," in *The Poems of Andrew Marvel* (London: G. A. Aitken, 1892), pp. 43–44.

90 **evacuation, and, lastly, excess passion:** Burton, *The Anatomy of Melancholy*, pp. 217, 250–330. On the Galenic nonnaturals, see L. J. Rather, "The 'Six Things Non-Natural': A Note on the Origins and Fate of a Doctrine and a Phrase," *Clio Medica* 3 (1968): 337–347; S. Jarcho, "Galen's Six Non-Naturals: A Bibliographic Note and Translation," *Bulletin of the History of Medicine* 44, no. 4 (1970): 372–377; P. H. Niebyl, "The Non-Naturals," ibid., 45, no. 5 (1971): 486–492; Chester R. Burns, "The Nonnaturals: A Paradox in the Western Concept of Health," *Journal of Medicine and Philosophy* 1, no. 3 (1976): 202–211.

90 **"the mind to rest":** Burton, *The Anatomy of Melancholy*, p. 250.

91 **malice, vengeance, ambition, and covetousness:** Ibid., pp. 250–330.

91 **turn them to laughter:** Thomas Wright (1601), *The Passions of the Minde in Generall: In Six Bookes* (London: Miles Flesher, 1630), pp. 3–5, 8.

91 **finally banished from England:** Arikha, *Passions and Tempers*, pp. 219–220.

92 **madness, vice, and warfare:** Wright, *The Passions of the Minde in Generall*, p. 13. Also see p. 69.

92 **against its sometimes frenzied invaders:** Edward Reynolds (1640), *A Treatise of the Passions and Faculties of the Soul of Man with the Severall Dignities and Corruptions Thereunto Belonging* (London: Robert Bostock & George Badger, 1650), p. 41.

92 **material, could affect each other?:** Kenneth C. Clatterbaugh, *The Causation Debate in Modern Philosophy: 1637–1739* (New York: Routledge, 1999).

93 **he had no idea:** René Descartes, *Descartes Philosophical Writings*, ed. N. K. Smith (New York: Modern Library, 1958), p. 252.

93 **the body ever mixed:** Gaukroger, *Descartes*, pp. 388–390.

93 **"observations as I," he declared:** Quote in Shorto, *Descartes' Bones*, p. 31. Gaukroger, *Descartes*, p. 228.

95 **not long for this earth:** Gaukroger, *Descartes*, pp. 15–16.

96 **provoked only ridicule and disgust:** Spinoza, *Ethics*, p. 53. Critiques of authors from Henry More to Nicholas Steno would seem to lend support to this claim.

96 **groups ravaged the body politic:** Hobbes, *Leviathan*, p. 475.

96 **"madness in the multitude":** Ibid., p. 50.

97 **"poor, nasty, brutish and short":** Ibid., p. 84.

97 **pursue their own selfish ends:** Ibid., pp. 48–49.

97 **"the power of witches":** Ibid., pp. 14, 463.

98 **to myths about biblical times:** Thomas Browne, *The Works of Sir Thomas Brown*, ed. Charles Sayle, vol. 1 (London: Grant Richards, 1904).

98 **"the many sorts of madness":** Hobbes, *Leviathan*, p. 54.

99 **"without shame or blame. . . .":** Ibid., pp. 16, 47.

PART II: THE ENGLISH MIND

101 **"kingdome is."—Edward Dyer:** Sir Edward Dyer, "My Mynd to Me a Kingdome Is," in *The Writings in Verse and Prose of Sir Edward Dyer* (n.p.: private publication, 1872), pp. 21–25.

5. "MYSELF IN A STORM"

103 **denizen of "great Bedlam England":** John Locke, *The Correspondence of John Locke*, trans. E. S. De Beer (Oxford: Clarendon Press, 1976), p. 42. Among Locke biographies, see the fascinating early account by Jean Le Clerc, *An Account of the Life and Writings of Mr. John Locke, Author of the Essay Concerning Humane Understanding* (London: John Clarke, 1713). Of recent biographies, see Maurice Cranston, *John Locke: A Biography* (Oxford: Oxford University Press, 1985).

104 **"found myself in a storm. . . .":** Cited Ian Harris, *The Mind of John Locke: A Study of Political Theory in Its Intellectual Setting* (Cambridge: Cambridge University Press, 1994), p. 49.

105 **would be considered an absurdity:** John W. Yolton, *Thinking Matter: Materialism in Eighteenth-Century Britain* (Minneapolis: University of Minnesota Press, 1983).

105 **everything from pimples to gonorrhea:** Kenneth Dewhurst, *John Locke (1632–1704), Physician and Philosopher: A Medical Biography; With an Edition of the Medical Notes in His Journals* (London: Welcome Historical Medical Library, 1963).

106 **authorities to secure Locke's position:** Cranston, *John Locke*, p. 93. The same story is related with some minor differences by Shaftesbury's grand-

son. See A. A. C. Shaftesbury, *The Life, Unpublished Letters, and Philosophical Regimen of Anthony Earl of Shaftesbury*, ed. B. Rand (London: Swan Sonnenchein, 1900), pp. 328–332.

106 **"the plot will run out"**: Cited in Kenneth Dewhurst, *Dr. Thomas Sydenham, 1624–1689: His Life and Original Writings* (Berkeley: University of California Press, 1966), p. 38.

107 **chemical presumptions cured no one**: Early in his career, Sydenham would be greatly opposed, but later on when Locke became famous, he successfully promoted his mentor; see Peter Anstey, "The Creation of the English Hippocrates," *Medical History* 55, no. 4 (2011): 457–478.

107 **construct the celebrated drainage pipe**: Dewhurst, *Dr. Thomas Sydenham, 1624-1689*, pp. 164–165, 223–224.

107 **compendium of clinical medicine**: Dewhurst, *John Locke (1632–1704)*, p. 41.

107 **a case of fraud**: Ibid., p. 148.

107 **Robert Boyle had addressed themselves**: Cranston, *John Locke*, p. 117. Some have argued that Robert Boyle helped spur on Locke's thought with ideas that Boyle made public in his 1681 *A Discourse of Things Above Reason*. He argued that even the greatest minds could never conceive of the soul; Robert Boyle, *Selected Philosophical Papers of Robert Boyle*, ed. M. A. Stewart (Indianapolis: Hackett, 1991), p. 217.

109 **the domain of ethics**: Hazard, *The Crisis of the European Mind*, p. 105.

110 **after his death in 1677**: Spinoza's influence or lack thereof has been a constant source of debate, which commenced soon after his death. Recently, strong claims for the import of his work have been made by Jonathan Israel. See, for example, his *Radical Enlightenment: Philosophy and the Making of Modernity, 1650–1750* (Oxford and New York: Oxford University Press, 2001). On the reception of Spinoza's 1670 *Theological-Political Treatise*, see Steven Nadler, *A Book Forged in Hell: Spinoza's Scandalous Treatise and the Birth of the Secular Age* (Princeton: Princeton University Press, 2011).

111 **made up of infinite, eternal substance**: Benedictus de Spinoza (1677), *Ethics*, trans. E. M. Curley (New York: Penguin Books, 1996), p. 32.

112 **make God's designs apparent**: On Spinoza and emotions, one of the best sources is Walther Riese, *La théorie des passions à la lumière de la pensée médicale du XVIIe siècle* (Bâle and New York: S. Karger, 1965).

112 **"occult quality of the Scholastics"**: Ibid., p. 128, 161–162.

112 **"Cartesian, and now an atheist"**: Israel, *Radical Enlightenment*, p. 604.

113 **structure was a democratic republic**: Ibid., p. 260.

113 **would go mostly unacknowledged**: Edward A. Driscoll, "The Influence of Gassendi on Locke's Hedonism," *International Philosophical Quarterly* 12, no. 1 (1972): 87–110. Also Lisa T. Sarasohn, *Gassendi's Ethics: Freedom in a Mechanistic Universe* (Ithaca: Cornell University Press, 1996), pp. 175–197.

114 **"powerfully produces the greatest mischief"**: Cited in Cranston, *John Locke*, p. 200. The date was May 16, 1681.

114 **matter, should He please**: Locke wrote this in 1686 while in exile in Utrecht. His exact phrases were "superadded with thinking immaterial substance" and "GOD can, if he pleases, superadd to matter a faculty of thinking." John Locke (1690), *An Essay Concerning Human Understanding*, ed. A. C. Fraser, vol. 2 (New York: Dover Publications, 1959), p. 193.

114 **studied through natural philosophy**: See ibid., vol. 1, pp. 196–197, on the possible materiality of the soul.

114 **extrapolator of Pierre Gassendi's thought**: Sarasohn, *Gassendi's Ethics*, p. 168.

115 **and most critically, "mind"**: On Epicurus in Montpellier, see Thomas M. Lennon, *The Battle of the Gods and Giants: The Legacies of Descartes and Gassendi, 1655–1715* (Princeton: Princeton University Press, 1993), pp. 66–155.

115 **"the marriage of true minds"**: William Shakespeare, *Shakespeare's Sonnets* (New York: Washington Square Press, 2004), p. 237. The sonnet is no. 116.

115 **"minister to a mind diseased:"** *Oxford English Dictionary*, pp. 797–800. Sir Edward Dyer, "My Mind to Me a Kingdom Is," in *The Writings in Verse and Prose of Sir Edward Dyer*, p. 21. William Shakespeare, *King Henry VI, Part II* (New York: Washington Square Press, 2008), p. 225, and *MacBeth* (New York: Random House, 2013), p. 249.

116 **would need to wonder**: Kenelm Digby, *Two Treatises* (London: John Williams, 1645). Digby became one of the founders of the Royal Society when he returned to England in 1660.

116 **one merged with matter**: Richard Burthogge, *The Philosophical Writings of Richard Burthogge,* ed. Margarel Landes (Chicago: Open Court Pub., 1921). Dr. Burthogge dedicated his later books to Locke and entered into a correspondence with him.

117 **theater of subjective experience**: In this claim, I am in agreement with Yolton, *Thinking Matter*, p. 3.

117 **mind, made it a thing**: In this claim that Locke was critical to the reification of the mind, I am in agreement with, among others, Charles Taylor, *Sources of the Self*, pp. 166–167. For a different view, see Macdonald, *History of the Concept of Mind*, pp. 334–338.

117 **the study of the Lord**: Macdonald, *History of the Concept of the Mind*, p. 109. A school of Cartesians led by Arnaud opposed Malebranche. See Kenneth C. Clatterbaugh, *The Causation Debate in Modern Philosophy: 1637-1739* (New York: Routledge, 1999).

117 **differed over those matters**: Locke, *An Essay Concerning Human Understanding*, Book I, p. 104.

117 **"the beginning of his soul"**: Ibid., pp. 127–128.

118 **perception—came from ideas**: Ibid., pp. 302–303.

118 **individual identity and self**: Ibid., p. 449.

119 unity to the same person: Ibid., pp. 458, 469.

119 acts of his sick self: Ibid., p. 461.

119 "together in any substance": Ibid., pp. 501, 525.

119 "the faculty of reasoning. . . .": Dewhurst, *John Locke (1632–1704)*, p. 70.

120 "either king or candle": Ibid., p. 71.

120 "wrong phansys they have taken": Locke discusses some who never can shake wrong impressions once they are made: "From whence one may see of what moment it is to take care that the first impression we settle upon our minds be comfortable to the truth . . . or else all our meditations and discourse there upon will be noe thing but perfect raveing"; ibid, p. 89.

120 "suggested it to me": Locke, *An Essay Concerning Human Understanding*, vol. 1 p. 528.

120 unaware of his elder's precedent: On Locke's seeming disinterest in citing precedents, see Driscoll, "The Influence of Gassendi on Locke's Hedonism," p. 87. On the history of the association of ideas, see David Rapaport, *The History of the Concept of the Association of Ideas* (New York: International Universities Press, 1974).

120 charge deep into adulthood: Locke, *An Essay Concerning Human Understanding*, p. 531. Thus, there is evidence that Locke both considered the imagination and passions to disrupt the mind's associative flow and also that it could occur without such instigation. On the former, see Louis Charland, "John Locke on Madness: Redressing the Intellectualist Bias," *History of Psychiatry*, 25, no. 2 (2014): 137–153.

121 when he saw the doctor: Locke, *An Essay*, vol. 1, p. 532.

121 "the most dangerous one": Ibid., pp. 534–535.

121 "intercourse with the Deity": Ibid., pp. 430–431.

121 "*judge and guide in everything*": Ibid., pp. 437–438.

122 mind as a natural object: Yolton, *Thinking Matter: Materialism in Eighteenth-Century Britain*, p. 5.

122 "writt by *one* man": Maurice Cranston, "John Locke and John Aubrey," *Notes and Queries* 195 (1950): 553.

123 could not be immortal: Samuel Clarke's 1704 and 1705 Boyle Lectures, "Demonstration of the Being and Attributes of God," and "Unchangeable Obligations of Natural Religion," can be found in *A Defense of Natural and Revealed Religion, Being an Abridgement of the Sermons* (London: D. Midwinter et al., 1739), pp. 81–179. On superadded matter, see p. 142. Also see Henry Lee, *Anti-Scepticism, or Notes Upon Each Chapter of Mr. Lock's Essay* (London: R. Cavel & C. Harper, 1702); Robert Jenkin, *The Reasonableness and Certainty of the Christian Religion* (London: Richard Sare, 1708); and Andrew Baxter, *An Enquiry into the Nature of the Human Soul* (London: James Bettenham, 1733).

123 "the Devil against Christianity": Anonymous, *The Procedure, Extent, and Limits of Human Understanding* (London: William Innys, 1729), p. 40.

123 **thinking matter was impossible:** Giacinto Gerdil, *L'immaterialité de l'âme demontrée contra Locke* (Turin: L'Imprimerie Royale, 1747). Andrew Baxter, *An Enquiry into the Nature of the Human Soul* (London: James Bettenham, 1733). See Yolton, *Thinking Matter*, pp. 24–25.

124 **created this new quality:** Anthony Collins (1707), *An Essay Conerning the Use of Reason* (New York: Garland Press, 1984). For the debates with Clarke over consciousness and other matters, see *The Clark-Collins Correspondance of 1707–1708*, ed. William Uzgalis (Buffalo: Broadview Edition, 2011).

124 **protectors of the faith:** Eustace Budgell, "Untitled," in Joseph Addison, Richard Steele, and Henry Morley, *The Spectator: A New Edition, Reproducing the Original Text* (London and New York: G. Routledge & Sons, 1891), vol. 2 (May 27, 1712), p. 389.

125 **"springs of the human body":** Voltaire, *Letters Concerning the English Nation* (London: C. Davis & A. Lyon, 1733), p. 98.

125 **Voltaire grasped the essential point:** Ibid., p. 103.

126 **"the mind's presence room":** Locke, *An Essay Concerning Human Understanding*, Book I, p. 149.

126 **morally responsible for himself:** See Charles Taylor, *Sources of the Self: The Making of the Modern Identity* (Cambridge: Harvard University Press, 1989), pp. 159–176 on Locke's self.

6. THE SAGACIOUS LOCKE

128 **no different than brutes:** Pierre Bayle (1697), *Dictionaire historique et critique,* vol 4 (Amsterdam: P. Brunel et al., 1730), p. 84.

128 **"celebrated" philosopher's life and thought:** *Biographia Britannica; or, The Lives of the Most Eminent Persons*, vol 5 (London: W. Meadows et al, 1747), pp. 2992–3009.

128 **Zedler's German *Universal-Lexicon*:** Denis Diderot and J. L. R. d'Alembert, *Encyclopédie ou Dictionnaire raisonné des sciences, des arts et des métiers* vol. 9 (Paris: Briasson, 1754–1772), pp. 625–627; Johann Zedler, *Universal-Lexicon* vol. 18 (Halle and Leipzig: J. Zedler, 1738-54), pp. 107–113. This rare work is available on www.zedler-lexikon.de. My thanks to Prof. Erik Midelfort for alerting me to Zaubler's extraordinary, single-authored compendium.

128 **ideas neatly followed Locke's:** Samuel Johnson, *A Dictionary of the English Language*, Entry for "Madness," 1755, http://johnsondictionaryonline.com.

128 **not a part of theology, but anthropology:** Roy Porter, *Enlightenment: Britain and the Creation of the Modern World* (London and New York: Allen Lane/Penguin Press, 2000), p. 170.

128 **he studied the human body:** Akihito Suzuki, "Anti-Lockean Enlightenment?: Mind and Body in Early Eighteenth–Century English Medicine,"

in *Medicine in the Enlightenment*, ed. Roy Porter (Atlanta: Rodopi, 1995), p. 307. Also see Akihito Suzuki, "Dualism and the Transformation of Psychiatric Language in the Seventeenth and Eighteenth Centuries," *History of Science* 33, no. 4 (1995): 417–447.

128 **owed much to Locke:** The soul was still conceived of as either a Cartesian immaterial substance or in the older tripartite scholastic manner, *Encyclopedia Britannica* (Edinburgh: A. Bell & C. Macfarquhar, 1771), pp. 247, 618.

128 **his model of reason:** J. Addison, Untitled, *The Spectator* 1, no. 110, July 6, 1711. Ibid, 3, no. 531, November 8, 1712. Unsigned, "Will's Coffee-house, July 11," *The Tatler* 40, July 12, 1709, pp 239–241.

128 **in the parlor reading Locke:** R. Steele, Untitled, *The Spectator* 2, no. 242, December 7, 1711.

128 **verse from the *Essay*:** J. Addison, "On the Pleasures of the Imagination," *The Spectator*, 3, no. 413, June 24, 1712, p. 42.

129 **"a cabinet empty and void":** Chistopher Smart, "The Furniture of a Beau's Mind," *Universal Visitor and Memorialist* 9 (September, 1756), pp. 429–430.

129 **later part of that century:** See P. Delany, *British Autobiography in the 17th Century* (London: Routledge, Kegan & Paul, 1969); M. Mascuch, *Origins of the Individualist Self: Autobiography and Self-Identity in England, 1591–1791* (London: Blackwell, 1997); and Elspeth Graham et al., *Her Own Life: Autobiographical Writing by Seventeenth-Century Englishwomen* (London: Routledge, 1989).

129 **crisis and eventual rebirth:** M. H. Abrams, *Natural Supernaturalism: Tradition and Revolution in Romantic Literature* (New York: W. W. Norton, 1971), p. 48. On Augustine, see Eric Auerbach, *Mimesis: The Representation of Reality in Western Literature*, trans. W. R. Trask (Princeton: Princeton University Press, 1953), pp. 66–74.

130 **by taking an inward journey:** Gerrard Winstanley, *The Complete Works of Gerrard Winstanley,* eds. Thomas N. Corns et al. (Oxford: Oxford University Press, 2009). Also see Abrams, *Natural Supernaturalism*, pp. 51–53.

130 **that made her individual:** Margaret Cavendish, *The Life of William Cavendish, to Which Is Added the True Relation of My Birth, Breeding, and Life* (London: John Nimmo, 1886), pp. 275–318.

130 **and keeping a journal:** Samuel Johnson's diaries, cited in Allen Ingram, ed., *Patterns of Madness in the Eighteenth Century* (Liverpool: Liverpool University Press, 1998), pp. 107–111.

130 **dissection of his own mind:** Claire Tomalin, *Samuel Pepys: The Unequalled Self* (New York: Vintage Books, 2002), p. xxx.

130 **"may God forgive me":** Samuel Pepys, *Passages from the Diary of Samuel Pepys*, ed. Richard Le Gallienne (New York: Modern Library, 1921), p. 188.

132 **growth of their own consciousness:** M. Mascuch, *Origins of the Individualist Self*, p. 13.

132 **"other sources of prejudice whatsoever":** Laurence Sterne (1759–1767), *The Life and Opinions of Tristram Shandy: Gentleman* (Middlesex, Eng.: Penguin, 1978), p. 39.

132 **the fate of one's soul:** Roy Porter, *London: A Social History* (Cambridge: Harvard University Press, 1994), p. 184.

133 **appeared in December of 1689:** John Locke (1690), *Two Treatises on Government,* ed. Peter Laslet (Cambridge: Cambridge University Press, 2003).

133 **in a silly manner:** John Locke, *A Letter Concerning Toleration: Humbly Submitted,* trans. William Popple (London: Printed for A. Churchill, 1689).

133 **"every man's self," he wrote:** Ibid., p. 33.

134 **deemed to be mad:** John Locke, *A Second Letter Concerning Toleration* (London: Awnsham & John Churchill, 1690), p. 27.

135 **compel assent from others:** See Barbara J. Shapiro, *Probability and Certainty in Seventeenth-Century England: A Study of the Relationships Between Natural Science, Religion, History, Law, and Literature* (Princeton: Princeton University Press, 1983).

135 **worship for Nonconformists sprang up:** Michael Heyd, *Be Sober and Reasonable: The Critique of Enthusiasm in the Seventeenth and Early Eighteenth Centuries* (Leiden and New York: E. J. Brill, 1995), p. 212.

135 **different for varied people:** J. Addison, *The Spectator,* 3, no. 531, November 8, 1712.

135 **society would also be intolerable:** Locke (1689), *A Letter Concerning Toleration,* pp. 34–36. Atheists would probably be considered mad, Locke believed.

136 **what made the blood pulse:** Locke, *An Essay Concerning Human Understanding,* Book I, pp. 313–350. Interestingly, he did not note that the same charge could have been levied against thinking matter.

136 **"fools are the only freemen":** Ibid., p. 347. Men and women sought to choose well, but they often misread their best interests. Shortsighted hedonists embraced pleasure now at the cost of long-standing pain, and others hurried away from a bit of pain despite its long-term rewards; see ibid, pp. 356–369.

137 **found in natural law:** Reason had been given to men to exercise it, and life had been given to humans so as to preserve it. The refusal to reason and self-destruction, including most obviously suicide, were absolute evils; see John Locke, *Two Treatises of Government,* II, 6; also Locke, *An Essay Concerning Human Understanding,* Book I, pp. 100–105. On ethics, see Taylor, *Sources of the Self,* pp. 234–247. On suicide, see Michael MacDonald and Terence R. Murphy, *Sleepless Souls: Suicide in Early Modern England* (Oxford: Clarendon Press, 1990).

137 **God was an analogy:** Anonymous, *The Procedure, Extent and Limits of Human Understanding* (London: William Innys, 1729), p. 40. John Toland, *Christianity Not Mysterious* (London: Sam Buckley, 1696).

137 **reason test all Christian beliefs**: Porter, *Enlightenment*, p. 120. Anthony Collins, *An Essay Concerning the Use of Human Reason*, 1707; John Trenchard, *Natural History of Superstition*, 1709; Matthew Tindal *Christianity as Old as Creation*, 1730.

138 **it announced Locke's death**: *Journal de Trévoux*, June 1705, p. 1090.

138 **"Business of Mankind in general"**: Harris, *The Mind of John Locke*, p. 260.

138 **good or bad character**: John Locke (1693), *Some Thoughts on Education* (London: A. & J. Churchill, 1712).

138 **sixteen French editions by 1800**: Porter, *Enlightenment*, p. 340.

139 **"cured as any," delusion**: J. Locke, *Of the Conduct of the Understanding* (New York: Maynard, Merrill, & Co., 1901), p. 114.

139 **imperil the moral order**: Ibid., pp. 124–132. Also see Louis Charland, "John Locke on Madness: Redressing the Intellectualist Bias," *History of Psychiatry* 25 (2014): 137–153.

139 **universal morality in Locke**: Thomas Burnett, *Remarks Upon an Essay Concerning Humane Understanding* (London: M. Wotton, 1697).

140 **"not the madness of people"**: Locke, *The Correspondence of John Locke*, vol. 4, Isaac Newton to John Locke, June 30, 1691, p. 290.

140 **word of his own outburst**: Letters of September 16, 1693, and October 15, 1693, ibid., pp. 727, 732.

141 **absolute morality and divine reason**: On Henry More's influence, see John Henry, "A Cambridge Platonist's Materialism," *Journal of the Warburg Institute*, 1986; Like Glanvill, More supported his argument for God by arguing for the spirits and witches, something Newton gradually abandoned.

141 **"life and reason, is . . . credulous"**: Andrew Baxter, *An Enquiry into the Nature of the Human Soul* (London: James Bettenham, 1733), p. 299.

142 **"had the least control"**: A. A. C. Shaftesbury, *The Life, Unpublished Letters, and Philosophical Regimen of Anthony, Earl of Shaftesbury*, ed. B. Rand (London: Swan Sonnenschein, 1900), pp. 296, 403–405, 413–417. Also see Jerrold E. Seigel, *The Idea of the Self: Thought and Experience in Western Europe Since the Seventeenth Century* (New York: Cambridge University Press, 2005), p. 90, and Robert Voitle, *The Third Earl of Shaftesbury, 1671–1713* (Baton Rouge: Louisiana State University Press, 1984).

143 **published his "Letter Concerning Enthusiasm"**: Shaftesbury gave a Lockean twist to Burton's equating of enthusiasm with a form of melancholy. Passion shackled the reason of these zealots, who caused intense panic to spread. An example of such mass panic was religion.

143 **wrote on June 3, 1709**: A. A. C. Shaftesbury, *The Life, Unpublished Letters, and Philosophical Regimen of Anthony Earl of Shaftesbury*, p. 403. This letter is to Michael Ainsworth.

144 **"WHATEVER IS, IS RIGHT"**: Alexander Pope, *Essay on Man* (Oxford: Clarendon Press, 1879), p. 36.

144 **perfect of all possible worlds:** Voltaire, *Candide, Zadig, and Selected Stories* (New York: Signet, 1961). Scholars see Pope's writing and Voltaire's satire as directed to Gottfried Leibniz as well.

145 **nothing more than a ruse:** B. De Mandeville (1711), *A Treatise of the Hypochondriack and Hysterick Passions* (New York: Arno Press, 1976).

145 *Private Vices, Publick Benefits:* Bernard Mandeville (1723), *The Fable of the Bees: Or, Private Vices, Publick Benefits*, ed. Frederick Benjamin Kaye, 2 vols. (Oxford: Clarendon Press, 1957).

145 **high-minded ideals were commonplace:** See Lionel Trilling, *Sincerity and Authenticity* (Cambridge: Harvard University Press, 1972).

145 **adages of "la Morale":** For Mandeville's debt to La Rochefoucauld, see Mandeville, *The Fable of the Bees*, vol. 1, pp. 213, 230. Also see Anthony Levi, *French Moralists: The Theory of the Passions, 1585 to 1649* (Oxford: Clarendon Press, 1964).

145 **"only vices in disguise":** François La Rochefoucauld, *Collected Maxims and Other Reflections*, ed. E. H. Blackmore, A. M. Blackmore, and Francine Giguère (Oxford and New York: Oxford University Press, 2007), p. 3.

146 **simply flattered the species:** Mandeville, *The Fable of the Bees*, vol. 2, pp. 212, 230.

147 **"refuted by his own Character":** Ibid., vol. 2, pp. 378, 439.

147 **aid for the impoverished:** See George Bluet's 1725 critique collected in ibid., vol. 2, p. 409. Also see Harold John Cook, "Bernard Mandeville and the Therapy of 'the Clever Politician,' " *Journal of the History of Ideas* 60, no. 1 (1999): 101–124.

147 **"the Subject will admit":** Cited in Roger Smith, *The Norton History of the Human Sciences* (New York: W. W. Norton, 1997), p. 243.

148 **man might otherwise perish:** A. A. C. Shaftesbury, *The Life, Unpublished Letters, and Philosophical Regimen of Anthony Earl of Shaftesbury*, p. 404.

148 **could not *all* be true:** Ann Thomson, *Bodies of Thought: Science, Religion, and the Soul in the Early Enlightenment* (Oxford; New York: Oxford University Press, 2008), p. 147.

148 **soul had been simultaneously exploded:** While perhaps the most successful, Voltaire's *Letters Concerning the English Nation* (London: C. Davis & A. Lyon, 1733), expanded in French as *Lettres philosophiques* (Amsterdam: E. Lucas, 1734), was neither the first nor the only work to extoll Locke and the English. See for example, Louis de Muralt (1725), *Lettres sur les Anglais et les Français* (Berne: Steiger, 1897).

149 **headache for Locke's translators:** Locke, *An Essay Concerning Human Understanding*, Book I, pp. 448–449.

149 **defenders of the faith:** Samuel I. Mintz, *The Hunting of Leviathan; Seventeenth-Century Reactions to the Materialism and Moral Philosophy of Thomas Hobbes* (Cambridge: Cambridge University Press, 1962), pp. 147–152.

7. BEDLAM IN BRITANNIA

150 **this competing mental paradigm:** Regarding Foucault, the late Roy Porter among others has been convincing on the following points: (1) moral treatment and psychiatry began far before 1800, when Foucault and others mark a paradigm shift; (2) there was no Great Confinement during the years of 1660–1800 in England, France, or Germany, nor in Spain, Russia, Poland, or Ireland; (3) Porter rightly concludes: "Psychiatry was thus not just—probably not even primarily—a discipline for controlling the rabble"; (4) Foucault's claims of a great rupture in 1790 with Samuel Tuke and Phillipe Pinel, seems overstated; and (5) his view of the freedom enjoyed by the mad before the Age of Reason was highly romancitized. See, by Roy Porter, "The Rage of Party: A Glorious Revolution in English Psychiatry?" *Medical History* 27 (1983): 35–50, and *Mind-Forg'd Manacles: A History of Madness in England from the Restoration to the Regency* (Cambridge: Harvard University Press, 1987). Quote on p. 9. For a devastating review of the historical errors in Foucault's work on madness, see Andrew T. Scull, "Scholarship of Fools: The Frail Foundations of Foucault's Monument," *Times Literary Supplement*, March 23, 2007, pp. 3–4.

151 **civil toleration or criminal punishment:** Locke, *A Second Letter Concerning Toleration*, p. 41.

152 **"now reckon'd idle stories":** Cited in Porter, *Mind-Forg'd Manacles*, p. 81.

152 **"Love, Hate, Grief, Covetousness, Despair":** Thomas Tryon, *The Way to Health, Long Life, and Happiness* (London: Printed by H.D. for D. Newman, 1691), p. 234.

152 **that of a whole army?:** See his 1697 "Tale of the Tub" and its digression on madness, in Jonathan Swift, *Gulliver's Travels, and Other Writings*, ed. Miriam Kosh Starkman (Toronto and New York: Bantam Books, 1981), pp. 366–377.

153 **this more open society:** The term "mentalist" is employed here and elsewhere to simply denote the theory that psychic phenomena are the result of the mind. The term has other connotations, including the idealist claim that the mind controls the physical and bodily realm. That is not the intended meaning here.

153 **soul died with the body:** Cited in Akihito Suzuki, *Mind and Its Disease in Enlightenment British Medicine* (Ph.D. diss., University College London, 1992), pp. 182–184.

153 **still hesitated before Locke's mind:** Nicholas Robinson, *A New System of Spleen, Vapors, and Hypochondriack Melancholy* (London: A. Bettlesworth, W. Innys & C. Rivington, 1729), pp. 34, 51–52. Also see Suzuki, *Mind and Its Disease in Enlightenment British Medicine*, p. 194.

154 **hospital-worth of the mad:** Gideon Harvey, *The Third Edition of the Vanities of Philosophy and Physick* (London: A. Roper & R. Basset, 1702).

155 **a reasoned man was not:** See Anne Digby, *Madness, Morality, and Medicine: A Study of the York Retreat, 1796–1914* (Cambridge; London; Melbourne: Cambridge University Press, 1985).

155 **"it may blaze and expire":** Samuel Johnson, *Selected Writings*, ed. Patrick Cruttwell (Harmondsworth, Eng.: Penguin, 1986), pp. 535, 254.

155 **"deeper commiseration than any other":** Adam Smith (1759), *The Theory of Moral Sentiments* (New York: Penguin Books, 2009), pp. 16–17.

155 **"they outvoted me," he wrote:** Cited in Samuel Taylor Coleridge (1817), *Biographia Literaria* (London: J. M. Dent, 1975), pp. 148–149.

156 **"die first at the top":** Victoria Glendinning, *Jonathan Swift: A Portrait* (New York: Henry Holt, 1998), p. 265.

156 **his sad premonition had come true:** Ibid., pp. 271–275.

156 **the mind and its ills:** Akihito Suzuki's research helped inform the revisionist work of Jonathan Andrews and Andrew Scull, who argued that MacAlpine and Hunter and others overstated the impact of Locke on doctors. Most did not accept this new model between 1700 and 1750. See Suzuki, *Mind and Its Disease in Enlightenment British Medicine*.

156 **generally kill the poor:** Christopher Smart, *The Poetical Works of Christopher Smart*, vol. 4, *Miscellaneous Poems, English and Latin* (Oxford: Clarendon Press, 1987), p. 263.

156 **prescribed by expensive academic physicians:** Harold John Cook, *The Decline of the Old Medical Regime in Stuart London* (Ithaca: Cornell University Press, 1986).

157 **Nerve Fotus for frenzy and madness:** Anonymous, *A Treatise of Diseases of the Head, Brain, and Nerves* (London: n.p., 1727).

157 **attack poor Dr. James:** Christopher Smart, *The Annotated Letters of Christopher Smart*, eds. B. Rizzo and R. Mahoney (Carbondale: Southern Illinois University Press, 1991), pp. 56–68. Smart's father-in-law distributed James's concoctions.

157 **the teachings of Jesus Christ:** Harold John Cook, "Boerhaave and the Flight from Reason in Medicine," *Bulletin of the History of Medicine* 74, no. 2 (2000): 229–233; John P. Wright, "Boerhaave on Minds, Human Beings, and Mental Diseases," *Eighteenth-Century Culture* 20 (1990), pp. 289–302; and Peter J. Koehler, "Neuroscience in the Work of Boerhaave and Haller," in *Brain, Mind, and Medicine: Essays in Eighteenth-Century Neuroscience*, ed. Harry A. Whitaker, C. U. M. Smith, and Stanley Finger (New York: Springer, 2007).

158 **the King of Prussia:** Giorgio Baglivi, *The Practice of Physick, Reduced to the Ancient Way of Observations . . . Together with Several New and Curious Dissertations; Particularly of the Tarantula, and the Nature of Its Poison* (London, 1723). Frédéric Hoffmann, *La Médecine raisonnée de M. Fr. Hoffmann*, trans. Jacques-Jean Bruhier (Paris: Briasson, 1739).

158 **controlled mental and bodily functions:** L. S. King, "Stahl and Hoff-

mann: A Study in Eighteenth Century Animism," *Journal of the History of Medicine and Allied Sciences* 19 (1964): 118–130.

158 **humoral disruption or a soul-sickness:** Gideon Harvey, *The Third Edition of the Vanities of Philosophy and Physick* (London: A. Roper & R. Basset, 1702), and John Purcell, *A Treatise of Vapours or Hysterical Fits* (London: Nicholas Cox, 1702).

158 **kept mum about thinking matter:** Some exceptions included John Quincy's introduction to Sanctorius, *Medicina statica: Being the Aphorisms of Sanctorius*, trans. John Quincy (London: W. & J. Newton, 1723).

159 **soul's actions on the body:** Robinson, *A New System of Spleen, Vapors, and Hypochondriack Melancholy.*

160 **save his own:** Archibald Pitcairn, *The Works of Archibald Pitcairn* (London: E. Curll & J. Pemberton, 1715), p.16. See Anita Guerrini, "Archibald Pitcairne and Newtonian Medicine," *Medical History* 31 (1987): 70–83.

160 **younger doctor to his knees:** George Cheyne, *The English Malady; or, a Treatise of Nervous Diseases of All Kinds* (London: G. Strahan & J. Leake, 1733). On Cheyne, see Anita Guerrini, *Obesity and Depression in the Enlightenment: The Life and Times of George Cheyne* (Norman: University of Oklahoma Press, 2000). Suzuki, "Anti-Lockean Enlightenment?: Mind and Body in Early Eighteenth-Century English Medicine."

161 **matters without a priest's sanctity:** Edward Strother, *An Essay on Sickness and Heath in Which Dr. Cheyne's Mistaken Opinions in his Late Essay Are Occasionally Taken Notice Of* (London: Charles Rivington, 1725), p. 417.

162 **"less innocently mad than They":** Thomas Fitzgerald, "Bedlam," in *Poems on Several Occasions* (London: J. Watts, 1736), p. 11.

163 **rogue and a virtuous heroine:** Daniel Defoe (1722), *The Fortunes and Misfortunes of the Famous Moll Flanders*, ed. Juliet Mitchell (Harmondsworth, Eng.: Penguin Books, 1978).

163 **could veer out of control:** George Lillo (1731), *The London Merchant* (Lincoln: University of Nebraska Press, 1965).

163 **their brains and nerves:** Anonymous, *Two Discourses Shewing the Fatal Consequences of the Habitual Drinking of Distilled Spiritous Liquors* (n.p., 1736). Anonymous, *A Physical Account of the Nature of All Distilled Spiritous Liquors and the Malignant Effects They Have Upon Human Bodies* (n.p., 1736). Thomas Wilson, *Distilled Spirituous Liquors: The Bane of the Nation* (London: J. Roberts, 1736).

163 **help dampen one's ardor:** *Onania; or, the Heinous Sin of Self-Pollution: And All Its Frightful Consequences, in Both Sexes Consider'd* (London: Printed for the author, and sold by J. Isted . . . 1737), p. 54.

163 **Hell, but terrible decay:** John Wesley (1747), *Primitive Physic; or, an Easy and Natural Method of Curing Most Diseases* (London: Barr & Co., 1843).

164 **found guilty as charged:** See Paul Seaver, ed. *History of Suicide in England,* vol. 1 (Pickering & Chatto, 2012), p. 5.

164 **mad acts understood by medicine:** MacDonald and Murphy, *Sleepless Souls,* pp. 120–125.

164 **"Addison approved Cannot be wrong":** Ibid., pp.107, 149.

8. SYMPATHY, IDEA, NERVE

166 **any other in the world:** See Steven Shapin, "The Audience for Science in Eighteenth Century Edinburgh," *History of Science* 12, no. 2 (1974): 95–121. J. R. Christie, "The Origins and Development of the Scottish Scientific Community, 1680–1760," ibid., p. 122–141. Christopher Lawrence, "The Nervous System and Society in the Scottish Enlightenment," in *Natural Order: Historical Studies of Scientific Culture,* ed. Barry Barnes and Steven Shapin (Beverly Hills, Calif.: Sage Publications, 1979), pp. 19–40.

167 **virtuous and vicious behavior:** Francis Hutcheson, *An Essay on the Nature and Conduct of the Passions and the Affections with Illustrations on the Moral Sense* (London: James & John Knapton, 1730), p. xii.

167 **charity and remorse from deceit:** Ibid., p. 58.

167 **both personal and social harmony:** Ibid., pp. 54, 181.

168 **reason accounted for morality:** David Hume (1738), *A Treatise on Human Nature* (Oxford: Clarendon Press, 1896).

168 **thanks to shared, natural sentiments:** Smith, *The Theory of Moral Sentiments.* Also see Mandeville, *The Fable of the Bees,* vol. 2, p. 414.

168 **"my various conduct," he wrote:** James Boswell, *Boswell's London Journal: 1762–1763* (London; Melbourne: W. Heinemann, 1950), p. 39.

169 **These were innate and pathological:** Francis Hutcheson, *An Essay on the Nature and Conduct of the Passions and Affections,* pp. 54, 181. Also see R. A. Houston, *Madness and Society in Eighteenth-Century Scotland* (Oxford and New York: Clarendon Press, 2000). Andrew T. Scull, "The Peculiarities of the Scots? Scottish Influences on the Development of English Psychiatry, 1700–1980," *History of Psychiatry* 22, no. 4 (2011): 403–415.

169 **sympathy, sentiments, and the nerves:** I. Waddington, "The Struggle to Reform the Royal College of Physicians, 1767–1771: A Sociological Analysis," *Medical History* 17, no. 2 (1973): 107–126. Lawrence, "The Nervous System and Society in the Scottish Enlightenment," p. 34.

169 **different parts of the body:** E. H. Ackerknecht, "The history of the discovery of sympathetic nervous system," *Medical History* 18 (1974): 1–8.

170 **force infused all of Nature:** Robert Whytt, *An Essay on the Vital and Other Involuntary Motions of Animals* (Edinburgh: Hamilton, Balfour & Neill, 1751), p. 266.

170 **fits could be similarly contagious:** Robert Whytt, *Observations on the Nature, Causes, and Cure of Those Disorders Which Have Been Commonly*

Called Nervous, Hypochondriac, or Hysteric (Edinburgh: T. Becket and P. A. de Hondt, 1765), p. 219.

171 **"apply himself to the Mind":** William Cullen, *Institutions of Medicine: Part 1, Physiology for the Use of Students* (Edinburgh: Charles Eliot, 1775), p. 143. Also see Julius Rocco, "William Cullen (1710–1790) and Robert Whytt (1714–1766) on the Nervous System," in *Brain, Mind, and Medicine: Essays in Eighteenth-Century Neuroscience*, ed. Harry A. Whitaker, C. U. M. Smith, and Stanley Finger (New York: Springer, 2007), pp. 85–98.

171 **with matter, Dr. David Hartley:** James Boswell, *Boswell's London Journal: 1762–1763,* ed. Frederick Albert Pottle (London and Melbourne: W. Heinemann, 1950), p. 312.

171 **the author himself greatly suffered:** See Richard Allen, *David Hartley on Human Nature* (Albany: State University of New York Press, 1999), p. 53.

171 **through the interweaving of ideas:** John Gay,"Preliminary Dissertation Concerning the Fundamental Principle of Virtue or Morality," in William King, *An Essay on the Origin of Evil* (London: W. Thurlbourn, 1731).

172 **take charge of actions, including moral choices:** This was psychophysics *avant la lettre*. See Robert B. Glassman and Hugh Buckingham, "David Hartley's Neural Vibrations and Psychological Associations," in *Brain, Mind, and Medicine: Essays in Eighteenth-Century Neuroscience*, eds. Harry A. Whitaker et al. (New York: Springer, 2007), pp. 177–190, and Corinna Delkeskamp, "Medicine, Science, and Moral Philosophy: David Hartley's Attempt at Reconciliation," *Journal of Medicine and Philosophy* 2, no. 2 (1977): 162–176.

172 **Sin, Hell, and eternal damnation:** W. B. Trigg, "The Correspondence of Dr. David Hartley and Rev. John Liste," *Transactions of the Halifax Antiquarian Society* (1938), p. 237.

173 **divine body of Jesus Christ:** Ibid., p. 251.

173 **errors of the mind:** David Hartley, *Prayers and Religious Meditations* (Cambridge, Mass.: Hilliard & Brown, 1829), p. 32. Also see Trigg, "The Correspondence of Dr. David Hartley and Rev. John Liste," p. 236. Delkeskamp, "Medicine, Science, and Moral Philosophy," p. 168.

173 **he couldn't fully convince himself:** David Hartley, *Observations on Man, His Frame, His Duty, and His Expectations* (London: T. Tegg & Son, 1834), pp. 347–364.

173 **privately confessed, "I am mechanical":** Trigg, "The Correspondence of Dr. David Hartley and Rev. John Liste," p. 254.

173 **analogy he considered very objectionable:** Ibid., p. 255.

173 **known to sometimes concede:** J. B. Priestly, "Introduction" to Hartley, *Observations on Man, His Frame, His Duty, and His Expectations,* p. xx.

174 **approach the mind's problems:** R. Hoeldtke, "The History of Associationism and British Medical Psychology," *Medical History*, 11, no. 1 (1967): 48.

174 **only Hartley's psychology intact:** J. B. Priestly, "Introduction" to Hartley, *Observations on Man, His Frame, His Duty, and His Expectations,* p. 2.

174 **Alfred Binet and Sigmund Freud:** Roger Smith, "The Background of Physiological Psychology in Natural Philosophy," *History of Science* 11, no. 2 (1973): 75–123.

174 **such bodily and mental troubles:** Hartley, *Observations on Man, His Frame, His Duty, and His Expectations,* p. 234.

175 **"considerable light from this theory. . . .":** Ibid., p. 236.

175 **fight that made him famous:** This story is recounted in John H. Jesse, *Memoirs of Celebrated Etonians* (London: Richard Bentley & Son, 1875), pp. 18–23. Battie's diminutive stature was mocked in Anonymous, *The Battiad: Canto the First* (London: G. Smith, 1750), p. 3.

177 **"Doctor turns to low Buffoon":** Ibid., p. 4.

177 **Bedlam like a stern reproach:** Battie has not found a biographer, but much on his life and thought can be found in Jonathan Andrews and Andrew T. Scull, *Undertaker of the Mind: John Monro and Mad-Doctoring in Eighteenth-Century England* (Berkeley: University of California Press, 2001).

177 **William Battie opened its doors:** Leonard D. Smith, *Lunatic Hospitals in Georgian England, 1750–1830* (New York: Routledge, 2007), pp. 8–10.

178 **"(almost) to a single Person":** *Reasons for the Establishing and Further Encouragement of St. Luke's Hospital for Lunaticks* (London: J. March, 1786), pp. 3–5.

178 **book in English on madness:** William Battie, *A Treatise on Madness* (London: J. Whiston & B. White, 1758). For Battie's views on mental illness, also see his *Aphorismi de cognoscendis et curandis morbis* (London: n.p., 1760), pp. 61–74.

178 **doors for advancement and learning:** Ibid., p. v.

178 **attack on all royal hospitals:** Andrews and Scull, *Undertaker of the Mind,* p. 46.

178 **in madness were "extremely delusive":** Battie, *A Treatise on Madness,* p. 16.

179 **an out-of-control animal:** Ibid., p. 32.

179 **all driven by "shaping fantasies":** William Shakespeare, *A Midsummer's Night Dream* (New York: Washington Square Press, 1993), p. 143.

179 **Whytt, on sympathetic reflexes:** On Haller and Whytt, see Suzuki, *Mind and Its Disease in Enlightenment British Medicine,* pp. 221–268.

179 **ideas that solidified into insanity:** Battie, *A Treatise on Madness,* pp. 26, 43.

180 **"ought strictly to be forbidden":** Ibid., pp. 68–69.

180 **great indebtedness to Locke:** See Locke, *Of the Conduct of the Understanding,* pp. 130.

180 **quite plausible counterarguments:** See Paul Laffey, "Psychiatric Therapy in Georgian Britain," *Psychological Medicine* 33, no. 7 (2003): 1289.

181 **the head to encourage perspiration:** T. Smollett, "Review of William

Beattie's 'Treatise on Madness,'" *The Critical Review; or, Annals of Literature.* 4 (1758), pp. 513, 516.

181   *of Sir Launcelot Greaves*: T. Smollett (1762), *Adventures of Sir Launcelot Greaves; with the Author's Preface, and an Introduction* (New York: Jenson Society, 1907); and Richard A. Hunter and Ida Macalpine, "Smollett's Reading in Psychiatry," *Modern Language Review* 51, no. 3 (1956). Also James Boswell, "The Hypochondriack. No. Lxiii.," *London Magazine; or, Gentleman's Monthly Intelligencer* (1782).

182   *The London-Citizen Exceedingly Injured*: A. Cruden, *The London-Citizen Exceedingly Injured: Or a British Inquisition Display'd* (London: T. Cooper & Dodd, 1739). Also see Julia Keay's biography of Cruden, *Alexander the Corrector* (London: HarperCollins, 2004).

182   **"bird upon the wing"**: Cruden, *The London-Citizen Exceedingly Injured*, p.13.

182   **to dine with the Pope:** Andrews and Scull, *Undertaker of the Mind*, pp. 7–8.

184   **of course, William Battie:** John Monro, *Remarks on Dr Battie's Treatise on Madness* (London: John Clarke, 1758), pp. 16, 29.

184   **I have seen what cures:** Ibid., p. 20. These claims of cure were also positioned against a category of incurable "original madness," postulated by William Battie, which Monro claimed did not exist.

185   **"without the shadow of experience":** Haller to Tissot, December 3, 1759; in *Albrecht Hallers Briefe an August Tissot, 1754–1777* (Bern: Huber, 1977), p. 87.

185   **long enough to be acquitted:** Andrews and Scull, *Undertaker of the Mind*, p. 71.

186   **Socrates' medicine that was required:** George Baker, "On the Affections of the Mind and the Diseases Arising from Them," in Hunter and Macalpine, *Three Hundred Years of Psychiatry*, pp. 399–400.

186   **one observer the "Antimaniac physicians":** Ibid., pp. 463–465.

186   **right all the wrong associations:** William Perfect, *Cases of Insanity: The Epilepsy, Hypochondriacal Affection, Hysteric Passion, and Nervous Disorders, Successfully Treated* (Rochester, Eng.: T. Fisher, 1780). Also see Jonathan Andrews and Andrew T. Scull, *Customers and Patrons of the Mad-Trade: The Management of Lunacy in Eighteenth-Century London: With the Complete Text of John Monro's 1766 Case Book* (Berkeley: University of California Press, 2002), p. 85.

187   **now rested on medical ground:** Thomas Withers, *Observations on the Abuse of Medicine* (London: J. Johnson, 1775), and his *Observations on Chronic Weakness* (York, Eng.: A. Ward, 1777). William Pargeter, *Observations on Maniacal Disorders* (Reading, Eng.: Smart & Cowslade, 1792). Andrew Harper, *A Treatise on the Real Cause and Cure of Insanity* (London: C. Stalker, 1789). James Adair in Hunter and Macalpine, *Three Hundred Years of Psychiatry*, pp. 489–490.

187 **filial piety of John Monro:** Tobias Smollett, Review of John Monro's "Remarks on Dr. Battie's Treatise on Madness," *Critical Review* 5 (1758): 226.

9. THE CURE OF A LUNATIC KING

188 **"oppressive tyranny makes him so":** Roy Porter, *Mind Forg'd Manacles*, pp. 148–152. Also Andrew T. Scull, *The Most Solitary of Afflictions: Madness and Society in Britain, 1700–1900* (New Haven: Yale University Press, 1993), p. 24.

189 **found no signs of illness:** Andrews and Scull, *Undertaker of the Mind*, pp. 50–54.

189 **custodial restraint, management with medicine:** Leonard Smith, *Lunatic Asylums in Georgian England, 1750–1830*, pp. 21–47.

190 **was determined to be different:** Thomas Arnold, *Observations on the Nature, Kinds, Causes, and Prevention of Insanity*, vol. 1 (Leicester, Eng.: G. Ireland, 1782). Also see Macalpine and Hunter, *Three Hundred Years of Psychiatry*, pp. 467–471.

190 **"moral and medical Insanity":** Arnold, *Observations on Nature, Kinds, Causes and Prevention of Insanity, Lunacy or Madness*, p. 470.

191 **made ill by ideas:** Ibid., pp.47–53.

191 **restore that sufferer to health:** Smith, *Lunatic Hospitals in Georgian England, 1750–1830*, p. 3.

191 **tortured and even murdered:** John Ferrier (1792), *Medical Histories and Reflections* (Philadelphia: Thomas Dobson, 1816), p. 187.

191 **conversely, offered hope:** Harper, *A Treatise on the Real Cause and Cure of Insanity*, pp. 59–61.

192 **further delay declared him mad:** Jonathan Andrews and Andrew Scull, *Customers and Patrons of the Mad-Trade* (Berkeley: University of California Press, 2003). See cases C5, 79, 25. Macalpine and Hunter, *Three Hundred Years of Psychiatry*, p. 422.

192 **the parts on stage himself:** Neil Curry, *Christopher Smart* (Northvale, Eng.: British Council, 2005), p. 5.

192 **priest who recommended prayer:** Christopher Smart, *The Annotated Letters of Christopher Smart*, ed. B. Rizzo and R. Mahoney (Carbondale: Southern Illinois University Press, 1991), pp. 67–68.

193 **though not in harsh conditions:** This may have been one of William Battie's private hospitals; see Chris Mounsey, *Christopher Smart: Clown of God* (Lewisburg, Pa.: Bucknell University Press, 2001), p. 206. Also see Thomas Keymer, "Johnson, Madness, and Smart," in *Christopher Smart and the Enlightenment*, ed. Clement Hawes (New York: St. Martin's Press, 1999).

193 **"image sunk, defac'd and maim'd":** Christopher Smart, *Hymn to the Supreme Being* (London: J. Newbery, 1756), p. 9.

193 **noted for its enlightened care:** William Cowper, *Cowper: Verse and Letters,* ed. Brian Spiller (Cambridge: Harvard University Press, 1968), p. 20.

193 **"fleshy tomb . . . / Buried above ground":** Ibid., p. 54.

193 **King George III became insane:** For the influential argument that the king suffered from porphyria, see Ida Macalpine and R. A. Hunter, *George III and the Mad-Business* (New York: Pantheon Books, 1969). This diagnosis has been questioned recently; see T. J. Peters and D. Wilkinson, "King George and Porphyria: A Clinical Re-examination of the Clinical Evidence," *History of Psychiatry* 21 (2010): 3–19.

195 **merrily playing an imaginary fiddle:** Walter Sydney Sichel and Georgiana Spencer Cavendish Devonshire, *Sheridan: From New and Original Material; Including a Manuscript Diary by Georgiana Duchess of Devonshire* (Boston: Houghton Mifflin, 1909), vol. 2, p. 406.

195 **The king is insane:** Macalpine and Hunter, *George III and the Mad-Business,* pp. 14–35. Also on Baker, see Macalpine and Hunter, *Three Hundred Years of Psychiatry,* p. 399.

196 **the sovereign would never recover:** *Report from the Committee Appointed to Examine the Physicians Who Have Attended His Majesty During His Illness: Touching the State of His Majesty's Health* (London: J. Stockdale, 1789). The one holdout was Sir Lucas Pepys.

196 **catered to the well-to-do:** On Willis, see the account of his grandson in Francis Willis, *A Treatise on Mental Derangement* (London: Longman et al., 1823), and Macalpine and Hunter, *George III and the Mad Business,* pp. 269–276.

196 **patients might enjoy a hunt:** Sichel and Devonshire, *Sheridan,* vol. 2, p. 41.

197 **Fanny Burney, in her diary:** Fanny Burney, *The Diary and Letters of Frances Burney,* ed. Sarah Chauncey Woolsey (Boston: Little, Brown & Co., 1910), p. 97.

197 **blend intelligence with "placid self-possession":** Nathaniel William Wraxall, *Posthumous Memoirs of His Own Time* (London: R. Bentley, 1836), pp. 197–198.

197 **the "meanest" of individuals:** Wraxall, *Posthumous Memoirs of His Own Time,* p. 198.

198 **"first to be severe" with George:** Sichel and Devonshire, *Sheridan,* vol. 2, p. 404.

198 **pounce upon this imprudence:** Ibid., pp. 416–417.

198 **He is much worse:** Ibid., p. 421.

199 **the "gusts of passion":** *Report from the Committee Appointed to Examine the Physicians Who Have Attended His Majesty During His Illness,* p. 81.

199 **document these success stories:** Ibid., pp. 13, 28, 29, 40.

200 **Pitt squashed any such discussion:** Sichel and Devonshire, *Sheridan,* p. 413.

200 **and too little rest:** Ibid., p. 42.

200 **tried his hand at Lear:** Ibid., p. 76.

200 **"his thus, Sir—thus!":** Macalpine and Hunter, *George III and the Mad-Business*, p. 272. Also see F. Reynolds, *The Life and Times of Frederick Reynolds Written by Himself*, vol 2 (London: Henry Colburn, 1826), pp. 23–24. The notion that the eye by its very emanations could fascinate another has a history in magical practices; see Keith Thomas, *Religion and the Decline of Magic* (New York: Charles Scribners' Sons, 1971), p. 578.

201 **"he manages his Madness":** Sichel and Devonshire, *Sheridan,* vol. 2, p. 413.

201 **"principal means used for recovery":** Anonymous, "Détails sur l'établissement du Docteur Willis, pour la guérison des aliénés," *Bibliothèque britannique* 1 (1796): 759–773. Quote on p. 770.

201 **the disturbed made chains unnecessary:** William Pargeter, *Observations on Maniacal Disorders* (Reading, Eng.: Smart & Cowslade, 1792).

201 **"a furious madman to be":** Ibid., pp. 49–53.

201 **settle into fixed delusions:** Macalpine and Hunter, *George III and the Mad-Business*, pp. 78–79, 87.

202 **"Britons Rejoice Your King's Restored, 1789":** Ibid., p. 94.

203 **mental method for madness:** "Détails sur l'établissement du Dr. Willis," 759–773.

203 **their living filling this demand:** On the rise of consumer society and the professions, see Porter, *Mind-Forg'd Manacles*.

203 **states were known to pass:** Francis Willis, *A Treatise on Mental Derangement* (London: Longman, Hurst, Rees, Orme & Brown, 1823).

203 **get his own bearings:** Macalpine and Hunter, *George III and the Mad-Business*, p. 144.

204 **madman—was sent to Bethlem:** Porter, *Mind-Forg'd Manacles*, p. 116.

204 **"steady and effectual government":** *The History of the Rise and Progress of the York Lunatic Asylum* (York, Eng.: n.p., 1785), p. 1.

205 **waistcoats and even employed bloodletting:** Digby, *Madness, Morality, and Medicine*, pp. 263–265.

206 **a pillar of fire:** Ibid., p. 192.

206 **an inborn morality:** L. C. Charland, "Benevolent Theory: Moral Treatment at the York Retreat," *History of Psychiatry* 18, no. 1 (2007): 61–80.

206 **he had learned in Edinburgh:** Digby, *Madness, Morality, and Medicine*, p. 105.

206 **utopian penitentiary, the Panopticon:** On the panopticon, see Simon Schaffer, "States of Mind: Enlightenment and Natural Philosophy," ed. G. S. Rousseau, *The Languages of Psyche* (Berkeley: University of California, 1990), pp. 233–288. Also see Michel Foucault, *Discipline and Punish*, trans. Alan Sheridan (New York: Vintage Books, 1975).

207 moral engagement and no medicine: Francis Willis, *A Treatise on Mental Derangement*, pp. 37–38.

207 success of their establishment: Samuel Tuke, *Description of the Retreat, An Institution Near York for Insane Persons* (York, Eng.: W. Alexander, 1813).

208 "right a mind gone wrong: Digby, *Madness, Morality, and Medicine*, pp. 237–246.

PART III: FROM FRENCH *ESPRIT* TO ALIENATION

209 "reader is the book itself": Denis Diderot, *Eléments de physiologie*, ed. Jean Mayer (Paris: Librairie M. Didier, 1964), p. 423. "Voilà le livre. Mais où est le lecteur? Le lecteur est le livre même."

10. THE FRENCH SENSATIONALISTS

211 seditious notions regarding the soul: See Marc Fumaroli, *When the World Spoke French,* trans. Richard Howard (New York: New York Review Books, 2011). In 1750, D'Alembert touted French as a universal language.

212 suggested that matter could think: Abbé Macy, *Traité de l'âme des bêtes: Avec des réflexions phisiques et morales* (Paris: P. G. Le Mercier, 1737). Macy was likely the editor of this work.

212 mechanical operations to the soul: Jean-Baptiste Joseph Lallemant, *Essai sur le méchanisme des passions en général* (Paris: Pierre Alexandre Le Prieur, 1751), p. xxiii.

212 be able to cogitate: Cited in Aram Vartanian, *La Mettrie's L'Homme machine: A Study in the Origins of an Idea* (Princeton: Princeton University Press, 1960), p. 68.

212 Locke, Newton, and Shaftesbury: On the problems of translating Locke into French, see John Hampton, "Les traductions françaises de Locke au XVIII siècle," *Revue de littérature comparée* 29 (1955): 240–251, and Ann Thomson, "Locke, Stillingfleet et Coste: La philosophie en extraits," *Cromohs* 12 (2007): 1–16.

212 enlightened royals of Europe: Delphine Soulard, "Anglo-French Cultural Transmission: The Case of John Locke and the Huguenots," *Historical Research* 85, no. 227 (2012): 105–132.

213 taverns, cafés, and bookshops: Robert Darnton, *The Forbidden Best-Sellers of Pre-Revolutionary France* (New York: W. W. Norton, 1995).

213 "completely detached from matter!": *Thérèse philosophe* was translated and published in ibid. See especially pp. 261–262.

213 hedonism and bodily need: Ibid., pp. 92–93.

213 this endorsement to himself: Madame du Deffand et al., *The Unpublished Correspondence of Madame du Deffand*, 2 vols. (London: A. K. Newman,

1810), vol. 1, pp. 129–130. Madame du Deffand to d'Alembert, letter ca. 1753.

214 **functions of the body:** See Vartanian, *La Mettrie's L'Homme machine*, pp. 57–70, and Ann Thomson, "Introduction" in La Mettrie's *Machine Man and Other Writings* (Cambridge: Cambridge University Press, 1996), p. xiii.

214 **controversies over thinking matter:** M. Locke, *Essai philosophique concernant l'entendement humain,* trans. M. Coste (Amsterdam and Leipzig: J. Schreuder & Pierre Mortier, 1755). This is the corrected fifth edition; the first edition appeared in 1729.

214 **Locke's life and thought:** Jean-Baptiste Boyer d'Argens, *Mémoires secrets de la république des lettres* (Amsterdam: Neaulme, 1744). Also see Thomson, "Locke, Stillingfleet et Coste. La philosophie en extraits."

214 **illicitly published** *Philosophical Letters:* Voltaire's work was first published in a pirated English version, *Letters Concerning the English Nation* (London: C. Davis, 1733). In 1734, the expanded version was published in French as *Lettres philosophiques* (Amsterdam: E. Lucas, 1734).

214 **matter by the Divine Maker:** Voltaire, *Letters Concerning the English Nation.* p. 111.

215 **"to hide one's miracles":** Émilie du Chatelet, *Selected Philosophical and Scientific Writings,* trans. Judith P. Zinsser and I. Bour (Chicago: University of Chicago Press, 2009), pp. 202, 229–230.

216 **three hundred by the 1760s:** Isser Woloch, *Eighteenth-Century Europe: Tradition and Progress, 1715–1789* (New York: W. W. Norton, 1982), p. 260.

216 **to know what was modern?:** Darnton, *The Forbidden Best-Sellers of Pre-Revolutionary France,* p. xix.

216 **French words and their usages:** New editions of the *Dictionnaire de l'Académie française* appeared in 1718 and again in 1740, 1762, and 1798. See the University of Chicago's *Dictionnaires d'autrefois,* http://artfl.uchicago .edu.

216 **human sentiment and conviction:** John Locke (1690), *An Essay Concerning Human Understanding,* ed. A. C. Fraser, vol. 1 (New York: Dover Publications, 1959), pp. 448–449, and Locke, *Essai philosophique concernant l'entendement humain,* p. 270. In the fifth edition of this French work, Coste writes: "En François, nous n'avons à mon avis que les mots de sentiment et de conviction . . ." p. 264.

216 **man recognizes good from evil:** See the definition of *conscience* in *Dictionnarie de l'Académie francaise,* editions of 1694 and 1762. *Dictionnaires d'autrefois,* http://artfl.uchicago.edu.

217 **words for these English terms:** Soulard, "Anglo-French Cultural Transmission, p. 121.

217 **ghosts, revenants, and vampires:** Augustin Calmet, *Traité sur les apparitions des esprits et sur les vampires, ou les revenans, de Hongrie, de Moravie, etc.* (Paris: Debure, 1751).

217 *esprit humain*—the human spirit: See the 1765 entry on *esprit* in *Ency-clopédie, ou dictionnaire raisonné des sciences, des arts et des métiers, etc.,* eds. Denis Diderot and Jean le Rond d'Alembert (University of Chicago: ARTFL Encyclopédie Project (Spring 2013 Edition), ed. Robert Morrissey, http://encyclopedie.uchicago.edu/. Spirit in medicine referred to animal spirits, a subtle wind that coursed through the body; chemical spirits were the same as gases. *Esprit* could also signify qualities of the soul, like genius, fine taste, or good character. Adding to the semantic confusion, the word could refer to the cultural product of a period or time, as in the spirit of an age.

218 **term was fatally vague:** Voltaire (1764), *A Pocket Philosophical Dictionary,* ed. John Fletcher; Nicholas Cronk (Oxford and New York: Oxford University Press, 2011), p. 50.

218 **which concerned modern views:** See Jürgen Habermas, *The Structural Transformation of the Public Sphere,* trans. T. Burger and F. Lawrence (Cambridge: MIT Press, 1991).

220 ***The Spirit of the Laws:*** Charles-Louis de Montesquieu (1748), *Esprit des loix* (Paris: Firmin Didot Frères, 1862).

220 **formed by its environs:** Ibid., pp. 248, 252, 368, 389, 442. See Sharon Krause, "History and the Human Soul in Montesquieu," *History of Political Thought* 24 (2003): 235–261. She has forwarded the argument that the baron's work was intended to counter Spinoza and Hobbes.

220 **author would face intense hostility:** Helvétius, *Correspondance générale d'Helvétius,* vol. 3, ed. David Smith (Toronto: University of Toronto Press, 1991), p. 285. David Hume to Rev. Hugh Blair reports this in a letter dated April 1, 1767. Two far more critical letters supposedly written by Helvétius about Montesquieu were likely forgeries; see R. Koebner, "The Authenticity of the Letters on the *Esprit des Lois* Attributed to Helvétius," *Historical Research* 24 (1951): 19–43. F. M. Grimm reported that Helvétius was motivated to write in response to Montesquieu; see p. 26. Also see David Wooten, "Helvétius: From Radical Enlightenment to Revolution," *Political Theory* 28 (2000): 307–336.

221 **shockingly dodged, saying "who knows?":** Claude-Adrien Helvétius (1759), *De l'esprit* (Paris: Lavigne, 1843), pp. 1–12. In English, see Helvétius, *De l'esprit; or, Essays on the Mind and Its Several Faculties* (London: Dodfley & Co., 1759), and C. A. Helvétius, *De l'esprit; or, Essays on the Mind,* trans. W. Mudford (London: W. Mudford, 1807), p. 5. Also see Mudford's introduction, p. viii, on the influence of Montesquieu on his friend; and for the battles over this book, see D. W. Smith, "The Publication of Helvétius's *De l'esprit* (1758–9)," *French Studies* 18, no. 4 (1964): 337. Jonathan Israel considers this thinker along with d'Holbach, Diderot, and others, to be central to the radical philosophy that drove the French Revolution. See his *Revolutionary Ideas* (Princeton: Princeton University Press, 2014), pp. 18–23, 278–279.

222 **fig leaf for these deep demands:** Helvétius, *De l'esprit*, pp. 155–208.

222 **tear these bodies to shreds:** Voltaire, *A Pocket Philosophical Dictionary*, pp. 26–27.

222 **a steady underground best-seller:** Alan Dainard et al., eds., *Correspondance générale d'Helvétius*, vol. 2 (Toronto: University of Toronto Press, 1984), p. 241. David Hume to William Robertson, March 12, 1759. Voltaire's letter and poem on *Les philosophes* is dated June 7, 1760. See p. 281.

223 **refer to human "understanding":** Ibid., p. 289. Letter from Voltaire to Helvétius is dated August 13, 1760.

223 *Essays on the Mind*: Helvétius, *De l'esprit; or, Essays on the Mind and Its Several Faculties.*

223 **"haven't a clue, have you?":** Voltaire, *A Pocket Philosophical Dictionary*, p. 50.

223 **began to infiltrate French life:** On this semantic slippage, see Sergio Moravia, "The Enlightenment and the Sciences of Man," *History of Science* 18 (1980): 247–268, and "The Capture of the Invisible: For a (Pre)History of Psychology in 18th-Century France," *Journal of the History of the Behavioral Sciences* 19, no. 4 (1983): 370–378.

223 **unsigned work made the rounds:** Étienne Bonnot Condillac, *Essai sur l'origine des connoissances humaines*, 2 vols. (Amsterdam: Pierre Mortier, 1746).

224 **autonomous capacity for reflection:** Cited in H. Wildon Carr, "Introduction," in Étienne Bonnot Condillac, *Condillac's Treatise on the Sensations* (Los Angeles: University of Southern California Press, 1930), p. xxi.

225 **the hatred of pain:** The notion of an inner movement, an inner sense of inquietude, like Locke's inner uneasiness, was critical to the arguments of how human will worked.

225 **"not the same with man?":** Étienne Bonnot Condillac, *Traité des sensations*, vol. 2 (Londres: DeBure, 1754), p. 264.

225 **only end in apostasy:** Denis Diderot, *Lettre sur les aveugles* (Londres: n.p., 1749), and *Lettre sur les sourds et muets* (n.p., 1751). For an English translation, see Denis Diderot, *Diderot's Early Philosophical Works*, trans. M. Jourdain (New York: AMS Press, 1973).

226 **"it realizes it is free":** Condillac, *Traité des sensations*. vol. 2, p. 277. In English, see Condillac, *Condillac's Treatise on the Sensations*, p. 247.

226 **eyes and ears and mouth:** Charles Bonnet, *Essai analytique sur les facultés de l'âme* (Copenhague et Genève: Cl. Philibert, 1769), pp. 10, 15.

226 **faculty to be immaterial soul:** Charles Bonnet, *Essai de psychologie* (Londres: n.p., 1755).

226 **anatomical interrogations of a physician:** Bonnet, *Essai Analytique sur les facultés de l'âme*, p. xxi.

226 **be at times its equivalent:** G. L. Godart, *La physique de l'âme humaine* (Berlin: Aux dépens de la Compagnie, 1755). M. Le Cat, *Traité des sensations*

et des passions en général, et des sens en particulier (Collège de la Sainte Trinité de la Compagnie de Jésus: Vallat-La-Chapelle, 1767). "Les constitutions spirituelles," Le Cat claimed, "et passionnées sont a peu pres les mêmes" (p. 218).

227 **Empirical Psychology and Rational Psychology**: Christian Wolff, *Psychologie, ou Traité sur l'âme* (Amsterdam and Leipzig: J. Schneuder & P. Morties, 1756). This volume consists of both the 1732 and the 1734 tracts.

228 **credulous believe any old thing**: Voltaire, *A Pocket Philosophical Dictionary*, pp. 67–68.

228 **"I refute him *thus*"**: James Boswell (1791) *Life of Johnson* (London: Oxford University Press, 1998), p. 333.

228 **reason, and imagination, were erased**: Voltaire, *A Pocket Philosophical Dictionary*, p. 236.

228 **the impressions we have received"**: Helvétius, *De l'esprit; or, Essays on the Mind*, p. 31.

228 **"what I want," he offered**: Voltaire, *A Pocket Philosophical Dictionary*, p. 174.

229 **symbol of Enlightenment, the dictionary**: On the extraordinary Diderot, see the classic biography Arthur Wilson, *Diderot* (New York: Oxford University Press, 1972); and more recently, Gerhardt Stenger, *Diderot: Le combatant de la liberté* (Paris: Perrin, 2013), and Pierre Chartier, *Vie de Diderot*, 3 vols. (Paris: Hermann, 2013).

229 **Dictionary would be profitable**: R. James et al., *A Medicinal Dictionary: Including Physic, Surgery, Anatomy, Chymistry, and Botany, in All Their Branches Relative to Medicine: Together with a History of Drugs* (London: T. Osborne, 1743). On James and his friendship and collobaration with Samuel Johnson, see O. M. Brack and Thomas Kaminski, "Johnson, James, and the 'Medicinal Dictionary,'" *Modern Philology* 81, no. 4 (1984): 378–400.

230 **law-bound world could do that**: Denis Diderot, *Diderot's Early Philosophical Works* (New York: AMS, 1973), p. 31.

230 **"jewels" and lingered there evermore**: Denis Diderot, *Les bijoux indiscrets* (1748) in *Oeuvres Romanesques* (Paris: Garnier Frères, 1981).

230 **accidents of our senses**: Denis Diderot (1749) *Lettre sur les aveugles à l'usage de ceux qui voient*, in *Oeuvres philosophiques* (Paris: Garnier, 1990), pp. 75–164.

231 **"holy mysteries with scorn"**: Robert Darnton, *The Great Cat Massacre: And Other Episodes in French Cultural History* (New York: Vintage Books, 1984), pp. 185–186.

232 **list of desired illicit books**: Paul Henri Thiry d'Holbach (1770), *System of Nature*, trans. H. D. Robinson (Manchester: Clinamen Press, 1999). See Darnton, *The Forbidden Best-Sellers of Pre-Revolutionary France*, p. 63, and Alan Charles Kors, *D'Holbach's Coterie: An Enlightenment in Paris* (Princeton: Princeton University Press, 1976).

233 **contained more thoughts than words:** Letter of Montesquieu to d'Alembert dated Dec. 15, 1753, in Madame du Deffand et al., *The Unpublished Correspondence of Madame du Deffand*, vol. 1, p. 51.

233 **"physics of the soul (âme)":** Jean le Rond d'Alembert (1751), *Preliminary Discourse to the Encyclopedia of Diderot*, trans. Richard Schwab and Walter Rex (Indianapolis: Bobbs-Merrill, 1963), p. 84. For the French, see Jean le Rond d'Alembert, *Discours préliminaire*, in *Encyclopédie, ou dictionnaire raisonné des sciences, des arts et des métiers, etc.*, http://encyclopedie.uchicago.edu/.

234 **one word for the other:** d'Alembert, *Preliminary Discourse*, p. 46.

234 **comprehend rational and sensitive souls:** Ibid., pp. 10, 13, 52.

236 **sensing, and perceiving mind:** Ibid., pp. 10, 14, 26; also see Darnton, *The Great Cat Massacre*, pp. 194–203.

236 **soul would remain distinct:** D'Alembert, *Preliminary Discourse*, p. 29. Ernst Cassirer argued that this assumption of unity stemmed from Descartes: "The rationalistic postulate of unity dominated the minds of this age," Ernst Cassirer, *Philosophy of Enlightenment*, trans. C. A. Koeln and J. P. Pettegrove (Princeton: Princeton University Press, 1951), p. 23.

237 **Spinoza needed no friends:** Denis Diderot, "*Âme*," in *Encyclopédie, ou dictionnaire raisonné des sciences, des arts et des métiers, etc.*, http://encyclopedie.uchicago.edu/. (From here on, ARTFL Encyclopédie Project.)

11. VITALISM, THE MISSING LINK

239 **found for a dinner party:** On science and medicine during this period of French history, see Charles Gillispie, *Science and Polity in France at the End of the Old Regime* (Princeton: Princeton University Press, 1980). Jacques Léonard, *La médecine entre les savoirs et les pouvoirs: Histoire intellectuelle et politique de la médecine Française au XIXe siècle* (Paris: Aubier-Montaigne, 1981).

239 **the pia mater and dura mater:** Le Cat, *Traité des sensations et des passions en général, et des sens en particulier.*

239 **cerebral hemispheres, the corpus callosum:** Diderot, "*Âme*," ARTFL Encyclopédie Project, pp. 24–25; Mr. De La Peyronnie's, 1741 "Observationes par lesquelles on tache de Peyronniés, découvrir la partie du cerveau ou l'âme exerce ses functions" is discussed in Godart, *La physique de l'âme humaine*. 1755.

241 **Glisson had called irritability:** Sergio Moravia, "From Homme Machine to Homme Sensible: Changing Eighteenth-Century Models of Man's Image," *Journal of the History of Ideas* 39, no. 1 (1978): 45–60. Also Georges Canguilhem, *A Vital Rationalist: Selected Writings from Georges Canguilhem*, ed. François Delaporte (New York: Zone Books, 1993), pp. 179–202.

241 **seen in mechanical terms:** Hermann Boerhaave, *Institutions de médecine de M. Herman Boerhaave avec un commentaire par Monsieur* ★★★ (Paris: Huart &

Moreau, et al., 1750). On La Metttrie's commentary and translation, see Aram Vartanian, *La Mettrie's L'Homme machine: A Study in the Origins of an Idea* (Princeton: Princeton University Press, 1960), p. 79. On his conflict with Haller, see Hubert Steinke, *Irritating Experiments: Haller's Concept and the European Controversy on Irritability and Sensibility, 1750–90* (Amsterdam and New York: Rodopi, 2005), pp. 194–197.

242 **animals possessed degrees of intelligence:** S. A. D. Tissot, *Correspondance, 1754–1797* (Genève: Slatkine, 2007), p. 90. Letter of October 26, 1758, to Zimmerman.

242 **only due to sensations:** Anonymous, *"Logique," Encyclopédie,* ARTFL Encyclopédie Project.

242 **be but a machine:** M. Charp, *Histoire naturelle de l'âme,* trans. M. H★★★ (Oxford: Aux Dépends de l'Auteur, 1745). For an English version, see Julien Offray de La Mettrie, *Machine Man and Other Writings,* trans. Ann Thomson (Cambridge: Cambridge University Press, 1996), pp. 41–74.

243 **come to precisely opposite conclusions:** Charp, *Histoire naturelle de l'âme,* trans. M. H★★★ (Oxford: Aux Dépends de l'Auteur, 1747). This later edition is "augmentée de la letter Critique de M. de la Mettrie á Madame la Marquise du Châtelet."

243 **he published *Man-Machine*:** Julien de La Mettrie, *L'homme machine* (Leiden: Luzac, 1748). In 1751, La Mettrie changed the title of his first book from a *Natural History of the Soul* to a *Treatise on the Soul.*

243 **to be the most unforgivable:** On the book's reception, see Vartanian, *La Mettrie's L'Homme machine,* pp. 95–110. In private, Frederick himself toyed with the idea that the mind was a machine. In one letter, he teased a friend to "take care of that machine that gives you such good ideas." Fumaroli, *When the World Spoke French,* p. 158.

244 **"winds its own springs":** On this subject, see Ann Thomson, who correctly, I believe, insists that La Mettrie was a vitalistic materialist, not a mechanistic one; Ann Thomson "Mechanistic Materialism vs. Vitalistic Materialism?" in *La lettre de la maison française d'Oxford,* 14 (2001): 21–36. Also see Timo Kaitaro, "'Man Is an Admirable Machine'—a Dangerous Idea?" *La lettre de la maison française d'Oxford* 14 (2001): 105–122.

244 **mule pulling the cart:** Aram Vartanian, *Science and Humanism in the French Enlightenment* (Charlottesville, Va.: Rookwood Press, 1999), pp. 64–65.

244 **Lucifer, then at least by Lucretius:** Vartanian, *La Mettrie's L'Homme machine,* pp. 110–111.

246 **his soul-directed explanations:** Dr. Sauvages cited in Elizabeth A. Williams, *A Cultural History of Medical Vitalism in Enlightenment Montpellier* (Burlington, Vt.: Ashgate, 2003), p. 88.

246 **theories would be called vitalism:** See Roselyne Rey, *Naissance et développement du vitalism en France* (Oxford: Voltaire Foundation, 2000). Also see Georges Canguilhem, *A Vital Rationalist: Selected Writings from Georges*

Canguilhem (New York: Zone Books, 1994), in which the author argued that vitalism had been misunderstood and undervalued since the late 19th century, and Owsei Temkin, *The Double Face of Janus and Other Essays in the History of Medicine* (Baltimore: Johns Hopkins University Press, 1977), pp. 340–344.

247 **purpose, force, and intention:** See Williams, *A Cultural History of Medical Vitalism in Enlightenment Montpellier*, pp. 80–111. Also see Julian Martin, "Sauvages's Nosology: Medical Enlightenment in Montpellier," in *Medical Enlightenment of the Eighteenth Century*, ed. Andrew Cunningham and R. K. French (Cambridge and New York: Cambridge University Press, 1990).

247 **must stem from the soul:** Steinke, *Irritating Experiments*, p. 187. On the infiltration of this notion in aesthetic and scientific circles, see Jessica Riskin, *Science in the Age of Sensibility* (Chicago: University of Chicacgo Press, 2002).

247 **contact to the soul:** Albrecht von Haller, *Dissertation sur les parties irritables et sensibles des animaux* (Lausanne: Marc-Michel Bousquet, 1755). Also see Dominique Boury, "Irritability and Sensibility: Key Concepts in Assessing the Medical Doctrines of Haller and Bordeu," *Science in Context* 21, no. 4 (2008): 521–535.

248 **the Royal Society of Sciences in Göttingen:** Albrecht von Haller (1755), *A Dissertation on the Sensible and Irritable Parts of Animals,* trans. Owsei Temkin (Baltimore: Johns Hopkins Press, 1936).

248 **attached to sensibility:** Robert Whytt, *An Essay on the Vital and Other Involuntary Motions of Animals* (Edinburgh: Hamilton, Balfour & Neill, 1751).

248 **sensibility was exclusively human:** He thus had trouble explaining human reflex actions; see Owsei Temkin, "Introduction" to Haller, *A Dissertation on the Sensible and Irritable Parts of Animals*, p. 653. This debate was also influenced by the Swiss naturalist Abraham Trembley's 1744 discovery that polyps could be divided but still survive.

248 **"materialists, fatalists, Spinozists":** Steinke, *Irritating Experiments*, p. 188.

249 **the soul was a *thing*:** Ibid., p. 194.

249 **making a big move:** There are no biographies of Bordeu. On his life, see the introduction by Charles Lefeuve, "Bordeu," in Théophile Bordeu, *Recherches sur l'histoire de la médecine* (Paris: Ghio, 1882), and Théophile Bordeu, *Correspondance*, 4 vols. (Montpellier: Centre national de la recherche scientifique, 1977).

249 **getting one's grades at school:** Théophile Bordeu, *Correspondance*, vol. 1, pp. 87–91 and following pages.

250 **how to truly practice medicine:** Ibid., vol. 1, p. 65.

251 **exploited him for that purpose:** Ibid., vol. 2, pp. 113–121. He wrote: "Le médicine étoit un fol a metre aux petites maisons, et si fol enfin qu'il a imagine créer une médicine et faire un livre pour cela . . . et c'est ce qui l'atachoit a moi."

251 **had tried to enslave him:** Ibid., p. 114. Bordeu to his mother complained: "Il prit un tel empire sur moi." Also see Lacaze to Bordeu, p. 120.

251 **Lucretius and no author's name:** Louis de La Caze, *Idée de l'homme physique et moral: Pour servir d'introduction à un traité de médecine* (Paris: H. L. Guerin & L. F. Delatour, 1755). Also see Bordeu, *Théophile Bordeu, Correspondance*, vol 1, p. 70.

251 **the physical and the moral:** See François Azouvi, "Physique and Moral," in *Psyche and Soma: Physicians and Metaphysicians on the Mind-Body Problem from Antiquity to Enlightenment*, ed. John P. Wright and Paul Potter (Oxford: Clarendon Press, 2000). Also Moravia, "The Capture of the Invisible: For a (Pre)History of Psychology in 18th-Century France."

252 **sympathetic and antagonistic actions:** La Caze, *Idée de l'homme physique et moral*, pp. 74–75. Also see Jean-Jacques Menuret de Chambaud, *Éloge historique de M. Venel, professeur en mèdecine dans l'université de Montpellier* (Grenoble: J. Cuchet, 1777), p. 20.

252 **humans in sickness and in health:** La Caze, *Idée de l'homme physique et moral*, p.1.

252 **the entire bodily system:** Ibid., p. 309.

252 **one's choices and voluntary actions:** Ibid., p. 361.

252 **sensation and then willful action:** Ibid., p. 382.

252 **heart rate, and the skin:** Ibid., p. 401.

252 **Individual's sensibilities determined their character:** Ibid., p. 412.

253 **conversely, its excessive restraint:** See Philippe Huneman, "Montpellier Vitalism and the Emergence of Alienism in France (1750–1800): The Case of the Passions," *Science in Context* 21(2008): 615–647. Dominique Boury, "Irritability and Sensibility: Key Concepts in Assessing the Medical Doctrines of Haller and Bordeu," ibid., p. 532.

253 **freely pursue mental therapeutics:** Antoine Le Camus, *Médicine de l'esprit: Ou l'on traité des dispositions et des causes physiques qui, en conséquence de l'union de l'âme avec le corps, influent sur les opérations de l'esprit*, 2 vols. (Paris: Ganeau, 1753), vol. 1, p. 15.

254 **"the Medicine of Spirit!":** Voltaire wrote: "vous n'avez pas fait avec esprit la Médecine de l'esprit." See his *Dictionnaire philosophique* in *Oeuvres complètes* (Paris: Garnier Frères, 1879), vol. 4, p. 180.

254 **declared himself a faithful dualist:** Vartanian, *La Mettrie's L'Homme machine*, pp. 90–92.

254 **based on the animal economy:** T. Bordeu, *Recherches anatomiques sur la position des glandes et leur action* (Paris: Quillau, 1752). Also see Charles T. Wolfe and Motoichi Terada, "The Animal Economy as Object and Program in Montpellier Vitalism," *Science in Context* 21 (2008), pp. 537–579. Also see Elizabeth L. Haigh, "Vitalism, the Soul, and Sensibility: The Physiology of Théophile Bordeu," *Journal of the History of Medicine and Allied Sciences* 31, no. 1 (1976): 37.

255 **work of Bordeu and Lacaze:** Venel, "Irritabilité," 8:909, and M. Fouquet, "Sensibilité, Sentiment,"15:38–52, in the *Encyclopédie*, ARTFL Encyclopédie Project.

255 **mind needed to be breached:** Menuret de Cambaud, "Oeconomie animale," 11:360–366, in *Encyclopédie*, ARTFL Encyclopédie Project.

255 **"on moral life and happiness":** Ibid.

255 **burning sadness, and lost love:** Menuret de Chambaud, "Manie," 10:31–
34, in *Encyclopédie*, ARTFL Encyclopédie Project 1765. He was also known
as Jean-Joseph Menuret.

255 **to slowly regulate and heal:** Ibid.

256 **"both morally and physically":** Théophile de Bordeu, *Correspondance*,
vol. 4, p. 67. La Marquise de la Vaupalière wrote on July 3, 1776: "O mon
cher Théophile, quel mal fait votre absence moralement et physiquement!"

256 **founding a truly philosophical medicine:** Bordeu, *Recherches sur l'histoire
de la médecine*, p. 261.

256 **to ground their theories:** Ibid., p. 242.

256 **based on sensibility and sentiment:** Ibid., pp. 247–248.

257 **called the "circle of action":** La Caze, *Idée de l'homme physique et moral*, pp.
66–68.

257 **difference to delirium to laughter:** Louis Poinsinet de Sivry, *Traité des
causes physiques et morales du rire relativement à l'art de l'exciter* (Amsterdam:
Marc-Michel Rey, 1768).

258 **persuaded him of their position:** Some have taken Diderot to be a reductive mechanist, something any reading of *Jacques the Fatalist* should confound. I am in agreement with Martin Staum, Sergio Moravia, and others
who assert that Diderot was the *philosophe* closest to vitalism; see for example, Moravia, "The Capture of the Invisible, p. 375, and Jean-Paul Jouary,
Diderot et la matière vivante (Paris: Messidor, 1992). On Bordeu and Diderot,
see Alexandre Wenger, *Le médecin et le philosophe* (Paris: Hermann, 2012).
On Diderot's vitalism, see Dominque Lecourt, *Diderot: Passions, sexe, raison*
(Paris: Presses universitaires de France, 2013).

258 **heavily on contributors from Montpellier:** Diderot relied mostly on the
polymath Jaucort, who was Boerhaavian, and the vitalists Fouquet and
Menuret; See Caroline Warman, "Charts and Signposts: Following Vitalism and Mechanism Through the Encyclopédie Méthodique (1787–1830)
and the "Dictionaire des sciences médicales (1812–1822)," *La lettre de la
maison française d'Oxford* 14 (2001), pp. 85–104.

259 **"high that it would":** Denis Diderot, *Jacques the Fatalist*, trans. David
Coward (Oxford: Oxford University Press, 2008), p. 150.

259 **which was active consciousness:** Denis Diderot, *Rameau's Nephew, and
D'Alembert's Dream*, trans. L. Tancock (Harmondsworth, Eng.: Penguin,
1966), pp. 209–210.

259 **physical and moral makeup?:** Denis Diderot, "Réfutation suivie de l'ou-
     vrage d'Helvétius intitulé *L'Homme*," in *Oeuvres complètes de Diderot*, vol. 2,
     ed. J. Assezat (Paris: Garnier Fréres, 1875), pp. 276, 296.

259 **matter into a furry chick:** Ibid., p. 301.

260 **"reader is the book itself":** Denis Diderot, *Éléments de physiologie*, ed. Jean
     Mayer (Paris: Librairie M. Didier, 1964), p. 423. "Voilà le livre. Mais où est
     le lecteur? Le lecteur est le livre meme."

260 **thought, self, and consciousness:** See Kurt P. A. Ballstadt, *Diderot: Natural
     Philosopher* (Oxford: Voltaire Foundation, 2008).

260 **its use of philosophy:** J. L. Alibert, "Éloge historique de Roussel," in
     Pierre Roussel (1775), *Systéme physique et moral de la femme* (Paris: Caille &
     Ravier, 1809), p. x.

260 **offered vast philosophical opportunities:** Ibid., p. v.

261 **"force that governs animated beings":** Ibid., p. x1. Also see Anne C.
     Vila, "Sex and Sensibility: Pierre Roussel's *Système Physique et Moral de la
     Femme*," *Representations*, no. 52 (1995): 76–93.

261 **comprehend the lives of women:** Pierre Roussel (1775), *Systéme physique
     et moral de la femme* (Paris: Caille & Ravier, 1809). Also see Williams, *A
     Cultural History of Medical Vitalism in Enlightenment Montpellier*, pp. 226, 230.

261 **to study women after heartbreak:** Jean Louis Alibert, *Éloge historique de
     Pierre Roussel*, p. xxxi.

262 **figure to many Parisian *literati*:** Jacques Lordat, *Exposition de la doctrine
     médicale de P.-J. Barthez et mémoires sur la vie de ce médecin* (Paris: Gabon,
     1818), p. 8. On Barthez, see Alisa Schulweis Reich, "Paul Joseph Barthez
     and the Impact of Vitalism on Medicine and Psychology" (Ph.D diss., Uni-
     versity of California, 1995).

262 **as an "Astonishing Genius":** S. A. D. Tissot, *Correspondance, 1754–1797*
     (Genève: Slatkine, 2007), pp. 278–279. Zimmerman refers to this "Genies
     etonnans" in a letter to Tissot dated Feb. 27, 1765.

262 **coeditor of the *Journal des sçavans*:** Lordat, *Exposition de la doctrine médicale
     de P.-J. Barthez et mémoires sur la vie de ce médecin*, p. 15.

262 **chancellor of the university:** His lectures show him attacking clinical
     problems by weaving inner forces for illness like temperament and sen-
     sibility with external forces, such as diet and climate. See P. J. Barthez,
     Consultations de médicine, ed. Jacques Lordat (Paris: Michaud, 1810).

263 **would not ruin their friendship:** Haller applauded Barthez's dismissal of
     the fictions of Dr. Lacaze, but diminished Barthez's finding by attributing
     it to a host of others. Williams, *A Cultural History of Medical Vitalism in
     Enlightenment Montpellier*, pp. 259–261, and Lordat, *Exposition de la doctrine
     médicale de P.-J. Barthez et mémoires sur la vie de ce médecin*, p. 111.

264 **wisdom, and the good life:** P. J. Barthez, *Nouveaux éléments de la science de
     l'homme* (Montpellier: Jean Martel, 1778), p. i.

264 **the equation to make sense:** This point was made explicit in P. J. Barthez, *Nouvelle mécanique des mouvements de l'homme et des animaux* (Carcassonne: Pierre Polere, 1798), p. II.

264 **the Montpellier doctor cited approvingly:** Barthez, *Nouveaux éléments de la science de l'homme*, pp. 33–35.

264 **meant to delude and confuse:** Ibid., p. 95.

264 **what Barthez called a "synergy":** Ibid., p. 146.

264 **regulated the animal economy:** Ibid., pp. 249–250. He contended that bad habits augment or destroy sensitive forces in a way that makes the soul quake or fall into a torpor.

265 *of the Human Science:* Paul Joseph Barthez, *Nouveaux éléments de la science de l'homme* vol. 2 (Paris: Goujon & Brunot, 1806), p. 247.

12. HONEST JEAN-JACQUES AND THE MORALS OF SENSIBILITY

268 **the male sexual addict:** Paul Jacques Malouin, "Satyriasis," *Encyclopédie* 14:703–704. ARTFL Encyclopédie Project.

268 **the moderation of the emotions:** Menuret de Chambaud, "Manie," *Encyclopédie*, 10:31–34. ARTFL Encyclopédie Project. Jean-Joseph Menuret also was known as Menuret de Chambaud. See Reich, "Paul Joseph Barthez and the Impact of Vitalism on Medicine and Psychology," pp. 451–453. Also see Rey, *Naissance et développement du vitalisme en France*, pp. 88–109.

268 **nervous and mental disorders:** Barthez, *Nouveaux éléments de la science de l'homme*, vol. 1, pp. 293–300.

268 **rest cured the enervated:** Barthez and Lordat, *Consultations de médicine*, pp. 33–49. Treatments in this section range from 1763 to 1773.

269 **saddest period of his life:** On Tissot, see Antoinette Emch-Dériaz, *Tissot: Physician of the Enlightenment* (New York: P. Lang, 1992). For correspondence and an early account of his life, see Charles Eynard, *Essai sur la vie de Tissot* (Lausanne: Ducloux, 1839). On the "saddest period" of his life, see Antoinette Emch-Dériaz, ed. *Samuel-Auguste-André-David Tissot—Johann Georg Zimmermann: Correspondance 1754–1797* (Genève: Slatkine, 2007), p. 67. (Hereafter *Tissot—Zimmermann*.)

269 **one touched by genius:** Eynard, *Essai sur la vie de Tissot*, p. 56. This 1755 letter from A. Haller to C. Bonnet is cited here.

269 **thesis on mania and melancholia:** Emch-Dériaz, *Tissot: Physician of the Enlightenment*, pp.17–18.

269 **the *douceurs* of his life:** *Tissot—Zimmermann*, p. 768.

270 **to be a poet:** Ibid., pp. 86–87.

270 **his mark on the ages:** Ibid., p. 60.

270 **"dared to speak the truth":** Ibid., p. 69.

271 **nervous disorders were not one:** S. A. D. Tissot, *Advice to the People in*

General, with Regard to Their Health, trans. J. Kirkpatrick (Dublin: J. Hoey Senior, 1766). See Anne C. Vila, "Beyond Sympathy: Vapors, Melancholia, and the Pathologies of Sensibility in Tissot and Rousseau," *Yale French Studies* 92 (1997): 93, and her *Enlightenment and Pathology: Sensibility in the Literature and Medicine of 18th Century France* (Baltimore: Johns Hopkins University Press, 1998). Also see Patrick Singy, "The Popularization of Medicine in the Eighteenth Century: Writing, Reading, and Rewriting Samuel Auguste Tissot's *Avis Au Peuple Sur Sa Santé*," *Journal of Modern History* 8 (2010): 769–800.

271 **marked its difference:** This is explicitly noted by Tissot's English translator. See J. Kirkpatrick, "Introduction," in Tissot, *Advice to the People in General, with Regard to Their Health*, pp. iii–x.

271 **interesting aspect of their field:** *Tissot—Zimmermann*, pp. 31, 92.

271 **consider William Battie's mind cures:** Ibid., p. 87. Letter of Haller to Tissot, Dec. 3, 1759.

271 **years later, it caused panic:** S. A. D. Tissot, *L'onanisme* (Lausanne: Chapuis, 1760). The Latin version was published along with the tract on bilious fever in 1758.

271 **this book circulated widely:** Anonymous, *Onania or the Heinous Sin of Self Pollution And All its Frightful Consequences in Both Sexes Consider'd* (London: J. Isted, 1737).

272 **madness, and sudden death:** S. A. D. Tissot, *Three Essays: First, on the Disorders of People of Fashion: Second, on Diseases Incidental to Literary and Sedentary Persons . . . : Third, on Onanism; or, a Treatise upon the Disorders Produced by Masturbation*, trans. Francis Bacon et al. (Dublin: James Williams, 1772). Citations will be to this expanded 1772 edition. On the history of masturbation, see Thomas Laqueur, *Solitary Sex: A Cultural History of Masturbation* (New York: Zone Books, 2003).

272 **a drawn out act of suicide:** Tissot, *Three Essays*, p. v.

272 **nerves and the mind:** Ibid., p. 22.

272 **weakened the nervous system:** Ibid., p. 53.

272 **the freezing-cold bath:** Ibid, p.113. Nineteenth-century sexologists were confronted by the same quandary; they sought to pathologize masturbation but not intercourse, and hence turned to the strain on the imagination.

273 **"agitates the machine," he wrote:** Tissot, *Advice to the People in General, with Regard to Their Health*, p. 13.

273 **new medicine for madness:** *Tissot—Zimmermann*, p. 111. Letter dated July 13, 1759. Zimmermann would try and approach mental ills with a regimen for the *esprit* in a book, which he noted had the same goals as Tissot, if not the same approach. Ibid., p. 331. Letter dated May 22, 1766.

273 **imaginations to the breaking point:** This 1766 essay can be found in Tissot, *Three Essays*.

273 **abandon medicine to save himself?:** *Tissot—Zimmermann*, p. 622.

274 **crestfallen, then enraged:** Eynard, *Essai sur la vie de Tissot*, p. 192. *Tissot—Zimmermann*, pp. 503–520.

274 **Bavarian professor, Adam Weishaupt:** *Tissot—Zimmermann*, pp. 771, 789.

274 **Frederick the Great on his deathbed:** Johann Georg Zimmermann, *An Essay on National Pride*, trans. anon. (London: J. Wilkie, 1771).

274 **most accurate considerations of seizures:** S. A. D. Tissot, *Traité des nerfs et de leurs maladies: De la catalepsie, de l'extase, de l'anoesthesie, de la migraine, et des maladies du cerveau* (Genève: Grasset, 1783). Also see K. Karbowski, "Samuel Auguste Tissot (1728–1797)," *Journal of Neurology*, 248, no. 12 (2001): 1109–1110.

275 **Chaulnes, and sundry other royals:** André Guisan, *Le livre de malades du Dr. Tissot* (Genève: Georg, 1911).

275 **amuse his audience:** See the author's letter to his play's critics; Pierre Beaumarchias, *Le Barbier de Séville* (Paris; Ruault, 1775), p. 2.

275 **"his always irritated nerves":** Eynard, *Essai sur la vie de Tissot*, p. 28.

275 **he did in the grave:** Madame du Deffand et al., *The Unpublished Correspondence of Madame du Deffand*, vol. 1, p. 135. Letter of Madame du Deffand to Voltaire, 1753.

275 **his patients than to his books:** Voltaire, *Correspondence,* ed. T. Besterman (Genève: Institut et Musée Voltaire, 1965), vol. 80, letter 16402. Voltaire to David Louis de Constant Rebecque, Sept. 15, 1771.

275 **That patient was Jean-Jacques Rousseau:** On Rousseau's life, see Leopold Damrosch, *Jean-Jacques Rousseau: Restless Genius* (Boston: Houghton Mifflin Co., 2005), and Monique and Bernard Cottret, *Jean-Jacques Rousseau en son temps* (Paris: Perrin, 2005). The conception that Rousseau was uninformed about medicine, or wholly opposed to it, is incorrect. In fact, Montpellier medical theory was important to Rousseau's view of nature and his philosophy; see Marco Menin, "Jean-Jacques Rousseau vitaliste: La moralisation de l'hygiène médicale entre régime diététique et éthique alimentaire," *Nuncius* 27, no. 1 (2012): 81–109.

276 **"the malady of happy people":** Damrosch, *Jean-Jacques Rousseau*, pp. 139–140.

277 **out as his own:** Ibid., p. 304.

277 **debunked de Warens's herbalist potions:** Ibid., p. 187.

278 **enlightenment and never let up:** Ibid., pp. 213–214.

278 **did nothing but destroy morals:** Jean-Jacques Rousseau (1750/1760), *The First and Second Discourses*, ed. and trans., Roger D. Masters and Judith R. Masters (New York: St. Martin's Press, 1964), p. 50.

279 **self-torture he considered necessary:** Damrosch, *Jean-Jacques Rousseau*, p. 221. See Jean Starobinski, "The Illness of Rousseau," *Yale French Studies*, no. 28 (1961), pp. 64–74.

280 ***Sensibility; or, The Wiseman's Materialism:*** Rousseau's *La Morale sensitive ou le matérialisme du sage,* translated as "The Morals of Sensibility or the

Wiseman's Materialism," is discussed in Jean-Jacques Rousseau (1782), *The Confessions of Jean-Jacques Rousseau*, ed. J. M. Cohen (Harmondsworth, Eng.: New York: Penguin, 1979), p. 381. Also see Damrosch, *Jean-Jacques Rousseau*, p. 263.

280 **generosity was masked self-satisfaction:** François de la Rochefoucauld, *Collected Maxims*, trans. E. H. Blackmore et al. (Oxford: Oxford University Press, 2008), p. 75.

280 **"all the rest together":** Ibid., p. 223. Not particularly concerned with consistency, this author elsewhere dismissed the soul's troubles as nothing more than a change in the blood's temperature.

280 **consolidated into a personal style:** Jean de la Bruyère (1696), *Les Caractères*, ed. Emmanuel Bury (Paris: Librairie Générale Française, 1995), p. 411.

280 **"which they so often disturb?":** He wrote: "Que d'écarts on sauverait à la raison, que de vices on empêcherait de naître si l'on savait forcer l'économie animale à favoriser l'ordre moral qu'elle trouble si souvent!" Jean-Jacques Rousseau (1782) *Les Confessions* (Paris: Livre de poche, 1963), vol. 2, p. 129. I have modified the English translation by J. M. Cohen where "économie animale" is translated as "brute functions" and therefore loses its specific medical and philosophical meaning. See *The Confessions of Jean-Jacques Rousseau*, p. 381.

281 **he suddenly abandoned the project:** *The Confessions of Jean-Jacques Rousseau*, pp. 380–381, 478. *Les Confessions*. vol. 2, pp. 128–129.

281 **been clear, "I hate you":** *The Confessions of Jean-Jacques Rousseau*, p. 500. On the relationship between Rousseau and Voltaire, see Henri Gouhier, *Rousseau et Voltaire: Portrait dans deux miroirs* (Paris: Vrin, 1983).

282 **"pleasure of not being dead":** J.-J. Rousseau (1762), *Émile: Or, on Education*, trans. Alan Bloom (New York: Basic Books, 1979), p. 27.

282 **"daily through your diseased imagination. . . .":** Ibid., p. 54.

283 **"very sorry for you":** Ibid., p. 69.

283 **modesty, moderation, and benevolence:** Ibid., p. 73.

285 **scandalize priests and *philosophes* alike:** Damrosch, *Jean-Jacques Rousseau*, p. 342.

285 **bitter, small-minded sects:** Jean-Jacques Rousseau, *Profession de foi du Vicaire Savoyard* (Paris: Flammarion, 1996), pp. 97, 111.

286 **from their combined "general will":** J.-J. Rousseau (1762), *The Social Contract and Other Later Political Writings,* ed. Victor Gourevitch (Cambridge: Cambridge University Press, 2003). On the notion of the *volonté générale* and its usage from Diderot and to Helvétius, Condorcet and Rousseau, see Jonathan Israel, *Revolutionary Ideas*, p. 23.

286 **decried that crazy "little monster":** Jean-Jacques Rousseau, *Correspondance complète de Jean-Jacques Rousseau*, ed. R. A. Leigh (Genève: Institute et Musée Voltaire, 1970), vol. 12, pp. 21–22. Letter 1986, Voltaire to D'Alembert, dated July 12, 1762.

286 **excesses would land him:** Ibid., p. 106, letter 2035, Denis Diderot to Sophie Volland, dated July 25, 1762.

287 **the experience was transformative:** Ibid., p. 27, letter 1990, Tissot to Zimmermann, dated July 13, 1762.

287 **humble and honest:** Ibid., p.18, letter 1983, Tissot to Albrecht von Haller, dated July 11, 1762.

287 **"rights of men," the physician wrote:** Ibid., p. 33, letter 1994, Tissot to Dr. Johann Caspar-Hirzel.

287 **Albrecht von Haller:** Ibid., p. 152, letter 2059, Tissot to Zimmermann, dated August 4, 1762. Also see Letter 1983.

287 **a quite modest punishment:** Ibid., p. 55, letter 2009, from Haller to Tissot, dated July 19, 1762.

287 **soul, and its immortal life:** Ibid., pp. 140–141, letter 2052, from Tissot to Haller, dated August 2, 1762.

288 **for his opinion:** Ibid., pp. 50–51, letter 2006, from Charles Bonnet to Haller, dated July 17, 1762.

288 **fundaments of religion and government:** Ibid., pp. 153–154, letter 2060, from Charles Bonnet to Charles de Geer, dated August 4, 1762.

288 **probably take him in:** Ibid., pp. 185–186, letter 2074, from Charles Bonnet to Albrecht von Haller, dated August 13, 1762.

288 **called for his imprisonment:** Jean-Jacques Rousseau, *Correspondance complète de Jean Jacques Rousseau*, vol. 24 (Banbury, Eng.: The Voltaire Foundation, 1975), pp. 48–49, letter 4042, from Charles Bonnet to J-N-S Allamand, dated February 19, 1765; p. 107, letter 4073, from Charles Bonnet to John Turton, dated February 27, 1765; pp. 220–222, letter 4145, Charles Bonnet to H-S Gerdil, dated March 14, 1765.

288 **critics, detractors, and haters:** Darnton, *The Great Cat Massacre*, p. 181.

288 **delirium and black despair:** Jean-Jacques Rousseau (1782), *Les reveries du promeneur solitaire* (Paris: Gallimard, 1972), pp. 35–36.

288 *Advice to the People*: Tissot's archive contains over 1,300 letters of medical consultation, see Patrick Singy, "The Popularization of Medicine in the Eighteenth Century: Writing, Reading, and Rewriting Samuel Auguste Tissot's *Avis au peuple sur sa santé*," *Journal of Modern History*, vol. 82 (2010): 769–800.

289 **he suffered from himself:** Rousseau, *Correspondance*, vol. 12, pp. 82–83, letter 2022, Rousseau to Tissot, dated July 22, 1762. Also pp. 179–180, letter 2072, from Tissot to Rousseau, dated August 13, 1762.

289 **he begged the physician:** Rousseau, *Correspondance*, vol. 24, pp. 230–231. letter 4153, from Rousseau to Tissot, dated March 16, 1765.

289 **so as to discredit him:** Ibid., pp. 276–278, letter 4180, from Tissot to Alexandre de Golowkin, dated March 22, 1765.

290 **feed his melancholia:** Ibid., pp. 288–291, letter 4186, from Tissot to Rousseau, dated March 23, 1765.

290 Rousseau's moral and physical being: Eynard, *Essai sur la vie de Tissot*, pp. 116–117.

290 worried, but he was not: Rousseau, *Correspondance*, vol. 24, pp. 288–291, letter 4186, from Tissot to Rousseau, dated March 23, 1765.

290 Isabelle Guyenet had recovered: Ibid., vol. 25, pp. 2–3, letter 4227, from Rousseau to Tissot, dated April 1, 1765.

290 physical ills, his patient recoiled: See note written by Tissot in the "Notes Explicatives," ibid., p. 3.

290 grave disappointment in his friends: Ibid.

291 "the doctor of my soul!": Ibid.

291 "as had his Émile": Eynard, *Essai sur la vie de Tissot*, p. 120.

291 "Poor Jean-Jacques is mad": Rousseau, *Correspondance*, p. 70, letter 4264, from d'Alembert to Voltaire, dated April 9, 1765.

291 abandoned his own children: Damrosch, *Jean-Jacques Rousseau*, p. 390.

291 once doubted, miracles and medicine: Ibid., pp. 131–132. Rousseau, *Correspondance*, letter 4308, from Rousseau to Tissot, dated April 20, 1765.

291 make use of these insights: Rousseau, *Les rêveries du promeneur solitaire*, p. 187. "Mon Portrait" was written between 1755–62.

292 young women, and more: Rousseau (1782), *Les Confessions*. 2 Vols.

293 "Study wears out the machine": Tissot, *Three Essays*, p. 33.

293 his chronic urinary troubles: Ibid., p. 33.

293 "after having long been maddish": J. Y. T. Greig, ed., *The Letters of David Hume* (Oxford: Clarendon Press, 1969), vol. 2, pp. 1, 10. An avalanche of letters on Rousseau from Adam Smith, d'Alembert, Turgot, d'Holbach, and others were sent to Hume, see pp. 407–452.

293 the Academy of Lausanne: Rousseau, *Correspondance* vol. 37 (Oxford: Voltaire Foundation, 1980), pp. 3–5, letter 6520, Rousseau to Tissot, dated January 5, 1768. (This letter is misdated and was actually written in January of 1769).

293 "destination that will heal me": Ibid., pp. 5–6, letter 6521, Rousseau to Julie-Anne-Marie Boy de la Tour, dated January 1769.

294 that this doctor had inspired: Ibid., pp. 37–40, letter 6536, Rousseau to Tissot, dated February 1769.

295 taken *only* by doctors: J. F. Dufour, *Essai sur les operations de l'entendement humain* (Amsterdam: Merlin, 1770).

295 man's suffering in its whole: Anonymous, *A Philosophical Essay on Man Being an Attempt to Investigate the Reciprocal Influence of the Soul on the Body* (London: J. Ridley, 1773), p. ix. On Marat being run out of Paris, see Geoffrey Sutton, "Electric Medicine and Mesmerism," *Isis* 72 (1981): 390.

295 entrusted with public morality: M. D. T. de Bienville, *Nymphomania; or, A Dissertation Concerning the Furor Uterinus*, trans. E. S. Wilmat (London: J. Bew, 1775), pp. 28, 50. He considered nymphomania no longer as a uterine furor, but an excess of imagination and irritation of the "throne of love."

Dissertations from Montpellier during this period show that some medical students followed Dr. Tissot, that hero who revealed masturbation was not so much a sin as a terrible health hazard. One medical student concluded his dissertation with an ode in honor of that great man who "purged humanity from an hideous vice." Jean-François Sacombe, *Dissertatio medica de mastrupatione* (Montpellier: J. F. Picot, 1780), p 16.

296 **utter strangers called him:** See Darnton, *The Great Cat Massacre*, pp. 217, 251. On Rousseau mania, see Simon Schama, *Citizens: A Chronicle of the French Revolution* (New York: Knopf, 1989), pp. 145–162.

297 **"revolution in our minds":** George Sand (1847), *Historie de ma vie* (Paris: Libraire Générale Française, 2004), p. 64. Fumaroli, *When the World Spoke French*, pp. 173–174.

297 **Rousseau published in 1762:** Ibid., p. 179.

297 **beginnings of a new nation:** Rousseau in the *Confessions* and in *Reveries of a Solitary Walker*, claimed to be unique and authentic. See Rousseau, *Les Confessions*. vol. 1, p. 2, and *Les reveries du promeneur solitaire*, p. 74.

13. DR. MESMER'S INVISIBLE FIRE

299 **science and public health:** See T. D. Murphy, "The French Medical Profession's Perception of Its Social Function Between 1776 and 1830," *Medical History* 23, no. 3 (1979): 259–278.

300 **"a civilization, a people":** M. Tenon, *Memoirs sur les hôpitaux de Paris* (Paris: Méquignon, 1816), p. 1.

300 **"the Door to Heaven":** The inscription read: "C'est icy la Maison de Dieu et la Porte du Ciel." See Marcel Fosseyeux, *L'Hôtel-Dieu au XVII et au XVIII siècle* (Paris: Berger-Levrault, 1912). On French hospitals and their attempts to reform after 1789, see Erwin Ackerknecht, *Medicine at the Paris Hospital, 1794–1848* (Baltimore: Johns Hopkins University Press, 1967).

301 **a provincial French hospital:** Tenon, *Memoirs sur les hôpitaux de Paris*, p. 453.

301 **contaminating the whole city:** See L. S. Greenbaum, "'Measure of Civilization': The Hospital Thought of Jacques Tenon on the Eve of the French Revolution," *Bulletin of the History of Medicine* 49, no. 1 (1975): 49–52.

302 **this was a staggering figure:** Tenon, *Memoirs sur les hôpitaux de Paris*, p. 91. Erwin Heinz Ackerknecht, "Political Prisoners in French Mental Institutions Before 1789, During the Revolution, and Under Napoleon I," *Medical History* 19 (1975): 250–255.

302 **unabashedly opposed to them:** C. Jones, "The 'New Treatment' of the Insane in Paris: The Formation of the Lunatic Asylum Under the French Revolution," *History Today* 30 (1980): 8.

303 **an eager populace awaited him:** On Mesmer and animal magnetism, see Alan Gauld, *A History of Hypnotism* (Cambridge and New York: Cam-

bridge University Press, 1992); Adam Crabtree, *From Mesmer to Freud: Magnetic Sleep and the Roots of Psychological Healing* (New Haven: Yale University Press, 1993); and Robert Darnton, *Mesmerism and the End of the Enlightenment in France* (Cambridge: Harvard University Press, 1968). On Mesmerism and the French vitalists, see Williams, *A Cultural History of Medical Vitalism in Enlightenment Montpellier,* p. 306.

303 **subjects and, inadvertently, themselves:** Benjamin Franklin (1751), *Benjamin Franklin's Experiments,* ed. I. B. Cohen (Cambridge: Harvard University Press, 1941). On the "new Prometheus," see Stanley Finger, "Benjamin Franklin and the Electrical Cure for Disorders of the Nervous System," in *Brain, Mind, and Medicine: Essays in Eighteenth-Century Neuroscience,* eds. H. Whitaker, C. U. M. Smith, and S. Finger (New York: Springer, 2007), p. 247.

304 **paralyses, melancholias, and hysterias:** Finger, ibid., pp. 245–256.

304 **shocks might clear the blockage:** The claim that electrical fluid made up the body's nervous fluid was made as early as 1733 by Stephen Hales and peaked after Galvani's publication of 1791. See Eric T. Carlson and Meribeth M. Simpson (1969), "Models of the Nervous System in Eighteenth Century Psychiatry, *Bulletin of the History of Medicine* 43, no. 2 (1969): 111–113. Also see Roderick Home, "Electricity and the Nervous Fluid," *Journal of the History of Biology* 3, no. 2 (1970): 235–251.

304 **electrical cures for the masses:** See James G. Donat, "John Wesley on the Estimation and Cure of Nervous Disorders," in *Brain, Mind, and Medicine,* pp. 285–299.

304 **he employed his sizzling therapies:** Sutton, "Electric Medicine and Mesmerism," p. 381.

305 **stars to the human body:** Henri F. Ellenberger, *The Discovery of the Unconscious: The History and Evolution of Dynamic Psychiatry* (New York: Basic Books, 1970), pp. 57–70.

308 **cures but didn't know it:** On Gassner, see Erik Midelfort, *Exorcism and Enlightenment: Johann Joseph Gassner and the Demons of 18th-Century Germany* (New Haven: Yale University Press, 2005), and Ellenberger, *The Discovery of the Unconscious,* pp. 54–57. Unconvincingly, Ellenberger traces the origins of dynamic psychiatry to this encounter between "the physician" Mesmer and the "exorcist" Gassner.

308 **nervous forces and magnetism:** Franz Anton Mesmer, *Mémoire de F. A. Mesmer, docteur en médecine, sur ses découvertes* (Paris: Fuchs, 1799), p. 113.

308 **prancing and gesticulating being:** See Mesmer's account in his *Précis historique des faits relatifs au magnétisme-animal jusques an Avril 1781* (Londres: n.p, 1781), pp. 15–20.

309 **that "invisible fire" inside:** Mesmer, *Mémoire de F. A. Mesmer,* p. 108. Also Darnton, *Mesmerism and the End of the Enlightenment in France,* p. 10.

310 *chambres des crises,* **padded with mattresses:** See the description in *Rapport*

des commissaires de la Société Royale de Médecine, nommés par le roi pour faire l'examen du magnétisme animal (Paris: Moutard, 1784), p. 12.

311 **one cure, his own:** Franz Anton Mesmer, *Aphorismes de M. Mesmer* (Nice: Gabriel Floteron, 1785), p. 70.

313 **"use while it lasts":** Benjamin Franklin, *The Works of Benjamin Franklin,* ed. John Bigelow, vol. 10 (New York: G. P. Putnam's Sons, 1904), pp. 296–297. Letter to M. de la Condamine, March. 19, 1784.

313 **the hope of success:** Benjamin Franklin, *Benjamin Franklin's Experiments,* p. 347.

313 **fell into a furious fit:** *Rapport des commissaires chargés par le roi, de l'examen du magnétisme animal* (Paris: P. F. Didot, 1784), p. 27.

314 **"affectations of the *esprit*":** Ibid, p. 26.

314 **electrical cures were false:** Antoine Laurent de Jussieu, *Rapport de l'un des commissaires chargés par le roi de l'examen du magnétisme animal* (Paris: Herissant & Barrois, 1784), pp. 18–19, 33, 72.

315 **science, but rather seduction:** Actually, they produced three reports, one published, the other on methods, and the third, secret.

316 **preexisting increased nerve sensibility:** Pierre Pomme, *Traité des affections vaporeuses des deux sexes* (Paris: De l'imprimerie Royale, 1782), p. 72. On the politics of mesmerism, see the groundbreaking Robert Darnton's *Mesmerism and the End of the Enlightenment* (Cambridge: Harvard University Press, 1968).

316 **the true source of Mesmer's cures:** M. Sousselier de la Tour, *L'ami de la nature, ou manière de traiter les maladies par le pretend magnétisme animal* (Dijon: J. B. Capel, 1784).

317 **credulous approach to science:** Michel-Augustin Thouret, *Recherches et doutes sur le magnétisme animal* (Paris: Prault, 1784), pp. 3–4.

317 **not seriously evaluating anything:** M. Galart de Montjoye, *Lettre sur le magnétisme animal* (Philadelphie: P.J. Duplain, 1784), pp. 65–66.

318 **monopolies and protecting their pocketbooks:** See, for example, P. A. O. Mahon, *Examen sérieux et impartial du magnétisme animal* (Paris: Royez, 1784).

318 **object of government:** John Bell, *New System of the World and the Laws of Motion* (London: By the author, 1788), pp. 37–41, 49.

319 **energy behind sexual attraction:** M. Salaville, *Le moraliste mesmérien* (Londres: Belin & Brunet, 1784), p. 8.

319 **it is not my fault:** Pierre Choderlos de Laclos (1782), *Les liaisons dangereuses: Roman* (Paris: Éditions Larousse, 2007), p. 339.

320 **a bunch of magnets:** Pierpaolo Polzonetti, "Mesmerizing Adultery: 'Così fan tutte' and the Kornman Scandal," *Cambridge Opera Journal* 14, no. 3 (2002): 263–296.

320 **in his "Temple of Divinity":** Jean-Jacques Paulet, *Mesmer justifié* (Constance, Ger.: n.p., 1784), p. 2.

320 **Mesmer and his swooning patients:** See Gauld, *A History of Hypnotism,*

pp. 25–38. Also Polzonetti, "Mesmerizing Adultery: 'Così fan tutte' and the Kornman Scandal," p. 283.

321 **who was perfectly, completely blind:** Ellenberger, *The Discovery of the Unconscious*, pp. 66–67.

321 **to harness it:** E. Ogden, "Mesmer's Demon: Fiction, Falsehood, and the Mechanical Imagination," *Early American Literature* 47, no. 1 (2012): 143–170. Crabtree, *From Mesmer to Freud*, p. 17.

322 **Soon, his health returned:** Jacques Maxime Paul de Chastenet Puységur, *Rapport des cures opérées à Bayonne par le magnétisme animal* (Bayonne, Fr.: Prault, 1784), pp. 22–24.

322 **animal machines were wired together:** Mesmer, *Mémoire de F. A. Mesmer*, pp. 117–127.

323 **their confidence, and wreak havoc:** Puységur, *Rapport des cures opérées à Bayonne par le magnétisme animal*, p. 32.

323 **part of the mind:** Ibid., pp. 158–159, 392.

326 **into a magnetic crisis:** John Pearson, *A Plain and Rational Account of the Nature and Effects of Animal Magnetism* (London: W. & J. Startford, 1790), pp. 30–33.

326 **"crisis which may convulse mortality!":** Cited in Tim Fulford, "Conducting the Vital Fluid: The Politics and Poetics of Mesmerism in the 1790s," *Studies in Romanticism* 43, no. 1 (2004): 57.

327 **locked up in Bedlam:** Roy Porter, "Under the Influence: Mesmerism in England," *History Today* 35, no. 9 (1985): 28. Fulford, "Conducting the Vital Fluid," pp. 57–78.

327 **Mesmerism began to mix:** Natalie Zacek, "Medical Revolutionaries: The Enslaved Healers of Eighteenth-Century Saint Domingue," *Callallo* 32 (2009): 667–670. James E. McClellan, *Colonialism and Science: Saint-Domingue in the Old Regime* (Chicago: University of Chicago, 2010).

328 **the first magnetic revolution:** See Murphy, "The French Medical Profession's Perception of Its Social Function Between 1776 and 1830." Ogden, "Mesmer's Demon: Fiction, Falsehood, and the Mechanical Imagination."

328 **de Puységur landed in prison:** Ellenberger, *The Discovery of the Unconscious*, p. 73.

14. JOURNEY TO THE END OF REASON

330 **"he has revealed everybody's secret":** Cited in Alfred Pearce Dennis, "Our Changing Consitution," *The Atlantic* 95 (1905): 532. A slight variation on the quote is cited in the biographical introduction of Madame du Deffand et al., *The Unpublished Correspondence of Madame du Deffand*, vol. 1, p. 19. On Deffand, see Fumaroli, *When the World Spoke French*, pp. 216–239. Also Inès Murat, *Madame du Deffand: La lettre et l'esprit* (Paris: Perrin, 2003).

330 **pain dictated human actions:** On the *De l'esprit* affair, see *Correspondance*

générale d'Helvétius, vol. 3, which covers the years of the author's exile and demoralization.

332 **a resident of Auteuil:** On the likely forgeries that the Abbé created during the Terror, see R. Koebner, "The Authenticity of the Letters on the *Esprit des Lois*," *Historical Research*, 24 (1951): 19–43.

332 **asked him to move in:** Martin S. Staum, *Cabanis: Enlightenment and Medical Philosophy in the French Revolution* (Princeton: Princeton University Press, 1980), pp. 14–16.

332 **his home once a week:** On Auteuil, see Antoine Guillois, *Le Salon de Madame Helvétius: Cabanis et les Idéologues* (New York: Franklin, 1971); Guy de La Prade, *L'illustré société d'Auteuil 1772–1830, ou, la fascination de la liberté* (Paris: F. Lanore/F. Sorlot, 1989); and Jean-Paul de Lagrave, ed., *Madame Helvétius et la société d'Auteuil* (Oxford: Voltaire Foundation, 1999).

333 **" 'my hand: I forgive you' ":** Dorothy Moser Medlin, "Benjamin Franklin's Bagatelles for Madame Helvétius: Some Biographical and Stylistic Considerations," in *Early American Literature*, Spring 1980, p. 47.

333 **vengeance on their deceased spouses:** To what extent this 1780 piece was a witty charade remains a matter of debate. It was published as "Lettre de M. Franklin à Madame Helvétius," in *Correspondance littéraire, philosophique, et critique*, January 1780. See Benjamin Franklin, *The Works of Benjamin Franklin*, ed. Jared Sparks (Chicago: T. MacCoun, 1882), pp. 202–205, for the piece called "A Madame H," as well as his charming, "Très-Humble requête présentée à Madame Helvétius par ses chats," on pp. 206–219.

334 **reason, immorality, and hideous deceit:** Nicolas Chamfort, *Oeuvres complètes*, 2 vols. (Paris: Éditions du Sandre, 2009). Also see Sèbastien-Roch-Nicolas Chamfort, *Products of the Perfected Civilization: Selected Writings of Chamfort,* trans. W. S. Merwin (San Francisco: North Point Press, 1984).

334 **was like attending an execution:** As a Royalist, Chateaubriand's description cannot be simply taken at face value, but he called Chamfort "the most bilious literary man with whom I was acquainted." François-René Chateaubriand, *Memoirs of Chateaubriand: From His Birth in 1768, Till His Return to France in 1800* (London: Henry Colburn, 1849), p. 183.

335 **medical illnesses and statistical deviations:** Nicolas de Condorcet, *Tableau historique des progrès de l'esprit humain*, ed. J. P. Schandeler and P. Crépel (Paris: Institut National d'Études Démographiques, 2004). The historian, philosopher, and politician Constantin-François de Chasseboeuf, or Volney, was the author of, among other works (1791), *Les ruines: ou méditation sur les révolutions des empires* (Paris: Baudoin Frères, 1826).

336 **"happiness or of misery to mankind":** Thomas Paine, *Common Sense Addressed to the Inhabitants of America* (Lancaster, Pa.: Francis Bailey, 1776).

337 **make the world explode:** Honoré-Gabriel de Riqueti Mirabeau, *Oeuvres érotiques* (Paris: Fayard, 1984).

337 had the "spice of insanity": *Gentleman's Magazine*, vol. 158-159 (1835): 615.

338 happy to become one: Honoré-Gabriel de Riqueti Mirabeau, *Mirabeau's Letters During His Residence in England* 2 vols. (London: E. Wilson, 1832).

338 "it is the nation itself": Schama, *Citizens*, p. 301.

338 fine furniture, and precious portraits: Marquis de Sade, *Justine, Philosophy in the Bedroom, and Other Writings* (New York: Grove Weidenfeld, 1990), p. 144. Sade complains of his loss in a 1790 letter to Monsieur Gaufridy.

339 new France to be born: Chateaubriand, *Memoirs of Chateaubriand*, p. 208.

340 right as Emperor Julius Caesar: Schama, *Citizens*, p. 407. I am much indebted to Schama's brilliant account of the French Revolution.

341 squinting in the sunlight?: Edmund Burke (1790), *Reflections on the Revolution in France* (Baltimore: Penguin Books, 1969), pp. 90, 137, 173–174, 181–182, 185, 211.

341 "the nation had changed. . . .": Thomas Paine, *Rights of Man, Being an Answer to Mr. Burke's Attack on the French Revolution* (London: J. S. Jordan, 1791), p. 89.

341 Helvétius, Condillac, and Bonnet: Staum, *Cabanis*, p. 126.

342 a nervous, sick body: Mirabeau, *Mirabeau's Letters During His Residence in England*, p. 535.

342 excitement made on his body: Pierre-Jean-Georges Cabanis (1790), *Journal de la maladie et de la mort d'Honoré-Gabriel-Victor Riquetti Mirabeau*, in *Oeuvres complètes* (Paris: Bossange Frères, 1823), vol. 2, p. 11.

343 his own chambers, came apart: Ibid., pp. 18–33.

343 "Marat is dead, fuck": See Robert Darnton and Daniel Roche, eds. *Revolution in Print: The Press in France, 1775–1800* (Berkeley: University of California Press, 1989). On the rise of a radical press and Jean-Paul Marat's paper "*L'ami du people*," see Israel, *Revolutionary Ideas*, pp. 30–52, 79, 89, 129, 311–312. On Jacques Hébert and Le Père Duchesne, see ibid, pp. 164, 169, 296–297, and Hébert, *Le Père Duchesne, 1790–1794*, ed. Albert Soboul, vol. 8 (Paris, Edis, 1969), pp. 52, 62, 69. This volume of his writings alone contains the word *foutre*, or "fuck," on eighty pages.

344 abolition of the death penalty: Schama, *Citizens*, p. 578.

346 himself could hardly believe it: D. A. F. de Sade, *The 120 Days of Sodom; or, the Romance of the School for Libertinage* (Paris: Olympia Press, 1954).

347 "endured from my tyrants": Marquis de Sade, *Justine, Philosophy in the Bedroom, and Other Writings*, p. 138. Letter of 1783 to his wife. Also see Marquis de Sade, *Letters from Prison*, trans. Richard Seaver (New York: Arcade Pub., 1999).

348 one of his inspirations: Ibid., p. 185. On Sade's "philosophical anthropology" as a critique of Condillac and d'Holbach, see Henry Martyn Lloyd, "Philosophical Anthropology and the Sadean 'System'; Or Sade and the Question of Enlightenment Humanism," in *Representing Humanity in*

the Age of Enlightenment, ed. A. Cook, N. Curthoys, and S. Konishi (London: Pickering & Chatto, 2013), pp. 173–183.

348 **hedonism should guide France forward:** Ibid., pp. 296–339.

349 **saints' days were erased:** On the campaign to dechristianize France, see Israel, *Revolutionary Ideas,* pp. 479–502. François Furet, *Revolutionary France, 1770–1880* (Oxford: Blackwell, 1992), pp. 141–142.

350 **burn a statue of Atheism:** Schama, *Citizens*, pp. 771–774, and Israel, *Revolutionary Ideas*, p. 488.

350 **cage, where he soon perished:** The debates on the Terror are intense and politically charged. François Furet argued that this illiberal turn was intrinsic to the Revolution; see his *Revolutionary France, 1770–1880*. Recently, Israel has argued that this signified a shift from a radical democratic revolution to a discrete period of counterrevolution and authoritarian populism, one that prefigured modern fascism. See Israel, *Revolutionary Ideas*, pp. 28, 503–573, 694–702.

351 **transformed into political beheadings:** Thomas Paine, *The Age of Reason. Part the Second. Being an Investigation of True and of Fabulous Theology* (London: R. Carlile, 1818). The preface of Part II was written in October of 1795.

351 **"received with general approbation":** On Thermidor, see Israel, *Revolutionary Ideas*, pp. 574–634. The quote is cited in Schama, *Citizens*, p. 827.

352 **influenced, deluded, or ill:** In fact, common presumptions that guided thinkers like Diderot, Bordeu, and Tissot became foundational for the emergence of biology as a new discipline in France. Prior static notions of heredity were challenged by the theory that simple forces over generations formed complex organizations with new properties. Jean-Baptiste Lamarck, Mirabeau's friend, was a botanist from the Jardin des Plantes. A few years after the Revolution, Lamarck would put forward a historical model in which simple building blocks in living creatures were pressured over generations into more complex organizations with new, adaptive functions. Famously, he believed life experiences, including mental ones, might foster change so woven into an individual's body that they would be acquired by offspring. While geared toward the invertebrates he knew so well, Citizen Lamarck's theory also dispelled monarchist notions of superior heredity that helped buoy the old order.

15. CITIZENS AND ALIENISTS

354 *maisons de force* **in France:** See H. Mitchell, "Politics in the Service of Knowledge: The Debate over the Administration of Medicine and Welfare in Late Eighteenth-Century France," *Social History* 6, no. 2 (1981): 185–207. T. M. Adams, "Medicine and Bureaucracy: Jean Colombier's Regula-

tion for the French Dépôts de Mendicité," *Bulletin of the History of Medicine* 52, no. 4 (1978): 529–541.

355 **passed on to them:** Jean Colombier and François Doublet, *Instruction sur la manière de gouverner les insensés, et de travailler à leur guérison dans les asyles qui leur sont destinés* (Paris: De l'Imprimerie Royale, 1785). Also M. Paul Carrette, "François Doublet et la psychiatrie au temps de Louis XVI," *Annales médico-psychologiques* 2, no. 84 (1926): 119–131.

355 **"him and that nature commands":** Tenon, *Memoirs sur les hôpitaux de Paris*, p. 216, also p. 393.

356 **useless and counterproductive:** Vincenzo Chiarugi (1793), *On Insanity and Its Classification*, ed. and trans. George Mora (Canton, Mass.: Science History Publications/U.S.A., 1987). Also see George Mora, "Vincenzo Chiarugi (1759–1820)—His Contribution to Psychiatry," *Bulletin of the Isaac Ray Medical Library* 2 (1954): 50–104, and "Vincenzo Chiarugi (1759–1820) and His Psychiatric Reform in Florence in the Late 18th Century: On the Occasion of the Bi-Centenary of His Birth," *Journal of the History of Medicine and Allied Sciences* 14 (1959): 424–433.

357 **might no longer be needed:** Pierre-Jean-Georges Cabanis, *Observations sur les hôpitaux* (Paris: De l'Imprimerie Nationale, 1790), p. A4.

358 **individuals and the public:** See Staum, *Cabanis*, p. 137.

358 **the southwestern Tarn region:** On Pinel's biography, see the groundbreaking work, Dora B. Weiner, *Comprendre et soigner: Philippe Pinel, 1745–1826: La médecine de l'esprit* (Paris: Fayard, 1999). Also Jackie Pigeaud, *Aux Portes de la psychiatrie: Pinel, L'ancien et le moderne* (Paris: Aubier, 2001).

358 **immortality of the soul:** René Semelaigne, *Aliénistes et philanthropes: Les Pinel et les Tuke* (Paris: Steinheil, 1912), p. 12. On Pinel's early education, see Pierre Chabbert, "Les Années d'études de Philippe Pinel: Lavaur, Toulouse, Montpellier," *Monspeliensis Hippocrates* 3 (1960): 15–23.

358 **well-being of a nation:** Jean-Antoine-Claude Chaptal, *Mes souvenirs sur Napolèon*, ed. Emmanuel Anatole Chaptal de Chateloup (Paris: E. Plon, Nourrit & Cie, 1893), pp. 20–21.

358 **theses for lazy students:** Chabbert, "Les années d'études de Philippe Pinel: Lavaur, Toulouse, Montpellier," p. 21.

358 **Hippocrates, Plutarch, and Montaigne:** Weiner, *Comprendre et soigner*, p. 50, and Chaptal, *Mes souvenirs sur Napolèon*, pp. 18–21.

358 **tomb with the grieving widow:** Philippe Pinel, *Lettres de Pinel* (Paris: Librairie de V. Masson, 1859), p. 30.

359 **physiology, chemistry, and pharmacy:** Weiner, *Comprendre et soigner*, p. 57.

360 **immortality of the soul:** Philippe Pinel, *Traité médico-philosophique sur l'aliénation mentale, ou la manie* (Paris: Richard, Caille & Ravier, 1801), pp. 158–159.

360 **history as an extraordinary fraud:** Philippe Pinel's *Gazette* articles can be found in Jacques Postel, *Genèse de la psychiatrie: Les premiers écrits de Philippe Pinel* (Paris: Le Sycamore, 1981), pp. 101–157.

360 **Mesmer's passes and his *baquet*:** Jacques Postel, *Genèse de la psychiatrie*, pp. 103–155.

360 **the century of the *philosophes*:** Ibid., p. 139.

361 **realign the animal economy:** Weiner, *Comprendre et soigner*, pp. 43–44, 65, 80.

361 **shake off his despondency:** Pinel's son Scipion penned a short reminiscence of his father; see Gabriel Bollotte, "Documents sur Philippe Pinel," *L'information psychiatrique* 44, no. 9 (1968), p. 824.

362 **not medical consultants, but the police:** Philippe Pinel, *A Treatise on Insanity, in Which Are Contained the Principles of a New and More Practical Nosology of Maniacal Disorders*, trans. David Daniel Davis (Sheffield, Eng.: W. Todd, 1806), pp. 52–53. Also see J. Postel, "Un Manuscrit inédit de Philippe Pinel sur 'Les Guérisons opérées dans le 7ème emploi' de Bicêtre, en 1794," *Revue internationale d'histoire de la psychiatrie* 1, no. 1 (1983), pp. 79–82.

362 **coverage of mental maladies:** Postel, *Genèse de la psychiatrie: Les premiers écrits de Philippe Pinel*, pp. 161–213. On Arnold, see pp. 171–178.

362 **"that are more piously distinguished":** Ibid., pp. 192–196.

362 **immigrate to America:** Pinel, *Lettres de Pinel*, p. 7.

362 **"Teaching the Healing Art":** Pinel's 1790 manuscript is published in Gabriel Bollotte, "Pinel et la réforme de l'enseignement de l'art de guérir," *Information psychiatrique* 46, no. 7 (1970): 657–668. Pinel returned to this topic in 1793; see Philippe Pinel, *The Clinical Training of Doctors: An Essay of 1793*, ed. and trans. Dora B. Weiner (Baltimore: Johns Hopkins University Press, 1980).

363 **he was no Royalist:** Pinel, *Lettres de Pinel*, pp. 10–11. Also see Weiner, *Comprendre et soigner*, p. 87.

363 **lustily participated in the killing:** Schama, *Citizens*, pp. 634–635.

364 **former employer was arrested:** See Ackerknecht, "Political Prisoners in French Mental Institutions before 1789, During the Revolution, and under Napoleon I."

364 **the Bicêtre for eight years:** On Poussin and Pinel, see Jack Juchet, "Jean-Baptiste Pussin et Philippe Pinel à Bicêtre en 1793. Une Rencontre, Une Complicité, Une Dette," in *Philippe Pinel*, ed. Jean Garrabé (Paris: Les empêcheurs de penser en rond, 1994), pp. 55–69, and "Jean-Baptiste Pussin, 'Médecin des Folles,'" *Soins psychiatrie* 142/143 (1992). Also Dora B. Weiner, "The Apprenticeship of Philippe Pinel: A New Document, 'Observations of Citizen Pussin on the Insane,'" *American Journal of Psychiatry* 136, no. 9 (1979): 1128–1134, and her *Comprendre et soigner*, pp. 135–139, and pages 140–141 for admission diagnoses.

364 **straitjacket instead of chains:** Jacques Postel, et al., "Le myth revisité:

Philippe Pinel à Bicêtre de 1793 à 1795," in *Philippe Pinel*, ed. Jean Garrabé, p. 43.

365 **to break their spell:** Cited in Jan Goldstein, *Console and Classify: The French Psychiatric Profession in the Nineteenth Century* (Cambridge: Cambridge University Press, 1987), p. 110.

365 *Philosophy of Madness* **in 1791:** Joseph Daquin, *La philosophie de la folie* (Chambery: Gorin, père et fils, 1791). Also see Duccio Vanni, "Joseph Daquin, Piedmontese Savoyard Physician: A 'Not Well-Known Chiarugi,'" *Vesalius—Acta internationales historiae medicinae* 5, no. 1 (1999), pp. 30–40.

366 **cure those afflicted by insanity:** Ibid., pp. 112–116.

367 **he wrote beneath the image:** See E. H. Gombrich, "The Dream of Reason: Symbolism of the French Revolution," *Journal for Eighteenth-Century Studies* 2, no. 3 (2008): 187–205.

368 **the lens of natural history:** In Postel, *Genèse de la psychiatrie*, p. 233.

368 **qualities we might otherwise value:** Ibid, p. 234.

369 **"to restore distracted reason?" he demanded:** Ibid., p. 242. For this translation, see Dora B. Weiner, "Philippe Pinel's 'Memoir on Madness' of December 11, 1794: A Fundamental Text of Modern Psychiatry," *American Journal of Psychiatry* 149, no. 6 (1992): 730. Pinel calls it a "mysterious" silence in 1798, and in 1801 returns to it again as an "inhumane" secrecy.

369 **wall by heartless tyrants:** Postel, *Genèse de la psychiatrie*, p. 80.

370 **swinging it wildly into them:** Pinel, *Traité médico-philosophique sur l'aliénation mentale, ou la manie*.

370 **without leaving a scar:** Weiner, "Philippe Pinel's 'Memoir on Madness' of December 11, 1794," pp. 729–732.

371 **"to be happy, fuck?!":** Jacques-René Hébert, *Le Père Duchesne, 1790–1794*, ed. Albert Soboul, vol. 8 (Paris: Edhis, 1969), p. 2. See number 241, where he wrote, "Braves sans-coluttes, pourquoi avez-vous la revolution? N'est-ce pas pour être plus heureux, foutre?"

371 **Fury of the Gironde:** Elisabeth Roudinescu, *Madness and Revolution: The Lives and Legends of Théroigne de Méricourt* (London: Verso, 1991).

372 **discrete disease categories:** Philippe Pinel, *Nosographie philosophique, ou, la méthode de l'analyse appliquée à la médecine*, 2 vols. (Paris: Richard, Caille & Ravier, 1798). vol 1, p. xi.

372 **properties of sensibility and irritability:** Ibid., p. xxxii; also, vol 2, p. 364.

372 **secular land of France:** Pinel, *Nosographie philosophique*, vol 2, p. 394. Pinel concluded this work by writing: "et combine ces effects doivent devenir desormais sensibles dans un pays aussi Florissant que la France, et sous une gouvernement libre!"

373 **probably by buying them:** Staum, *Cabanis*, p. 97.

373 **its own logic and epistemology:** P. J. G. Cabanis (1798), *An Essay on the Certainty in Medicine*, trans. R. La Roche (Philadelphia: R. Desilver, 1823).

374 **man, including reason:** P. J. G. Cabanis, *Coup d'oeil sur les révolutions et sur la réforme de la médecine* (Paris: Crapart, Caille & Ravier, 1804). See George Rosen, "The Philosophy of Ideology and the Emergence of Modern Medicine in France," *Bulletin of the History of Medicine* 20 (1946), pp. 328–339. Also, Martin S. Staum, "Cabanis and the Science of Man," *Journal of the History of the Behavioral Sciences* 10, no. 2 (1974), p. 138.

374 **liberty, virtue, and happiness:** Cabanis, *Coup d'oeil sur les révolutions et sur la réforme de la médecine*, pp. 24, 335–336.

375 **a subset of zoology:** See Destutt de Tracy (1796), "Mémoires sur la Faculté de Penser," in *Mémoires de l'Institut National des Sciences et Arts* (Paris: Baudouin, 1798), pp. 323–326; and his (1801) *Élémens d'Idéologie* (Paris: Courcier, 1804), p. xiii.

376 *the Moral Aspects of Man:* P. J. G. Cabanis, *Rapports du physique et du moral de l'homme* (Paris: Crapart, Caille & Ravier, 1802). I will refer to the English translation, P. J. G. Cabanis (1802), *On the Relations Between the Physical and Moral Aspects of Man*, ed. George Mora, trans. M. Saidi 2 vols. (Baltimore: Johns Hopkins University Press, 1981). Cabanis published six memoirs in 1798 and twelve in 1802.

376 **of in private:** Staum, *Cabanis, in the French Revolution*, pp. 135–136.

376 **secure the new order:** Constantin-François Volney, *Catéchisme du citoyen français, ou la loi naturelle* (Paris: Dufart, 1798); Jean-François Saint-Lambert, *Le catéchisme universel*, in *Oeuvres philosophiques de Saint Lambert* (Paris: Agssem, 1801), vol. 2, p. 17. Also see Charles Hunter Van Duzer, *Contribution of the Ideologues to French Revolutionary Thought* (Baltimore: Johns Hopkins Press, 1935), pp. 59–65.

377 **"religion that replaces Christianity?":** François-René de Chateaubriand, *Essai historique, politique, et moral sur les révolutions* (Londres: J. Deboffe, 1797), pp. 649–653.

377 **manuals for behavior and didactic tracts:** Anonymous, *Manuel des Théophilanthropes, ou adorations de Dieu et amis des hommes* (Paris: Epinal, 1797). Also see Charles Lyttle, "Deistic Piety in the Cults of the French Revolution," *Church History*, 2, no. 1 (1933): 22–40, and Israel, *Revolutionary Ideas*, pp. 682, 686.

377 **Heaven and damnation in Hell:** Martin S. Staum, "The Enlightenment Transformed: The Institute Prize Contests," *Eighteenth-Century Studies* 19, no. 2 (1985): 153–179.

377 **"pronounced within these walls":** Martin S. Staum, "The Class of Moral and Political Sciences, 1795–1803," *French Historical Studies* 11, no. 3 (1980): 388.

378 **they would roguishly pursue it:** Cabanis, *On the Relations Between the Physical and Moral Aspects of Man*, vol.1, p. 18.

378 **Helvétius, Condillac, and Haller:** Ibid., pp. 9, 12, 32. On Haller, see pp. 83–84, 89.

378 Adam Smith, and Francis Hutcheson: Ibid., pp. 12, 68–69, 134.

378 criminal actions could be eradicated: Ibid. pp. 244, 354.

378 stomach churned out its juices: Ibid., p. 196.

379 the mind to impact the body: Ibid, p. 113.

379 book to be his Bible: Stendhal, *Souvenirs d'égotisme*, ed. Henri Martineau (Paris: Le Divan, 1927), p. 66, and his *Vie d'Henri Brulard* (Paris: Honoré & Edouard Champion, 1913), p. 12.

380 found in 1796: This translation is of Société Médicale d'Émulation de Paris. Of note, Barthez was a corresponding member.

380 the prophets of old: Philippe Pinel, "On Periodic or Intermittent Mania," *History of Psychiatry* 3, no. 11 (1992): 351–370. This paper was expanded into Section 1 of Pinel's *Traité*.

381 coming to his own conclusions: Alexander Crichton, *An Inquiry into the Nature and Origin of Mental Derangement. Comprehending a Concise System of the Physiology and Pathology of the Human Mind* (London: T. Cadell & W. Davies, 1798), vol. 1, p. v. On Pinel and Crichton, see Dora B. Weiner, "Mind and Body in the Clinic: Philippe Pinel, Alexander Crichton, Dominique Esquirol, and the Birth of Psychiatry," in *The Languages of Psyche: Mind and Body in Enlightenment Thought: Clark Library Lectures, 1985–1986*, ed. George S. Rousseau (Berkeley: University of California Press, 1990), pp. 331–390.

382 "advancement of a people's civilization": Pinel, *Traité médico-philosophique sur l'aliénation mentale, ou la manie* (1801), p. v.

382 fragmented and thus alienated: See M. H. Abrams, *Natural Supernaturalism: Tradition and Revolution in Romantic Literature* (New York: W. W. Norton, 1971), pp. 31, 147, 171.

382 referred to madness as an *alienatio mentis*: Pigeaud, *Aux portes de la psychiatrie*, p. 170.

382 language to make critical distinctions: Pinel, *Traité medico-philosophique sur l'aliénation mentale*, p. liv.

382 mind without the old "fetters": Ibid., pp. xliv, 45–46.

382 "of the Ideologists": Ibid., p. xxxv.

382 new nomenclature stand alone: The second edition is Philippe Pinel, *Traité médico-philosophique sur l'aliénation mentale* (Paris: J. A. Brosson, 1809). For the differences between editions see J. Postel, M. Postel, and P. Privat, "Les deux introductions au 'Traite medico-philosophique' de P. Pinel," *Annales Médico-psychologiques* 1, no. 1 (1971): 15–48.

383 them would be called alienists: Pinel, *Traité médico-philosophique sur l'aliénation mentale*, pp. 4, 491.

383 citizens by a despotic government: Pinel, *A Treatise on Insanity*, p. 89.

383 refused to try new treatments: Ibid., pp. 56–59.

384 "vicissitudes of public fortune": Ibid., p. 209.

384 "distinguished birthrights as rational beings": Ibid., p. 9.

384 **head was not his own:** Pinel referred to this patient as a silversmith and as a watchmaker: Ibid., pp. 26, 68.

385 **and were beheaded:** Ibid., pp. 61, 100, 103, 73, 143, 277. On the September massacres, see p. 155.

385 **Revolution, and, lastly, religious fanaticism:** Ibid., p. 113. Pinel confessed that his efforts to treat these fanatics generally failed. A missionary ready to murder for his God was incurable and in need of constant containment. Perhaps this reflected his clinical experience, but it may have also expressed his dread of a counterrevolution.

386 **existed in cases of idiotism:** Pinel, *A Treatise on Insanity,* pp. 112–120.

386 **old age—were equally incurable:** Idiotism was due to alcohol, trauma, tumors, masturbation, or being bled too much by one's doctor. Ibid., p. 167.

386 **pharmaceutical treatments were rubbish:** Ibid., p. 109.

386 **refused to reveal their methods:** Ibid., p. 4. Also see E. T. Carlson and N. Dain, "The Psychotherapy That Was Moral Treatment," *American Journal of Psychiatry* 117 (1960): 519–524.

387 **contrasted with nonsensical saints:** Ibid., pp. 66, 78.

387 **Consolation helped melancholics:** Ibid., p. 102.

387 **his nose and walked away:** Ibid., pp. 96–97.

387 **government's approach to its people:** Ibid., p. 228. The attacks on Pinel's legacy as not a liberator, but rather the representative of a new, more insidious form of state power, have been put forth by Michel Foucault, and further developed in works such as Robert Castel, *The Regulation of Madness: The Origins of Incarceration in France,* trans. W. D. Halls (Berkeley: University of California Press, 1988). This view has been challenged by, among others, Marcel Gauchet and Gladys Swain, in their *Madness and Democracy: The Modern Psychiatric Universe,* trans. Catherine Porter (Princeton: Princeton University Press, 1999).

388 **reached British shores:** On the reception of Pinel, see Jacques Postel, *Éléments pour une histoire de la psychiatrie occidentale* (Paris: l'Harmattan, 2007): 165–174. Also, Gladys Swain, "De Kant à Hegel: Deux époques de la folie," *Libre,* 1977, pp. 174–201.

388 **any in the world:** Pinel, *A Treatise on Insanity,* p. 288.

389 **mind from the Divine one:** François-Auguste Chateaubriand, *Le Genie du Christianisme* (Paris: Migneret, 1802). Also see *Memoirs of Chateaubriand: From His Birth in 1768 to his Return to France in 1800* (London: Henry Colburn, 1849).

389 **them as miserable materialists:** Karl Mannheim, *Ideology and Utopia* (New York: Harcourt, Brace & World, 1936), p. 72.

391 **boy's disabilities through mentalist means:** At this time, cases of abandoned children were not so rare. See, for example, the equally famed German case reported in Anselm von Feuerbach, *Caspar Hauser: An Account* (Boston: Allen & Ticknor, 1833).

392 **populate his empty mind:** The name was the *Société des observateurs de l'homme.*

392 **regulate himself within society:** Jean-Marc-Gaspard Itard (1807), *Rapports et mémoires sur le sauvage de l'Aveyron* (Paris: Bureau de Progrès médical, 1894). In English, see *The Wild Boy of Aveyron,* trans. George and Muriel Humphrey (New York: Appleton, Century, Crofts, 1962).

PART IV: THE SERPENT THAT ATE ITS TAIL

395 **"Mind being invisible Nature":** F. W. J. Schelling, *Ideen zu einer Philosophie der Natur* (Leipzig: Breitkopf & Härtel, 1797), p. 64. My thanks to David Levin for help with the translation of "Die Natur soll der sichtbare Geist, der Geist die unsichtbare Natur seyn." For alternatives, see F. W. J. Schelling (1797/1803), *Ideas for a Philosophy of Nature,* trans. E. Harris and P. Heath (Cambridge: Cambridge University Press, 1988), p. 42, who wrote: "Nature should be Mind made visible, Mind the invisible Nature." *Geist* is translated as "spirit," not "mind," in F. W. Schelling (1803), *Ideas on a Philosophy of Nature as an Introduction to the Study of Science,* in *Philosophy of German Idealism,* ed. Ernest Behler (New York: Continuum, 1987), p. 202.

16. KANT AND THE AGE OF SELF-CRITICISM

398 **a deep-seated despair:** See Angelica Goodden, *Madame de Staël: The Dangerous Exile* (Oxford: Oxford University Press, 2008), and Maria Fairweather, *Madame de Staël* (London: Constable and Robinson, 2006). Also see Lydia Maria Child, ed., *Memoirs of Madame De Staël and of Madame Roland* (New York: C. S. Francis & Co., 1847); Madelyn Gutwirth, "Madame De Staël, Rousseau, and the Woman Question," *Publications of the Modern Language Association of America* 86, no. 1 (1971): 100–109; and Jean Starobinski, "Suicide et melancholie chez Mme. De Staël," in *Madame de Staël et l'Europe* (Paris: Klincksieck, 1970), pp. 242–252.

398 **"make of her," she complained:** Tess Lewis, "The French Issue—Madame De Staël: The Inveterate Idealist," *Hudson Review* 54, no. 3 (2001), p. 420.

398 **who later mocked her:** Cited in Karyna Szmurlo, *The Novel's Seductions: Staël's Corinne in Critical Inquiry* (Lewisburg, Pa.: Bucknell University Press, 1999), p. 127.

398 **fear, liberty, and stability:** Anne-Louise Germaine de Staël, *De l'influence des passions sur le bonheur des individus et des nations* (Lausanne: Jean Mourer et al., 1796). *Essay on the Passions* was charged with the times. It was no miscue of passions for 24 million to rise up against the privileges of 200,000, she insisted. Nor was it crazed emotion that led aristocrats to resist Robespierre. Nonetheless, heated passions like vanity and envy had driven the

Revolution into a ditch. Orators became intoxicated with the crowd's roar, while mobs swelled with a shared animal power.

399 **"truly constitutes intellectual existence!"**: Madame de Staël, *Selected Correspondence,* trans. K. Jameson-Cemper (Dordrecht, Neth.: Kluwer Academic, 1974). Germain de Staël to Charles de Villers, Aug. 1, 1802, p. 135.

399 **"glimpse to all material clarity"**: Ibid., p. 139.

400 **prematurely refer to as Germany:** Baroness de Staël-Holstein (1810), *De L'Allemagne* (Paris: H. Nicolle, 1813). Lessing, Herder, and others already argued for a linguistic and cultural, if not a politically unified, Germany. My thanks to Sander Gilman for this point.

400 **the inspiring events in America:** Frederick C. Beiser, *Enlightenment, Revolution, and Romanticism: The Genesis of Modern German Political Thought, 1790–1800* (Cambridge: Harvard University Press, 1992), p. 23.

400 **theories of the Counter-Enlightenment:** On the debates surrounding the notions of Counter-Enlightenment, see the seminal work of Isaiah Berlin, *The Proper Study of Mankind: An Anthology of Essays* (New York: Farrar, Straus & Giroux, 1998), pp. 243–268, and the challenges posed by Zeev Sternhell, *The Anti-Enlightenment Tradition,* trans. David Maisel (New Haven: Yale University Press, 2010).

401 **society would descend into chaos:** On Kant's biography and the genesis of this essay, published in the *Berlinische Monatsschrift*, see Manfred Kuehn, *Kant: A Biography* (Cambridge: Cambridge University Press, 2001), pp. 288–292. Ironically, just prior to the famed essay on enlightenment, Kant published an essay on cosmopolitanism, which looked past state affiliations and challenged the Prussian state.

402 **"the most obedient character"**: See Baroness de Staël-Holstein, *De l'Allemagne,* p. 32, or *Germany* (London: J. Murray, 1813), vol.1, pp. 34–35. In an 1800 poem to his countrymen, Hölderlin accused his fellow Germans of being "rich in fancies" but "poor in deeds"; Friedrich Hölderlin, *Selected Verse,* trans. Michael Hamburger (London: Anvil Press Poetry, 1986), p. 72.

404 **beating back mystical, orthodox Lutherans:** See Manfred Kuehn, *Kant: A Biography,* pp. 100–188. Also see Paul Guyer, *Kant and the Claims of Knowledge* (Cambridge and New York: Cambridge University Press, 1987), pp. 26–61.

404 **"common man who knows nothing"**: Beiser, *Enlightenment, Revolution, and Romanticism,* p. 30.

404 **the limits of reason:** Kant explained this trajectory in Immanuel Kant (1781), *Critique of Pure Reason.* trans. Norman Kemp Smith (London: Macmillan, 1929). Also see Kant (1783), *Prolegomena to Any Future Metaphysics,* trans. J. W. Ellington (Indianapolis: Hackett Publishing Co., 1985), p. 5.

405 **understand the real thing:** Ibid., p. 6.

405 **Olympian assurance, "is impossible"**: Ibid., p. 9.

405 "that of the celebrated Locke": Kant, *Critique of Pure Reason*, p. 8.

405 critiques as "world-crushing": Mendelssohn used the word "Weltzermalmend." See Allen Wood, "Rational Theology, Moral Faith, and Religion," in *The Cambridge Companion to Kant*, ed. Paul Guyer (Cambridge: Cambridge University Press, 1992), p. 397. On the soul and German psychology, see Gary Hatfield, "Empirical, Rational, and Transcendental Psychology: Psychology as Science and as Philosophy," in ibid., pp. 200–227.

406 the Age of Reason: Kant, *Critique of Pure Reason*, p. 32.

407 this kind of semantic slippage: *Verstand* literally means "reason," but can also connote mind, *Gemüt* also could mean "soul" or "spirit," but it too over time was used for a natural seat of interiority, one that could sicken or die. On this term, see Cheryce Kramer, *A Fool's Paradise: The Psychiatry of Gemüt in a Biedermeier Asylum* (Ph.D diss., University of Chicago, 1998).

408 existed *during* life, not afterward: Immanuel Kant, *Prolegomena to Any Future Metaphysics*, p. 76.

408 a person could know: Ibid., pp. 37, 78.

408 rational doctrine of the "soul": Kant, *Critique of Pure Reason*, pp. 338–340, 67, 331, 366.

408 free will and human morality: Kant, *Prolegomena to Any Future Metaphysics*, pp. 27, 30.

410 essence; that truth was unavoidable: Hoke Robinson, "Two Perspectives on Kant's Appearances and Things in Themselves," *Journal of the History of Philosophy* 32, no. 3 (1994): 411–441.

411 philosophy over the next decades: J. G. Fichte (1794), *The Science of Knowledge*, trans. Peter Heath and John Lachs (Cambridge: Cambridge University Press, 1982), p. 13, 10. Also see Terry P. Pinkard, *German Philosophy, 1760–1860: The Legacy of Idealism* (Cambridge: Cambridge University Press, 2002), and B. Sassen, "Critical Idealism in the Eyes of Kant's Contemporaries," *Journal of the History of Philosophy* 35, no. 3 (1997): 421–455.

411 scientific physiology and psychology: Jakob Friedrich Fries and Johann Friedrich Herbart looked to the empirical Kant. See David Leary, "Immanuel Kant and the Development of Modern Psychology," in *The Problematic Science: Psychology in Nineteenth-Century Thought*, ed. William Woodward and Mitchell Ash (New York: Praeger, 1982), pp. 17–41.

412 descending into useless rumination: LeeAnn Hansen, "From Enlightenment to 'Naturphilosophie': Marcus Herz, Johann Christian Reil, and the Problem of Border Crossings," *Journal of the History of Biology* 26 (1993): 50–51.

412 excesses of the "philosophical *medici*": Immanuel Kant (1798), *Anthropology from a Pragmatic Point of View,* trans. Robert B. Louden (Cambridge: Cambridge University Press, 2006), p. ix.

413 religious enthusiasm and spiritualism: Kant, *Anthropology from a Pragmatic Point of View*, p. 54.

413 **soul, but rather a mind:** Ibid., pp. 96, 106, 113.

413 **only come from Kantian anthropologists:** Ibid., p. 108.

413 **collapse and lead to atheism:** Klaus Dorner, *Madmen and the Bourgeoisie: A Social History of Insanity and Psychiatry*, trans. J. Neugroschel and J. Steinberg (Oxford, Eng.: B. Blackwell, 1981), pp. 184–185.

414 **mental illness was incurable:** Kant, *Anthropology from a Pragmatic Point of View*, pp. 108, 111.

414 **the march in France:** Kuehn, *Kant,* pp. 340–343.

414 **increased freedom and equality:** LeeAnn Hansen, "Metaphors of Mind and Society: The Origins of German Psychiatry in the Revolutionary Era," *Isis* 89, no. 3 (1998): 394.

415 *Magazine for Empirical Psychology:* *Magazin zur Erfahrungseelenkund* was first published in 1783. On the fascinating but underappreciated Moritz, the best available study remains Mark Boulby, *Karl Philipp Moritz: At the Fringe of Genius* (Toronto: University of Toronto Press, 1979).

415 **dreams, and lost childhood memories:** Ibid., pp. 124–125. Moses Mendelssohn's article in the first volume compares the mind to the ruler of a well-ordered state, in which ideas were in harmony like good subjects. See Hansen, "Metaphors of Mind and Society," p. 406.

415 **Kantian philosophy and medicine:** Hansen, "From Enlightenment to 'Naturphilosophie,'" pp. 39–64. One of these efforts, a 1791 essay on vertigo, was sent to Kant, who apparently placed it unread on his shelf, saying he would not read it because he was not dizzy. See Kuehn, *Kant,* p. 320.

416 **how might it relieve suffering?:** Marcus Herz, *Versuch über den Schwindel* (Berlin: Voss, 1791). On this text, see Hansen, "From Enlightenment to 'Naturphilosophie,'" p. 56. In a second edition of his book, Herz confidently announced that the mind consisted of three tiers in which material ideas existed in between both immaterial ideas and the brain. This pseudosolution made little impact on others.

416 **physiology based on Kantian principles:** Johann Christian Reil, ed., *Archiv für die Physiologie* 1, no. 1 (1796). The title page reads 1796, but publication occurred in 1795. Reil's new journal was one of many: some seventy German medical journals were founded in the 1790s alone.

416 **the living from the dead:** Johann Christian Reil, "Von der Lebenskraft," *Archiv für die Physiologie* 1 (1796): 8–188. There is some argument about the positions that Reil took in this complex paper. Hansen convincingly reads it as the work of materialistic vitalism. See "From Enlightenment to 'Naturphilosophie'" pp. 39–64. Also see Timothy Lenoir, *The Strategy of Life: Teleology and Mechanism in Nineteenth-Century German Biology* (Chicago: University of Chicago Press, 1982), pp. 35–37.

417 **complaints into their objective determinants:** Thomas Hoyt Broman,

The Transformation of German Academic Medicine, 1750–1820 (Cambridge and New York: Cambridge University Press, 1996), pp. 86–90.

418 **poem was simply entitled "Buonaparte":** Hölderlin, *Selected Verse*, p. 11.

418 **"Come Rousseau, and be my guide!":** T. C. W. Blanning, *The Romantic Revolution: A History* (New York: Modern Library, 2010), p. 29.

419 **"vilified as drunks and lunatics":** Johann Wolfgang von Goethe (1774), *The Sorrows of Young Werther,* trans. David Constantine (Oxford and New York: Oxford University Press, 2012), p. 41, 7, 12.

419 **the hero in crazed despair:** Ibid., p. 42.

419 **save him were futile:** Ibid., p. 47.

419 **being misread in many ways:** See George di Giovanni and H. S. Harris, *Between Kant and Hegel: Texts in the Development of Post-Kantian Idealism* (Albany: State University of New York Press, 1985). Di Giovanni wrote, "Few philosophers were as badly misunderstood by their contemporaries as Kant was," (p. 3).

419 **metaphysics became psychology:** On Karl Reinhold, see George di Giovanni, "The Facts of Consciousness," in *Between Kant and Hegel*, pp. 3–50, and Kuehn, *Kant*, pp. 351–353.

420 **without ever coming onstage:** J. G. Fichte (1801), "A Crystal Clear Report to the General Public Concerning the Actual Essence of the Newest Philosophy," in Fichte, Jacobi, and Schelling, *Philosophy of German Idealism*, ed. Ernst Behler (New York: Continuum, 1987), pp. 50–51, 55. Also see J. G. Fichte (1794), *The Science of Knowledge*, trans. Peter Heath and John Lachs (Cambridge: Cambridge University Press, 1982).

420 **the core of human subjectivity:** Robert J. Richards, *The Romantic Conception of Life Science and Philosophy in the Age of Goethe* (Chicago: University of Chicago Press, 2002), pp. 72–80.

421 **"the character of reality":** Ibid., p. 51. On Fichte's theory of subjectivity, see Frederick Neuhouser, *Fichte's Theory of Subjectivity* (Cambridge: Cambridge University Press, 1990).

422 **devouring its own tail:** Coleridge used this phrase with regard to narrative understanding. See M. H. Abrams, *Natural Supernaturalism: Tradition and Revolution in Romantic Literature* (New York: W. W. Norton, 1971), p. 141.

422 **barely glimpsed inner being:** The origins and definition of "romantic" have long been controversial. According to Welleck, in one of the first references, Villers in 1810 referred to the small spiritual sect that emerged in Germany, which he praised for valorizing "la Romantique." René Wellek, "The Concept of 'Romanticism' in Literary History. I. The Term 'Romantic' and Its Derivatives," *Comparative Literature* 1, no. 1 (1949): 8.

422 **"excursion into infinity":** Germaine de Staël, *Germany*, vol. 1, p. 224.

424 **"from Bacon, Newton, and Locke":** Cited in Blanning, *The Romantic Revolution*, p. 87.

17. RHAPSODIES FOR PSYCHE

427 **complaint thirty years earlier:** Johann Wolfgang von Goethe (1809), *Elective Affinities: A Novel*, trans. David Constantine (Oxford and New York: Oxford University Press, 1994), p. 140.

427 **mavericks agitated for a republic:** On the generation of 1790, see T. Lenoir, "Generational Factors in the Origin of Romantische Naturphilosophie," *Journal of the History of Biology*, 11 no. 1 (1978): 57–100.

427 **denounced him as a traitor:** For the letters of Caroline Böhmer Schlegel Schelling to her circle, see www.carolineschelling.com. Letter of Nov. 1792 from Friedrich to Wilhelm Schlegel.

428 **her way to Jena:** Richards, *The Romantic Conception of Life Science and Philosophy in the Age of Goethe*, pp. 36–42.

428 **proclaimed, was the German Hamlet:** On the genesis of the different editions and the reception of Faust, see the commentary in Johann Wolfgang von Goethe, *Faust*, trans. Walter Arndt (New York: W. W. Norton, 2011).

428 **Then, Mephistopheles descended:** Goethe, *Faust*, pp. 33, 43.

428 **Medicine was a straight swindle:** Ibid., pp. 50–53. Madame de Staël, *De l'influence des passions sur le bonheur* (Lausanne: Jean Mourer, 1796), p. 558.

429 **came under Jena's sway:** Philippe Lacoue-Labarthe and Jean-Luc Nancy, *The Literary Absolute: The Theory of Literature in German Romanticism*, trans. P. Barnard and C. Lester (Albany: State University of New York, 1988). They claim the Jena thinkers created the first modern avant-garde.

429 **moment of "God in us":** de Staël-Holstein, *Germany* vol. 3, p. 388.

429 **Fichte, stuck to their beliefs:** On Goethe's politics, see W. Daniel Wilson, "Goethe and the Political World," in *Cambridge Companion to Goethe*, ed. Lesley Sharpe (Cambridge: Cambridge University Press, 2002), pp. 207–218.

430 **"off on the other side":** Cited in Richards, *The Romantic Conception of Life Science and Philosophy in the Age of Goethe*, p. 83. On the three Nature philosophies—transcendental, romantic, and metaphysical—see Timothy Lenoir, "The Göttingen School and Development of Transcendental Naturphilosophie in the Romantic Era," *Studies in History of Biology* 5:111–205, 1981.

430 **"means of an infinite approximation. . . .":** Lacoue-Labarthe, *The Literary Absolute*, p. 132.

431 **the foundations of science:** Ibid., p. 81.

431 **a new theory of life:** Richards, *The Romantic Conception of Life Science and Philosophy in the Age of Goethe*, pp. 116–126..

431 **"separates himself from himself":** F. W. Schelling (1803), *Ideas on a Philosophy of Nature as an Introduction to the Study of Science,* in *Philosophy of German Idealism*, ed. Ernest Behler (New York: Continuum, 1987), pp.

168–169. For an alternative translation, see Harris and Heath's wording in Schelling, *Ideas for a Philosophy of Nature*, p. 10.

432 **"Mind being invisible Nature"**: Schelling, *Ideas for a Philosophy of Nature*, pp. 40–42.

433 **"the pure gift of rendering. . . ."**: Friedrich Schlegel to Caroline Schlegel. Letter 203, dated Sept., 9 or 16, 1798. www.carolineschelling.com. Schelling himself was not afraid to admit that he had benefited from the study of Renaissance animist thinkers, something Coleridge pointed out to his readers in 1817; see Coleridge, *Biographia Literaria*, p. 87.

433 **"the granite, find a granitesse?"**: Friedrich Schlegel to Caroline Schlegel. Letter 207, dated Oct. 29, 1798. www.carolineschelling.com.

433 **"which proceeds only from identity"**: Schelling, *Ideas on a Philosophy of Nature as an Introduction to the Study of Science*, p. 169.

434 **"the current know this?"**: Ibid., p. 172.

434 **rather than mere representations**: Ibid., pp. 174–175.

434 **won Caroline Schlegel's heart**: Richards, *The Romantic Conception of Life Science and Philosophy in the Age of Goethe*, p. 195.

434 *Naturphilosophie* **were physicians and scientists**: Broman, *The Transformation of German Academic Medicine, 1750–1820*, pp. 92–98.

434 **doctors in the German lands**: F. W. J. Schelling to his parents. Letter 213a, dated Dec. 29, 1798. www.carolineschelling.com.

435 **therefore hastened her end**: G. B. Risse, "Schelling, 'Naturphilosophie,' and John Brown's System of Medicine," *Bulletin of the History of Medicine* 50, no. 3 (1976): 333.

435 **philosophy and a medical doctor**: See the cover page of F. W. J. Schelling, *Ideen zu einer Philosophie der Natur, als Einleitung in das Studium diser Wissenschaft* (Landshut, Ger.: Phillip Krüll, 1803).

435 **scientists, chemists, and clinicians**: F. W. J. Schelling, "On Medicine and the Theory of Organic Nature," *Journal of Speculative Philosophy* 15 (1881): 1–8; and F. W. J. Schelling, "Vorrede," *Jahrbücher der Medicin als Wissenschaft* 1, no. 1 (1805): vi.

436 **would provide answers**: G. B. Risse, "Kant, Schelling, and the Early Search for a Philosophical 'Science' of Medicine in Germany," *Journal of the History of Medicine and Allied Sciences* 27, no. 2 (1972): 145.

436 **"what he called "Instinct"**: Risse, "Schelling, 'Naturphilosophie,' and John Brown's System of Medicine," p. 327.

436 **matter to qualities of experience**: I have used the translation of Priscilla Hayden-Roy in Schelling, *Ideas on a Philosophy of Nature*, in *Philosophy of German Idealism*, p. 178. For an alternative translation, see Schelling, *Ideas for a Philosophy of Nature*, p. 20.

437 **organized whole structures**: To call this a vital force, he remarked, would be to posit a contradiction, since all forces must be opposed. Hence any vital force would necessarily contain a destructive one. This idea was even-

tually embraced by Sigmund Freud, who countered Eros with Thanatos, or the death drive. The relation of Schelling to Freud's unconscious has been explored in Matt ffytche, *The Foundation of the Unconscious: Schelling, Freud, and the Birth of the Modern Psyche* (Cambridge: Cambridge University Press, 2012).

437 **object together in true knowledge:** Ibid., p. 202.

438 **"produced designedly and as purposes":** Immanuel Kant (1790), *Critique of the Power of Judgment,* trans. Paul Guyer and Eric Matthews (Cambridge: Cambridge University Press, 2000), p. 275.

438 **not the Word, but rather the Deed:** Schelling, *Ideas on a Philosophy of Nature*, p. 171.

438 **Leipzig, Heidelberg, and Erlangen:** M. K. Amdur, "The Dawn of Psychiatric Journalism," *American Journal of Psychiatry*, no. 100 (1943): 206.

439 **Henrik Steffens, had moved to Halle:** On the underappreciated Reil, see Henrich Steffens, *Johann Christian Reil; Eine Denkschrift* (Halle: Curt, 1815); LeeAnn Hansen Le Roy, "Johann Christian Reil and 'Naturphilosophie' in Physiology" (Ph.D. diss., University of California, Los Angeles, 1985); Robert J. Richards, "Rhapsodies on a Cat-Piano, or Johann Christian Reil and the Foundations of Romantic Psychiatry," *Critical Inquiry* 24, no. 3 (1998): 700–736.

439 **that patient was himself:** On Goldhagen's delusion, see Richards, "Rhapsodies on a Cat-Piano," p. 712.

439 **a friend of science:** Ibid.

440 **brutalized by their keepers:** On Johann Peter Frank, see Amdur, "The Dawn of Psychiatric Journalism," p. 208. Also see the firsthand report by Reil's colleague, A. A. Kayssler, "Mein Besuch bey den Irren und Wahnsinnigen in der Charité zu Berlin," in *Magazin für die psychische Heilkunde* 1, no. 1 (1805): 115–173.

440 **modern forms of restraint:** Dorner, *Madmen and the Bourgeoisie*, p. 215. Horn's modern methods, as we shall see, would themselves end in disaster.

440 **state to prevent such abuses:** Ibid., pp. 170–172.

441 **appeared, nonetheless, in 1803:** Johann Christian Reil, *Rhapsodieen über die Anwendung der psychischen Curmethode auf Geisteszerrüttungen* (Halle: Curt, 1803). (Hereafter, *Rhapsodieen*).

441 **passions and regain their equanimity:** Little has been written on Langermann. See E. H. Ackerknecht, *Short History of Psychiatry*, trans. S. Wolff (New York, Hafner, 1968), pp. 34–39 and Klaus Doerner, *Madmen and the Bourgeoisie*, pp. 211–215.

442 **as his rotating machine:** Dorner, *Madmen and the Bourgeoisie*, p. 213–216.

442 **different from everyday experience:** Nicolai's account can be found in the collection of primary texts assembled in Shane McCorristine, ed., *Spiritualism, Mesmerism, and the Occult*, 5 vols. (London: Pickering & Chatto, 2012), vol 1, pp. 9–22. This first-person account was published in a Ger-

man journal of natural philosophy, then translated and widely read in English.

443 **French arrogance in medicine:** See Reil, *Rhapsodieen*, pp. 30–31. Reil considered Pinel's writings to be in parts excellent, but poor in systematic treatment, and without originality. He also unfairly criticized Pinel's therapeutics for having no basis in theory. See pp. 268–269.

443 **called him the German Pinel:** Richards, "Rhapsodies on a Cat-Piano," p. 703.

443 **these deep inner causes:** Anonymous, "Begriff der psychischen Medicin als Wissenschaft," in *Magazin für die Psychische Heilkunde*, vol. 1 (1805): 76. The first issue of the journal contains only unsigned articles. This one is likely by Reil.

443 **"ocean of the large world":** Reil, *Rhapsodieen*, pp. 7–8. I have employed the translation in Richards, *The Romantic Conception of Life Science and Philosophy in the Age of Goethe*, p. 264.

443 **Newton, Bacon, and Leibniz:** Reil, *Rhapsodieen*, p. 8.

444 **the *Seele* would be lost:** Reil, *Rhapsodieen*, pp. 8–9. Reil wrote: "with every limb, with every means of sensation, a part of our soul is amputated."

444 **psychic illnesses and cures:** Ibid., pp. 38–39.

444 **psychical medicine and science:** In 1805, Reil and Kayssler's journal contained a long article, likely by the former, on establishing psychical medicine as a science, Anonymous, "Begriff der psychischen Medicin als Wissenschaft," *Magazin für die Psychische Heilkunde,* vol.1, 1805, pp. 45–77.

444 **the emergence of mental capabilities:** Reil wrote: "The normal dynamic relationship of the brain is grounded in ideas, and it must be rectified through the ideas when it is disturbed." Cited in Le Roy, "Johann Christian Reil and 'Naturphilosophie' in Physiology," p. 183.

445 **"insofar as it is representable":** Reil, *Rhapsodieen*, p. 55. This translation is from Robert Richards, *The Romantic Conception of Life Science and Philosophy in the Age of Goethe*, p. 268.

446 **categories might contain multitudes:** Reil, *Rhapsodieen*, pp. 306–462.

446 **return him to inner peace:** Ibid., p. 345.

446 **"himself and therefore about himself":** Ibid., p. 344.

447 **philosophy professor, Anton Adalbert Kayssler:** Reil and Kayssler, *Magazin für die Psychische Heilkunde,* vol.1 (1805). Also see Amdur, "The Dawn of Psychiatric Journalism," p. 207. Reil and Kayssler were not alone; the same year, a competitor, the *Archiv für Gemüths-und Nervenkrankheiten*, appeared thanks to the efforts of Dr. August Winkelmann, a former student in Jena.

448 **the new journal appeared:** Johann Christian Reil and Johann Christoph Hoffbauer, *Beyträge zur Beförderung einer Kurmethode auf psychischem Wege* (Halle: Curt, 1808).

449 **of what once was the soul:** Ibid,. vol 1, no 2, pp.161–279. See especially pp. 168–169.

18. THE PROMISE OF PHRENOLOGY

451 **penned rhapsodies on psychical topics:** For example, see the contents of J. B. Friedreich's *Magazin für die philosophische, medicinische und gerichtliche Seelenkunde*, vol. 1 (1829).

452 **this grey, wrinkled flesh:** Edwin Clarke and L. S. Jacyna, *Nineteenth-Century Origins of Neuroscientific Concepts* (Berkeley: University of California Press, 1987), p. 220.

454 **insisted, was not his problem:** On Gall, see Erwin Ackerknecht and Henri Vallois, *Franz Joseph Gall, Inventor of Phrenology and His Collection* (Madison: Department of History of Medicine, University of Wisconsin Medical School, 1956). On his theories, see Robert Young, *Mind, Brain, and Adaptation in the Nineteenth Century* (New York: Oxford University Press, 1990), pp. 9–53. Of the more recent scholarship, I have benefited most from John Van Wyhe, "The Authority of Human Nature: The Schädellehre of Franz Joseph Gall," *British Journal for the History of Science* 35 (2002): 17–42.

454 **somnambulism, and childhood visions:** F. J. Gall, *Works in Six Volumes,* trans. Winslow Lewis (Boston: Marsh, Capen & Lyon, 1835), vol. 2, p. 282.

454 **intrusion on his freedom:** Ackerknecht and Vallois, *Franz Joseph Gall, Inventor of Phrenology,* p. 7.

454 **his day by gardening:** Gall, *Works in Six Volumes*, vol. 2, p. 282.

454 *Healthy State of Man*: F. J. Gall, *Philosophisch-Medicinische Untersuchungen über Natur und Kunst im Kranken und Gesunden Zustande des Menschen* (Vienna: Rudolph Gräffer, 1791).

454 **between these quite different positions:** Isaiah Berlin argued that Hamann was *the* central thinker for German Romanticism and the Counter-Enlightenment, see Isaiah Berlin, *The Roots of Romanticism* (Princeton: Princeton University Press, 1999), p. 47. Debates over the influence of Herder often reflect divisions over the nature of German Romanticism. In *Enlightenment, Revolution, and Romanticism: The Genesis of Modern German Political Thought, 1790–1800,* Beiser convincingly positioned Herder between Hamann and Kant. Some disagree and see Herder as a purely Anti-Enlightenment figure; see Zeev Sternhall, *The Anti-Enlightenment Tradition*, pp. 80, 93, 105, 115.

455 *Philosophy of the History of Man*: J. G. Herder (1784–1791), *Outlines of a Philosophy of the History of Man*, trans. T. Churchill 2 vols. (London: J. Johnson, 1803). Sternhell dated the beginning of the Anti-Enlightenment to the summer of 1774 when Herder wrote this book. See his *The Anti-Enlightenment Tradition*, p. 10.

455 **called the "Counter-Enlightenment":** This phrase is Isaiah Berlin's. See his "The Counter-Enlightenment," in *The Proper Study of Mankind* (New York: Farrar, Straus, & Giroux, 1998), pp. 243–268.

455 **"scarcely see three more letters?":** Cited in Sternhall, *The Anti-Enlightenment Tradition*, p. 142.

455 **he privileged this inner will:** Berlin, *The Proper Study of Mankind*, p. 560.

455 **modified by the environment:** See the excellent work by Jerrold E. Seigel, *The Idea of the Self: Thought and Experience in Western Europe Since the Seventeenth Century* (New York: Cambridge University Press, 2005), p. 332.

457 **"erected a valuable science":** J. G. Herder, *Outlines of a Philosophy of the History of Man*, vol. 1, pp. 137–142. For Herder's influence, see Clarke and Jacyna, *Nineteenth-Century Origins of Neuroscientific Concepts*, p. 230.

458 **keep telling fibs:** See Gall, *Works in Six Volumes*. vol. 4, pp. 14–15. This story of origins was repeated numerous times by phrenologists. See, for example, Nahum Capen, *Reminiscences of Dr. Spurzheim and George Combe* (New York: Fowler & Wells, 1881), pp. 62–70.

459 **diminished in this manner:** Erna Lesky, *The Vienna Medical School of the 19th Century* (Baltimore: Johns Hopkins University Press, 1976), pp. 10–11.

459 **dangerous time to be a genius:** Nahum Capen, "Biography of Dr. Gall," in Gall, *Works in Six Volumes*, vol. 1, p. 15.

460 **learn from brain anatomy:** Haller's conclusion that the white matter was all equally sensitive supported his antilocalization theories; see Clarke and Jacyna, *Nineteenth-Century Origins of Neuroscientific Concepts*, pp. 214–217.

462 **Herder, Cabanis, and Reil:** Ibid., p. 226.

463 **grandiosity or suicidal self-hatred:** Capen, "Biography of Dr. Gall," p. 16.

463 **society to recognize that:** Ibid., p. 9. Gall's letter to Joseph Fr. Von Retzer dated Oct. 1, 1798, can be found in Capen, *Reminiscences of Dr. Spurzheim and George Combe*, pp. 70–86.

463 **"appreciated the *a priori*":** Ibid.

463 **"lose their heads":** Ackerknecht and Vallois, *Franz Joseph Gall*, p. 9.

464 **brought down the house:** Richards, *The Romantic Conception of Life Science and Philosophy in the Age of Goethe*, p. 277. Also see Van Wyhe, "The Authority of Human Nature," pp. 35–36.

465 **man's inner spirit and reality:** Georg Wilhelm Friedrich Hegel, *The Phenomenology of Mind,* trans. J. B. Baillie (New York: Harper & Row, 1967), pp. 338–372.

466 **"strikingly developed":** A. M. Fosati of Paris reported this, as cited in Capen, *Reminiscences of Dr. Spurzheim and George Combe*, p. 58.

466 **number would have been eighteen:** F. J. Gall, *Introduction au cours de physiologie du cerveau, ou discours pronouncé par le M. le docteur Gall* (Paris: Firman Didot, 1808). This public lecture was delivered on January 15, 1808. Since Gall began his brain studies in 1790, he had been working on this for eighteen years, not thirty.

466 **sovereign, Napoleon, a vast genius:** Ibid., p. 10.

466   **They scorned organology:** Maine de Biran, *Oeuvres* (Paris: F. Alcan, 1924), vol. 5, pp. 69–129.

467   **what was and wasn't science:** On Cuvier, see Dorinda Outram, *Georges Cuvier: Vocation, Science, and Authority in Post-Revolutionary France* (Manchester, Eng.: Manchester University Press, 1984).

467   **"divisible matter and the indivisible Me":** F. J. Gall and G. Spurzheim, *Recherches sur le système nerveux en général, et sur celui du cerveau en particulier, Mémoire présenté a l'Institut de France, Mars 14, 1808* (Paris: F. Schoell & S. Nicolle, 1809), p. 4. Also see Dora B. Weiner, *Comprendre et soigner: Philippe Pinel, 1745–1826*, p. 187.

468   **blue skies and green trees?:** Gall and Spurzheim, *Recherches sur le système nerveux en général*, p. 8.

468   **worked through its organization:** Anonymous, *Some Account of Dr. Gall's New Theory of Physiognomy . . . , with Critical Strictures of C. W. Hufeland, M.D.* (London: Longman, Hurst, Rees & Orme, 1807), pp. 142, 163.

469   **"we please to call it. . . .":** Anonymous, *Some Account of Dr. Gall's New Theory of Physiognomy*, p. 26.

470   **skull malformations were present:** Philippe Pinel, *Traité médico-philosophique sur l'aliénation mentale, ou la manie*, p. 167. See Plates 1 and 2.

470   **any alteration in brain structure:** Weiner, *Comprendre et Soigner*, pp. 95–97.

470   **"synonymous with ignorant and stupid":** J. G. Spurzheim, *The Physiognomical System of Drs. Gall and Spurzheim* (London: Baldwin, Cradock & Joy, 1815), p. 554.

470   **watchmaker who sought perpetual motion:** See, for example, the numerous clinical examples of Pinel's used in Gall, *Works in Six Volumes*, vol. 1, pp. 324–332.

470   **a thief for no reason:** Ibid., vol. 2, pp. 286–287.

470   **the Viennese doctor noted:** Ibid., p. 289.

470   **delineate kinds of mania:** Ibid., p. 282.

472   **palpated hundreds of heads:** J. B. Demangen, *Physiologie intellectuelle ou développement de la doctrine du Professeur Gall* (Paris: Delance, 1806).

473   **"to prevent future crimes":** Anonymous, *Some Account of Dr. Gall's New Theory of Physiognomy*, pp. 137, 147–177.

19. THE MIND ECLIPSED

476   **had become a festooned thug:** See S. T. Coleridge's *Biographia Literaria*, p. 122, where Napoleon is characterized as a vulture.

476   **deceased king's brother, Louis XVIII:** Ibid., p. 77.

478   **his model of inner life:** Ibid., pp. 259–261.

478   **be degraded but never destroyed:** P. J. G. Cabanis, *Lettre de Cabanis sur les causes premières*, ed. F. Bérard (Paris: Gabon, 1824). Also see F. Colonna

d'Istria, "La religion d'apres Cabanis," *Revue de métaphysique et de morale* 23 (1916): 455–471.

478 **rooted in the soul:** On psychology in France during this period and the role of Victor Cousin, see Jan Goldstein, *The Post-Revolutionary Self: Politics and Psyche in France, 1750–1850* (Cambridge: Harvard University Press, 2005), pp. 122–142.

478 **the face of the soul:** Jean-Philibert Damiron, *Cours de philosophie: première partie, psychologie* (Paris: Hachette, 1837), vol. 1, pp. 3–5.

480 **social order would be imperiled:** Pierre Flourens, *Examen de la phrénologie* (Paris: Paulin, 1842). On Pierre Flourens, see Clarke and Jacyna, *Nineteenth-Century Origins of Neuroscientific Concepts*, pp. 244–267. Also see Robert Young, *Mind, Brain, and Adaptation in the Nineteenth Century* (New York: Oxford University Press, 1990), p. 46.

480 **one would find four atheists:** The expression in Latin—"tres medici, quatuor Athei . . ."—was attributed to Sylvain Maréchal. See L. S. Jacyna, "Medical Science and Moral Science: The Cultural Relations of Physiology in Restoration France," *History of Science* 25, no. 68 (1987): 113.

481 **brain physiology and the soul:** Goldstein, *The Post-Revolutionary Self*, pp. 257–262. Ironically, the course, meant to be friendly to the new authorities, was shut down in the wide sweep of the medical school in 1820.

481 **Jean-Étienne-Dominique Esquirol:** According to Goldstein, only 3 of Esquirol's 19 students turned to this spiritualist position. See ibid., p. 262. On Esquirol, see Goldstein's account as well as Jacques Postel, *Éléments pour une histoire de la psychiatrie occidentale* (Paris: Harmattan, 2007), pp. 187–220; G. Mora, "On the Bicentenary of the Birth of Esquirol (1772–1840), the First Complete Psychiatrist," *American Journal of Psychiatry* 129 (1972): 562–567; E. Szapiro, "Pinel et Esquirol: Quelques commentaires sur les débuts d'une amitié," *Annales médico-psychologiques* 2, no. 1 (1976): 59–61; Georgette Legee, "Jean-Étienne-Dominique Esquirol (1772–1840). La Personnalité d'un elève de Philippe Pinel," *Histoire des sciences médicales* 22, no. 2 (1988): 159–166. Michel Caire, "Esquirol en 1805: Titres, travaux, services rendus," ibid., 31, no. 1 (1997): 45–51. R. Huertas, "Between Doctrine and Clinical Practice: Nosography and Semiology in the Work of Jean-Étienne-Dominique Esquirol (1772–1840)," *History of Psychiatry* 19, no. 2 (2008): 123–140.

481 **passions as causes of illness:** E. Esquirol, *Des passions considerées commes causes* (Paris: Didot Jeune, 1805).

482 **diagnostic system for mental maladies:** When Sir Alexander Morison visited Esquirol in March of 1818, he was astonished to find the doctor surrounded by 200 plaster casts of mentally ill faces as well as some 600 skulls. Hunter and Macalpine, *Three Hundred Years of Psychiatry, 1535–1860*, p. 738. However, in François Leuret's *Du traitement moral de la folie* (Paris: J. B. Baillière, 1840), pp. 49–50, this acolyte of the French doc-

tor recounted Gall's disastrous visit to the Salpêtrière, where a skeptical Esquirol challenged the Viennese doctor to diagnose illnesses from craniums, which he failed to do. My thanks to Edward Brown for pointing out this testimony.

483 **some form of monomania:** Goldstein, *The Post-Revolutionary Self*, p. 154.

483 **mental causes and cures:** See his monumental work, E. Esquirol, *Des maladies mentales*, 3 vols. (Paris: J. B. Baillière, 1838).

483 **isolation to alter bad habits:** Claude Quétel and Yves Roumajon, *La loi de 1838 sur les aliénés. Ferrus, Falret, Esquirol, Faivre* (Paris: Ed. Frénésie, 1988), vol. 1, pp. 127–130.

483 **treat the mentally ill:** *La loi de 1838 sur les aliénés. L' Application* (Paris: Edition Frénésie, 1988), vol. 2, p. 17. On Foucault and the police function of doctors, see Goldstein, *The Post-Revolutionary Self*, p. 276, also see pp. 276–321.

484 **Madness was a meningeal disease:** A. L. J. Bayle, *Traité des maladies du cerveau et de ses membranes* (Paris: Gabon, 1826).

484 **Bayle drifted away from medicine:** E. M. Brown, "French Psychiatry's Initial Reception of Bayle's Discovery of General Paresis of the Insane," *Bulletin of the History of Medicine* 68, no. 2 (1994): 235–253.

484 **and the ruptures of alienation:** Jacques-Joseph Moreau, *Du Hachisch et de l'aliénation mentale* (Paris: Fortin, Masson, 1845). Also see F. Ledermann, "Pharmacie, Médicaments et Psychiatrie Vers 1850: Le Cas De Jacques-Joseph Moreau de Tours," *Revue d'histoire de la pharmacie* 35, no. 276 (1988): 67–76, and Tony James, *Dream, Creativity, and Madness in Nineteenth-Century France* (Oxford: Clarendon Press, 1995), pp. 98–129.

485 **attributed to minorities like Jews:** On the large literature on degeneration, see especially Ian Dowbiggin, *Inheriting Madness: Professionalization and Psychiatric Knowledge in Nineteenth-Century France* (Berkeley: University of California Press, 1991).

485 **tamed them with reason:** Erased from history was the true instigator of these changes, his assistant Pussin, as well as the decidedly unheroic straitjackets that replaced the chains. See Dora B. Weiner, "The Apprenticeship of Philippe Pinel: A New Document, 'Observations of Citizen Pussin on the Insane,'" *American Journal of Psychiatry* 136, no. 9 (1979): 1133.

485 **and values, seemed vindicated:** Beiser, *Enlightenment, Revolution, and Romanticism*, pp. 281–302.

486 **history, art, law, and politics:** Hegel's great work has been translated as *The Phenomenology of Mind*, trans. J. B. Baillie (New York: Harper & Row, 1967), as well as *Phenomenology of Spirit*, trans. A. V. Miller (Oxford: Oxford University Press, 1976).

487 **Romantic notions of inner conflict:** Johann F. Herbart, *Psychologie als Wissenschaft*, 2 vols. (Königsberg: August Wilhelm Unzer, 1824–1825).

Also see Karl G. Neumann, *Psychologie, ober Lehre von dem Nervenleben des Menschen* (Berlin: E. G. Flittner, 1818).

487 **dialectical materialism and revolution:** While some German philosophers continued to pursue psychology, that realm of study included, in the case of Jakob Friedrich Fries, a soul divorced from the body; J. Friedrich Fries, *Handbuch der psychischen Anthropologie* (Jena: Cröker, 1820).

487 **Hegel's auditorium overflowed:** Arthur Schopenhauer (1819), *The World as Will and Representation*, trans. E. F. J. Payne (New York: Dover Publications, 1969), vol. 1, and (1844), *The World as Will and Representation*, trans. E. F. J. Payne (New York: Dover Publications, 1969), vol. 2. Also see Rüdiger Safranski, *Schopenhauer and the Wild Years of Philosophy* (Cambridge: Harvard University Press, 1990), p. 252.

488 **were in part created there:** J. Müller (1833), *Elements of Physiology*, trans. W. Baly (London: Taylor & Walton, 1838).

488 **back to mechanistic models:** On the so-called School of Helmholtz or the Biophysics Movement of 1847 and its multiple historical narratives, see the excellent work of Laura Otis, *Müller's Lab* (Oxford: Oxford University Press, 2007). Also, P. F. Cranefield, "The Philosophical and Cultural Interests of the Biophysics Movement of 1847," *Journal of the History of Medicine* 21 (1966): 1-4.

488 **not be true in German labs:** Owsei Temkin, *The Double Face of Janus and Other Essays in the History of Medicine* (Baltimore: Johns Hopkins University Press, 1977), pp. 340–344.

489 **the efforts of J. G. Langermann:** While the humanitarian attitudes of Pinel, Chiarugi, Tuke, and Reil were applauded, brutish treatment of the mentally ill continued to predominate. Even alienists aware of moral and psychological theories simply incorporated them into their methods, as remedies applied not just to the body but to a recalcitrant self. At Sonnenstein, the asylum in Saxony, the latest in moral treatment was eagerly employed alongside tortures with names like the "Palisades Chamber" and "Hollow Wheel." Dorner, *Madmen and the Bourgeoisie*, pp. 212, 215–223.

490 **Heinroth called for "psychical doctors":** Johann Christian August Heinroth, *Textbook of Disturbances of Mental Life: or, Disturbances of the Soul and Their Treatment,* trans. J. Schmorak, 2 vols. (Baltimore: Johns Hopkins University Press, 1975). The term Heinroth employed was "psychiche Arzt."

490 **soon-to-be disgraced Ernst Horn:** Johann Christian Heinroth, *Lehrbuch der Anthropologie* (Leipzig: Vogel, 1822). His historical appraisals of the field are in *Textbook of Disturbances of Mental Life*, vol. 1, pp. 64–98.

490 **a casket called "the box":** Heinroth, *Textbook of Disturbances of Mental Life*, vol. 2, pp. 291–298.

491 **paralysis, epilepsy, and hysteria:** Albert Mathias Vering, *Psychische Heilkunde*, 2 vols. (Leipzig: Johann Ambrosius Barth, 1817).

491 **all in the title:** F. E. Beneke, *Beiträge zu einer reinseelenwissenschaftlichen Bearbeitung der Seelenkrankheitkunde* (Leipzig: Recalm, 1824).

491 **his disgraced predecessor, left behind:** See for example, Karl Ideler, *Grundriss der Seelenheilkunde*, 2 vols. (Berlin: Enslin, 1835–1838).

491 **virtuous people could go crazy:** J. B. Friedreich, *Historisch-kritische Darstellung der Theorien über das Wesen und der Sitz der psychischen Krankheiten* (Leipzig: Wigand, 1836). Also see this excellent article: Otto Marx, "German Romantic Psychiatry," in *History of Psychiatry and Medical Psychology*, Edwin R. Wallace and John Gach, eds. (New York: Springer, 2008), p. 328.

492 **exclusively on the diseased brain:** This esteemed editor of journals, like the *Zeitschrift für Anthropologie* (1823–1826), taught the great Romantic biologist Johannes Müller.

493 **commenced in England and Scotland:** E. P. Thompson, *The Making of the English Working Class* (New York: Vintage Books, 1966), pp. 181, 197.

493 **might endanger public morals:** Erasmus Darwin, *The Collected Letters of Erasmus Darwin*, ed. Desmond King-Hele (Cambridge: Cambridge University Press, 2007), pp. 91–97.

494 **its station in the brain:** Erasmus Darwin, *Zoonomia; or, the Laws of Organic Life* (London: J. Johnson, 1801). Also see his *The Temple of Nature; or, the Origin of Society* (London: J. Johnson, 1803), Canto I, Section 24–25.

494 **Jacobin, and a miserable poet:** N. Garfinkle, "Science and Religion in England, 1790–1800: The Critical Response to the Work of Erasmus Darwin," *Journal of the History of Ideas* 16 (1955): 376–388.

494 **emancipate mankind from all religions:** Alan Richardson, *British Romanticism and the Science of the Mind* (Cambridge and New York: Cambridge University Press, 2001), p. 28.

494 **"one great state prison":** Owsei Temkin, "Basic Science, Medicine, and the Romantic Era," *Bulletin of the History of Medicine* 37, no. 2 (1963): 97–129, and Richard Holmes, *The Age of Wonder: How the Romantic Generation Discovered the Beauty and Terror of Science* (New York: Vintage Books, 2010), p. 308.

494 *The New Prometheus:* This debate was characterized—incorrectly, as Temkin pointed out—as a debate of vitalists and mechanists, when it was actually a debate between these two forms of vitalism. Much has been written on the genesis of *Frankenstein*. See for example, Maurice Hindle, "Vital Matters: Mary Shelley's Frankenstein and Romantic Science," *Critical Survey* 2, no. 1 (1990): 29–35.

495 **deemed to impugn the Scriptures:** On Bentham's panopticon, see the influential reading by Michel Foucault in *Discipline and Punish: The Birth of the Prison,* trans. Alan Sheridan (New York: Vintage Books, 1995). On Lawrence's fate, see Owsei Temkin, "Basic Science, Medicine, and the

Romantic Era," p. 109, and Alan Richardson, *British Romanticism and the Science of the Mind*, p. 29.

496 **nonmedical moral treatment:** Samuel Tuke, *Description of the Retreat, an Institution Near York for Insane Persons* (York: W. Alexander, 1813). Also see R. Hunter and I. Macalpine, "Samuel Tuke's First Publication on the Treatment of Patients at the Retreat, 1811," *British Journal of Psychiatry* 111, no. 477 (1965).

496 **employ his machine, the Tranquillizer:** On Cox's swing and Morison's rotary machine, see Hunter and Macalpine, *Three Hundred Years of Psychiatry, 1535–1860*, pp. 596–600.

496 **fright, and too much study:** Ibid., p. 646.

496 **the physical roots of ideas:** Robert Young, *Mind, Brain, and Adaptation in the Nineteenth Century*, p. 98.

497 **integrating these would recede:** After his death in 1827, Brown's lectures appeared as *A Treatise on the Philosophy of the Human Mind*, 2 vols. (Cambridge: Hilliard & Brown, 1827). The first book took up the physiology of the mind and the second, emotions. Schopenhauer considered Brown boring and dismissed him. The effort would gain vigor at the end of the 19th century with the discovery of the neuron and renewed hope, again without evidence, that perhaps an idea could be housed in an individual nerve cell.

497 **was critical for medicine:** Hunter and Macalpine, *Three Hundred Years of Psychiatry, 1535–1860*, pp. 801–804. Also see John Haslam, *Sound Mind; or Contributions to the Natural History and Physiology of the Human Intellect* (London: Longman, Hurst et al., 1819), p. ix.

497 **the health of Americans:** Ibid., pp. 810–811, 821–825.

497 **the outside looking in:** William Bynum, "Rationales for Therapy in British Psychiatry, 1780–1835," in *Madhouses, Mad-Doctors, and Madmen*, ed. Andrew Scull (Philadelphia: University of Pennsylvania Press, 1981), p. 46.

499 **"theory of the human mind":** R. J. Cooter, "Phrenology and British Alienists, c. 1825–1845," *Medical History* 20, no. 1 (1976): 1–21, and 20, no. 2: 135–151.

499 **accounts of this new craze:** Richardson, *British Romanticism and the Science of the Mind*, pp. 23–24.

500 **would win over many:** Thomas Carlyle to Robert Mitchell, dated March 31, 1817, *The Carlyle Letters Online*, http://carlyleletters.dukejournals.org.

500 **"their varieties, eternal in duration":** Thomas Carlyle to James Johnston, dated Dec. 20, 1823, ibid.

500 **Phrenological Society was established:** Geoffrey Cantor and Steven Shapin, "Phrenology in Early Nineteenth-Century Edinburgh: An Historiographical Discussion," *Annals of Science* 32 (1975): 195–218.

500 **nymphomaniac could not stop herself:** In America, leading progressive
     alienists including Benjamin Rush, Amariah Brigham, Samuel Woodward,
     and Pliny Earle all took an interest in phrenology. Isaac Ray enthusiasti-
     cally declared, "Phrenology delivers us, and presents in its place a rational
     and intelligible exposition of the mental powers." Norman Dain, *Concepts
     of Insanity in the United States, 1789–1865* (New Brunswick, N.J: Rutgers
     University Press, 1964), p. 62.
500 **based on Gall's new science:** W. A. F. Browne, *What Asylums Were, Are,
     and Ought to Be* (Edinburgh: Adam & Charles Black, 1837), pp. 10–49.
501 **supported the skull doctors:** Cantor and Shapin, "Phrenology in Early
     Nineteenth-Century Edinburgh," p. 202.

EPILOGUE

508 **he labeled World-Mysteries:** E. Du Bois-Reymond (1872) "Ueber die
     Grenzen des Naturkennens," in *Reden von Emil du Bois-Reymond* (Leipzig:
     Verlag Von Veit, 1886), pp. 105–130. Over the last three decades, impres-
     sive advances in computing and neuroimaging again have engendered the
     dream of eliminating the psyche. A flurry of new fields, such as neuro-
     aesthetics and neuroethics, hold out that promise. If history is to be our
     guide, their efforts will be long on promissory notes and not much else.
     For to date, there is no valid neuroscientific account for consciousness or
     human agency.
510 **the mind-body problem to others:** On this late 19th-century struggle
     with mind and brain in these different disciplines, see my *Revolution in
     Mind: The Creation of Psychoanalysis* (New York: HarperCollins, 2008), pp.
     9–84. Hughlings-Jackson adopted psychophysical parallelism, in which the
     mind and brain would be treated as causal streams that were parallel to
     each other, though the link between the two was in doubt. Wundt and
     Hughlings-Jackson recognized that there was no viable scientific model in
     which one could accommodate ideational causes and the neural basis for
     subjectivity. Of course, all of these disciplines have included members who
     would cross these boundaries, usually with regrettable results.
510 **secular humanists alike:** Histories of psychiatry often do not reflect this
     hybrid nature, but often seek to define the field as essentially either mind
     or brain. This has led to dueling histories that have confirmed presen-
     tist assumptions. During the heyday of psychoanalysis, Franz Alexander
     and Sheldon Selesnick penned *The History of Psychiatry* (New York: Harper
     & Row, 1966), an account biased toward mind-based illnesses and cures.
     Three decades later, Edward Shorter's *A History of Psychiatry: From the Era
     of the Asylum to the Age of Prozac* (New York: John Wiley & Sons, 1997)
     lurched in the opposite direction. For a sophisticated series of discussions
     on psychiatry's past, see Kenneth Kendler and Josef Parnas, eds., *Philosophi-*

cal Issues in Psychiatry III: The Nature and Sources of Historical Change (Oxford: Oxford University Press, 2015).

510 **which they cannot account:** Of note, recent efforts to bridge these divides have emerged in the exciting field of epigenetics, which offers a synthesis of the Nature and Nurture problem, and the still-aspirational fields of cognitive neuroscience and neuropsychoanalysis.

510 **one scientific and the other humanistic:** C. P. Snow, *The Two Cultures* (Cambridge: Cambridge University Press, 1993). For a much more sophisticated account of the conflicts between Nature and Culture in modernity, see Bruno Latour's extraordinary work, *We Have Never Been Modern*, trans. Catherine Porter (Cambridge: Harvard University Press, 1993).

Acknowledgments

THIS BOOK OWES its origins to my extraordinary father, Dr. Jack George Makari, who passed away in 2013. A passionate scientist, a writer, and a man of hard-won personal faith, he loved to examine the problems that are at the heart of this study. Thanks to my mother, Odette Makari, whose never-ending encouragement I cherish; due to her I developed a fascination with France, without which this book could not have materialized. My greatest debt of gratitude goes to my wife, Arabella Ogilvie, whose astonishing erudition is only outweighed by her warmth and humor. My children, Gabrielle and Jack, have been a constant infusion of delight. I hope this book answers some of their questions that stymied me over the dinner table.

I have been immensely lucky to have colleagues across numerous disciplines, from physics, psychiatry, and psychoanalysis, to history and literature. For over two decades, my intellectual home has been the DeWitt Wallace Institute for the History of Psychiatry in the Department of Psychiatry at Weill Medical College of Cornell University. My gratitude goes out to my steadfast chairman Jack D. Barchas, and my associates, including Nathan Kravis, Leonard Groopman, Robert Michels, Orna Ophir, Theodore Shapiro, Lawrence Friedman, Rosemary Stevens, and especially the always helpful

Megan Wolff. Thanks to Marisa Shaari, the gracious research librarian of the Oskar Diethelm Library, an astonishing collection that was indispensible for this work. In a time when such scholarly communities are rare, the DeWitt Wallace–Reader's Digest Fund of the New York Community Trust has continued its farsighted support of this unique institute and library. This is my attempt to reward their commitment.

My second home during the eight years in which I researched and wrote this book has been at the Center for Studies in Biology and Physics at Rockefeller University. There, I have benefited from discussions on the philosophy of science with Mitchell Feigenbaum and colleagues such as Nicola Khuri. Lastly, I would like to acknowledge my colleagues at the Columbia Psychoanalytic Center, who have encouraged me to consider mind-brain questions repeatedly over the last years.

This project coalesced after conversations in London with my superb literary agent, Sarah Chalfant. I am deeply fortunate to work with Sarah and everyone at The Wylie Agency. This manuscript was read and improved upon by Sander L. Gilman, Akihito Suzuki, Leonard Groopman, Noga Arikha, Siri Hustvedt, and Anthony Walton. Finally, my editor at W. W. Norton, Jill Bialosky, placed her faith in me and this project and has never wavered. Thank you to Jill, Fred Wiemer, Angie Shih, Elizabeth Riley, Maria Rogers, and the team at Norton for all their efforts.

Illustration Credits

Figure 1: *The Death of Socrates*, Jacques Louis David, 1787, The Metropolitan Museum of Art, New York, Catharine Lorillard Wolfe Collection, Wolfe Fund, 1931

Figure 2: "Marin Mersenne," line engraving by P. Dupin, 1765, Wellcome Library, London

Figure 3: "Pierre Gassendi," line engraving by Claude Mellan, n.d., Wellcome Library, London

Figure 4: 16th-century automaton, Kunst Historisches Museum Wien, Vienna

Figure 5: "René Descartes," line engraving by J. Suyderhoeff, after F. Hals, 1649, Wellcome Library, London

Figure 6: "Thomas Hobbes," line engraving by W. Humphrys, 1839, Wellcome Library, London

Figure 7: Thomas Willis, *Cerebri anatome* (Amsterdam: G. Schagen, 1664), Wellcome Library, London

Figure 8: *Bills of Mortality* (London: E. Cotes, 1665), Wellcome Library, London

Figure 9: Joseph Glanvill (1681), *Saducismus Triumphatus* (London: A. Baskerville, 1689), Oskar Diethelm Library, DeWitt Wallace Institute for the History of Psychiatry, Weill Cornell Medical College, New York

Figure 10: Robert Burton (1621), *The Anatomy of Melancholy* (London: Peter Parker, 1676), Oskar Diethelm Library, DeWitt Wallace Institute for the History of Psychiatry, Weill Cornell Medical College, New York

Figure 11: *The Ranters Ranting* (London: B. Alsop, 1650), The British Library

Figure 12: J. F. Senault (1641), *The Use of Passions* (London: John Sims, 1671), Oskar Diethelm Library, DeWitt Wallace Institute for the History of Psychiatry, Weill Cornell Medical College, New York

Figure 13: René Descartes, *De Homine* (Leiden: F. Moyard and P. Leffen, 1662), p. 82, Wellcome Library, London

Figure 14: "John Locke," line engraving by G. Vertue, 1738, Wellcome Library, London

Figure 15: "Benedictus Spinoza," stipple engraving by C. F. Riedel, Wellcome Library, London

Figure 16: "Samuel Pepys," color reproduction of oil painting, Wellcome Library, London

Figure 17: Bernard de Mandeville, *The Fable of the Bees* (London: J. Tonson, 1724), Oskar Diethelm Library, DeWitt Wallace Institute for the History of Psychiatry, Weill Cornell Medical College, New York

Figure 18: Giovanni Borelli (1685), *De moto animalium* (Neapoli: Typis Felicis Mosca, 1734), Prints and Photographs Division, Library of Congress, LC-USZ62-95253

Figure 19: William Hogarth, *A Rake's Progress* (London: Published by an Act of Parliament, 1735), Wellcome Library, London

Figure 20: "William Battie," oil portrait, Wellcome Library, London

Figure 21: "King George III," etching by W. Daniell, Wellcome Library, London

Figure 22: The goddess of health, Hygieia, holding a relief of King George III, after James Parker, 1789, Wellcome Library, London

Figure 23: C. A. Helvétius, *De L'esprit* (Paris: Durand, 1758), Oskar Diethelm Library, DeWitt Wallace Institute for the History of Psychiatry, Weill Cornell Medical College, New York

Figure 24: D. Diderot and J. d'Alembert, eds., *Encyclopédie, ou dictionnaire raisonné des sciences, des arts, et des métiers* (Geneva: Pellet, 1777–1779), vol. 1, Wellcome Library, London

Figure 25: Illustration of the nervous system from entry on "Anatomie," *Encyclopédie*, Wellcome Library, London

Figure 26: "Théophile Bordeu," stipple engraving by Lambert, Wellcome Library, London

Figure 27: "Paul Joseph Barthez," stipple engraving by Lambert, Wellcome Library, London

Figure 28: "Jean-Jacques Rousseau," line engraving, Wellcome Library, London

Figure 29: J. J. Rousseau, *Emile ou de l'Education* in *Collection Complete des Ouevres de J. J. Rousseau* (Geneva: 1782), vol. 4

Figure 30: "Animal Magnetism," engraving, 1802, Wellcome Library, London

Figure 31: "Les Effets Du Magnetisme . . . Animal," n.d., Oskar Diethelm

Library, DeWitt Wallace Institute for the History of Psychiatry, Weill
Cornell Medical College, New York

Figure 32: "Madame Helvétius," portrait, Louise-Elisabeth Vignée-
Lebrun, *The Memoirs of Mme. Vignée Lebrun*, trans. L. Strachey
(New York: Doubleday, 1903), Division of Rare and Manuscript
Collections, Cornell University Library, New York

Figure 33: "Mort de Louis XVI," print published circa 1890–1920, Prints
and Photographs Division, Library of Congress, LC-USZ62-124552

Figure 34: Tony Robert-Fleury, *Pinel Freeing the Insane from Their Chains*,
1876, Wellcome Library, London

Figure 35: Francisco Goya, *The Sleep of Reason Produces Monsters*, from *Los
Caprichos*, no. 43, 1797–1799, Prado Museum, Madrid

Figure 36: J. M. G. Itard, *Rapports et mémoires sur le sauvage de l'Aveyron*
(Paris: Bureau du Progres médical, 1894), Oskar Diethelm Library,
DeWitt Wallace Institute for the History of Psychiatry, Weill Cornell
Medical College, New York

Figure 37: "Immanuel Kant," stipple engraving by F. N. Bollinger,
Wellcome Library, London

Figure 38: "Madame de Staël," photographic print by Sophus Williams,
1884, Prints and Photographs Division, Library of Congress,
LC-USZ62-118849

Figure 39: Caspar David Friedrich, *Two Men Contemplating the Moon*,
1819/20, The Metropolitan Museum of Art, New York, Wrightsman
Fund, 2000

Figure 40: Reil and Kayssler, eds., *Magazin für die psychische Heilkunde*,
1805, Oskar Diethelm Library, DeWitt Wallace Institute for the
History of Psychiatry, Weill Cornell Medical College, New York

Figure 41: Johann Caspar Lavater, *Essays on Physiognomy* (London: William
Tegg, 1789), vol. 1, p. 208, Wellcome Library, London

Figure 42: "Le Dr. F. J. Gall, Mort à Paris, 22 Août, 1828," engraving,
1828, Oskar Diethelm Library, DeWitt Wallace Institute for the
History of Psychiatry, Weill Cornell Medical College, New York

Figure 43: J. E. D Esquirol, *Des maladies mentale* (Paris: Bailliere, 1838),
engraving by Ambroise Tardieu, Oskar Diethelm Library, DeWitt
Wallace Institute for the History of Psychiatry, Weill Cornell Medical
College, New York

Figure 44: Mary Wollstonecraft Shelley, *Frankenstein, or the New
Prometheus* (London: H. Colburn and R. Bentley, 1831). Engraving by
W. Chevalier, Wellcome Library, London

Figure 45: Anonymous, *Craniology Burlesqued in Three Serio-Comic Lectures*
(London: Effingham Wilson, 1818), Oskar Diethelm Library, DeWitt
Wallace Institute for the History of Psychiatry, Weill Cornell Medical
College, New York

Index

Page numbers in *italics* refer to illustrations.